Erastus Edgar Maryott

The New Medical World

Erastus Edgar Maryott

The New Medical World

ISBN/EAN: 9783741134463

Manufactured in Europe, USA, Canada, Australia, Japa

Cover: Foto ©Lupo / pixelio.de

Manufactured and distributed by brebook publishing software (www.brebook.com)

Erastus Edgar Maryott

The New Medical World

THE
NEW MEDICAL WORLD.

A BOOK FOR REFERENCE AND CONSULTATION

CONTAINING A

THOROUGH DESCRIPTION OF DISEASE

WITH THE LATEST AND BEST METHODS FOR ITS TREATMENT.

ALSO

POPULAR AND PRACTICAL DISCUSSIONS

ON MEDICAL PROGRESS, HEALTH, MARRIAGE,
MATERNITY, THE CARE OF CHILDREN,
NURSING OF THE SICK AND
MANY OTHER TOPICS OF

WORLD-WIDE INTEREST.

BY E. EDGAR MARYOTT, A.M., M.D.

ILLUSTRATED.

1897.
THE HAMPDEN PUBLISHING CO., PUBLISHERS,
SPRINGFIELD, MASS.

Copyright, 1897
BY HAMPDEN PUBLISHING CO.,
Springfield, Mass.

"I have often said, what profession is there equal in true nobleness to medicine? He that can abolish pain and relieve his fellow mortal from sickness, he is indisputably the usefulest of men. Him savage and civilized will honor; he is in the right, be in the wrong who may."—*Carlyle.*

AUTHOR'S PREFACE.

THE *title* of this book, "THE NEW MEDICAL WORLD," does not imply that a new system of medicine has been discovered; for this is no announcement of novel, or untried methods.

There have been, however, so many recent advances in the practice of medicine and surgery, as the result of bacteriological study, that it seems fitting to recognize them in a popular work. It is therefore believed that a book which delineates the *latest* and *best* in Medicine will be appreciated and accorded a favorable reception.

It has been the author's purpose to prepare a practical, modern and reliable work upon domestic medicine, which shall comprise the best known in medical literature suitable for the convenient use of the masses as a book of reference in health or sickness.

It contains a large amount of practical information, and will prove an earnest instructor and counselor to every one who possesses a thirst for medical knowledge; and when an emergency occurs it will enable one to act promptly, and to determine what course to pursue for the best interest of all.

It is not the purpose of the book to so instruct the masses that they will become experts in the healing art, for that would be impossible. It aims rather to be helpful by bringing into prominence many interesting and important facts; and hence it is essentially a book of *instruction* and *reference.*

It tells what to avoid and how to live in order to maintain good health. Directions for nursing the sick, advanced ideas upon the care and education of children are included; so that in this regard it is believed that it will be especially helpful to a large number of persons. The methods of treatment proposed are, for the most part, simple and efficient, such as can be understood by a mother, a nurse or any persons of ordinary intelligence. The prescriptions have been prepared with care, and are the result of experience and successful practice, and are of unusual value.

The treatment of all the more dangerous diseases could have been withheld, but this would have greatly marred the completeness and worth of the work. It is hardly to be expected that any person, without a suitable degree of medical knowledge, will desire to treat any except the more simple forms of disease, and yet it has seemed necessary to enter somewhat into details for the sake of information.

The work includes a brief discussion of many interesting and practical topics, closely allied to medicine, as healthy homes, food, clothing, climate, exercise, drainage, the water supply, the prevention of disease, necessary disinfection after contagious diseases, surgical hints upon fractures, hemorrhage and other emergencies. It attempts in this way to show the bearing of many topics not strictly medical to the conditions of health and disease, in order that correct living may be more easily attained.

Attention is also called to that part of the work which gives advice to those who *contemplate marriage.* The Chapter upon Marriage and Maternity contains many useful suggestions and directions.

It is designed to be a *safe* book for perusal or study, by young or old and with this end in view it has been examined and received the sanction of eminent clergymen and physicians. In so far as it has been deemed necessary to consider or discuss delicate topics, it conforms to good taste and will give satisfaction to the cultivated and those morally sensitive.

Technical language has been avoided so far as possible, with the belief that a medical work requiring constant reference to a dictionary would be of doubtful utility. The classification adopted is natural rather than scientific as a simple arrangement is more in accord with the general plan and purpose of the work.

The author has performed his task with scrupulous care, and believes that he has prepared a Medical book adapted to the every day need and use of the people.

E. E. MARYOTT.

SPRINGFIELD, MASS., July 1, 1897.

CONTENTS.

CHAPTER I.

		PAGE
INTRODUCTORY ARTICLES,		1
I. Medical Progress and X Rays,		1–4
II. Medical Study Fascinating,		6
III. Medicine a Popular Science,		7
IV. Medical Common Sense,		8
V. General Causes of Disease,		9
VI. Special Causes of Disease,		11
VII. Bacteria, or Germs in Disease,		12

CHAPTER II.

		PAGE
SANITARY SUBJECTS,		17
I. The Choice of a Home,		17
II. The House Furnishings,		20
III. Drainage and Sewerage,		21
IV. The Air and Ventilation,		24–26
V. The Water Supply,		29
VI. Food,		32
VII. Clothing,		36
VIII. Climate,		40
IX. Exercise,		43
X. Longevity,		47

CHAPTER III.

		PAGE
GENERAL TOPICS OF INTEREST IN MEDICINE,		52
I. Home Prescribing,		52
II. Strange Delusions,		53
III. Patent Medicines,		55
IV. Medicines,		57
V. Doses,		75
VI. Household Remedies,		80

CHAPTER IV.

		PAGE
POISONS AND THEIR ANTIDOTES,		88
I. Poisons in General,		88
II. The Mineral Acids,		91

		PAGE
III.	Oxalic Acid,	92
IV.	Carbolic Acid and Creosote,	92
V.	Acetic Acid,	93
VI.	Ammonia,	93
VII.	Prussic or Hydrocyanic Acid,	93
VIII.	Arsenic and its Preparations,	94
IX.	Copper, Mercury and Zinc Compounds,	95
X.	Tartar Emetic,	95
XI.	Lead Compounds,	96
XII.	Nitrate of Silver,	96
XIII.	Phosphorus,	96
XIV.	Opium and Morphine,	97
XV.	Chloral Hydrate,	97
XVI.	Strychnia,	98
XVII.	Aconite and Vegetable Poisons,	98
XVIII.	Poison Ivy,	98
XIX.	Poison Gases,	100

CHAPTER V.

The Use of Alcohol and other Dangerous or Narcotic Drugs, - - - - - 102

I.	Alcohol, its Use and Abuse,	102
II.	Chronic Alcoholism,	104
III.	The Morphine, Cocaine and Chloral Habits,	107
IV.	The Effects of Tobacco,	109

CHAPTER VI.

Accidents, - - - - - - 111

I.	Drowning,	111
II.	Fainting,	112
III.	Burns and Scalds,	113
IV.	Lightning Stroke,	116
V.	Sprains and Bruises,	116
VI.	Frost Bite,	119
VII.	Bites of Serpents,	120
VIII.	Stings of Insects,	121
IX.	Poisoned Wounds,	122
X.	Hemorrhage from Wounds and the Treatment of Wounds in General,	124
XI.	Incised Wounds,	126
XII.	Scalp Wounds,	127

CHAPTER VII.

General Subjects Preliminary to the Study of Disease, - - - - - - 128

I.	Health and Disease,	128

		PAGE
II.	The Two Great Types of Disease,	131
III.	Temperature in Disease,	133
IV.	Kissing in its Relation to Disease,	135
V.	Bathing in its Relation to Disease,	136
VI.	Symptoms of Disease, How to Read and Interpret Them,	137

CHAPTER VIII.

ANATOMY AND PHYSIOLOGY, INCLUDING THE BONES, JOINTS AND MUSCLES, - - - - 149

I.	Anatomy and Physiology,	149
II.	The Relation of Physiology to Anatomy,	151
III.	The Anatomy of the Bones,	153
IV.	The Bones of the Skull,	153
V.	The Bones of the Face,	155
VI.	The Spinal Column,	157
VII.	Injuries of the Spine,	159
VIII.	The Bones of the Upper Extremities, Chest and Pelvis,	160
IX.	The Bones of the Lower Extremities,	163
X.	The Joints,	166
XI.	The Muscles,	166
XII.	Nature's Effort to Prevent Injury,	168
XIII.	The Fracture of Bones,	171
XIV.	Dislocations.	176

CHAPTER IX.

THE BLOOD AND ITS DISEASES, - - - - 179

I.	Anæmia,	180
II.	Chlorosis,	182
III.	Leukæmia,	183
IV.	Septicæmia—Pyæmia. Blood Poisoning,	183

CHAPTER X.

THE LYMPHATIC SYSTEM AND GLANDULAR DISEASES, - 187

I.	The Lymphatic System,	187
II.	Scrofula,	189
III.	The Pancreas,	191
IV.	Diseases of the Pancreas,	192

CHAPTER XI.

THE SKIN—ITS ANATOMY, FUNCTIONS AND DISEASES, 194

I.	The Skin,	194
II.	Management of the Skin,	200

viii   CONTENTS.

		PAGE.
III.	Cosmetics,	202
IV.	General Observations on Diseases of the Skin,	202
V.	Disorders of the Sweat Glands,	205
VI.	Disorders of the Sebaceous Glands. 1. Seborrhea or Dandruff. 2. Wens or Tumors of the Scalp. 3. Baldness or Alopecia.	207
VII.	Acne and Comedo,	212
VIII.	Milium,	215
IX.	Prurigo, Itching or Pruritus	215
X.	Shingles or Herpes Zoster,	216
XI.	Eczema, Tetter, Milk Crust or Salt Rheum,	218
XII.	Urticaria, Hives or Nettle Rash,	220
XIII.	Psoriasis,	221
XIV.	Leprosy,	222
XV.	Lice or Pediculosis,	223
XVI.	Itch or Scabies,	224
XVII.	Ringworm or Tinea,	226
XVIII.	Favus,	227
XIX.	Freckles or Lentigo,	227
XX.	Moles,	228
XXI.	Warts,	229
XXII.	Corns or Clavus,	229
XXIII.	Bunions,	231
XXIV.	Scurvy.	231

CHAPTER XII.

THE BRAIN, CRANIAL NERVES, SPINAL CORD, NERVES, SYMPATHETIC NERVES AND THEIR DISEASES, — 233

I.	The Brain and Cranial Nerves,	233
II.	The Nerves and Spinal Cord,	238
III.	Hydrocephalus or Dropsy of the Brain,	240
IV.	Meningitis or Inflammation of the Brain,	241
V.	Neuralgia,	242
VI.	Headache,	245
VII.	Vertigo or Dizziness,	247
VIII.	Insomnia,	248
IX.	Insanity,	249
X.	Apoplexy,	251
XI.	Various Other Diseases of the Brain. 1. Abscess of the Brain. 2. Tumors of the Brain. 3. Aphasia. 4. Amnesia. 5. Numbness. 6. Hemiplegia. 7. Paraplegia. 8. Locomotor Ataxia. 9. Facial Paralysis. 10. Congenital Defects.	253–255

CHAPTER XIII.

The Eye, its Appendages and Diseases, - - 256

I. Description of the Eye. 1. The Orbits. 2. The Optic Nerves. 3. The Sclerotic. 4. The Choroid. 5. The Iris. 6. The Ciliary Muscle or Ligament. 7. The Ciliary Processes. 8. The Retina. 9. The Interior of the Eye. 10. The Appendages of the Eye. - - - - - 257–262
II. Examination of the Eyes. 1. Errors of Refraction. 2. Myopia or Near Sight. 3. Hypermetropia or Far Sight. 4. Presbyopia or Old Sight. 5. Astigmatism, - 262–264
III. The Use of Glasses, and Directions for Testing the Eyesight, - - - - 264–268
IV. Care of the Eyes, - - - - 268–270
V. Diseases of the Eye. 1. Ulcers. 2. Paralysis. 3. Twitching of the Lids. 4. Inflammation of the Eye. 5. Stye. 6. Blepharitis. 7. Wounds of the Eyelids. 8. Conjunctivitis or Ophthalmia. 9. Purulent Ophthalmia. 10. Granular Ophthalmia or Granular Lids, - - - - 270–273
VI. Foreign Bodies in the Eye, - - - 273
VII. Inflammations of the Cornea (Corneitis). 1. Ulcers of the Cornea. 2. Corneal Opacities. 3. Staphyloma, - - - - 273
VIII. Inflammation of the Iris or Iritis, - - 275
IX. Inflammation of the Choroid, - - - 276
X. Sympathetic Inflammation, - - - 276
XI. Glaucoma, - - - - - 276
XII. Inflammation of the Retina, - - - 277
XIII. Inflammation of the Optic Nerve, - - 277
XIV. Cataract, - - - - - 277
XV. Cross Eye, Squint or Strabismus, - - 279
XVI. Various Other Affections. 1. Growths. 2. Inflammation of the Tear Duct. 3. Abscesses of the Lachrymal Sac - - 279–280

CHAPTER XIV.

The Ear and its Diseases, - - - - 281

I. Description of the Ear. 1. The External Ear. 2. The Auditory Canal. 3. The Middle Ear or Tympanum. 4. The Eustachian Tube and the Ossicles. 5. The Internal Ear or Labyrinth, - - - 281–282

		PAGE
II.	Diseases of the Ear. 1. Deafness. 2. Impacted Wax or Cerumen. 3. Foreign Bodies in the Ear. 4. Inflammation of the Ear. 5. Polypi.	282
III.	Diseases of the Middle Ear. 1. Rupture of the Drum. 2. Acute and Chronic Catarrh of the Middle Ear or Otitis Media. 3. Inflation of the Middle Ear. 4. Congenital Defects of the Ear,	285
IV.	Mastoid Disease.	287

CHAPTER XV.

THE NOSE AND ITS DISEASES,		289
I.	Description of the Nose,	289
II.	Acute Coryza or Cold in the Head,	290
III.	Ulcers in the Nasal Cavity.	291
IV.	Other Affections. 1. Warts. 2. Polypi. 3. Tumors, etc.,	292
V.	Hemorrhage from the Nose,	292
VI.	Chronic Nasal Catarrh,	293
VII.	Hay Fever, Rose Cold or Summer Catarrh,	295

CHAPTER XVI.

THE MOUTH AND ITS APPENDAGES,		298
I.	Description of the Mouth and its Appendages. 1. The Mouth. 2. The Upper and Lower Jaw. 3. The Mucous Membrane. 4. The Lips. 5. The Cheeks. 6. The Glands. 7. The Tongue. 8. The Gums. 9. The Antrum. 10. The Palate. 11. The Teeth,	298–301
II.	Diseases of the Mouth, Tongue and Vicinity. 1. Alveolar Abscess or Gum Boil. 2. Catarrhal Stomatitis. 3. Canker or Aphthous Sore Mouth. 4. Gangrenous Stomatitis or Cancrum Oris. 5. Toxic Stomatitis. 6. Other Minor or Rare Affections. a. Calculus of the Ducts. b. Salivary Fistula. c. Growths. d. Hare Lip. e. Hypertrophy of the Lips. 7. Diseases of the Tongue. a. Tongue Tie. b. Enlargement of the Tongue or Hypertrophy. c. Inflammation of the Tongue or Glossitis,	301–305

CHAPTER XVII.

THE THROAT, LARYNX AND THEIR DISEASES, - - 306
    I. Description of the Throat and Larynx. 1. The Throat. 2. The Larynx, - - 306
    II. Affections of the Throat. 1. Getting Choked. 2. Taking Cold, - - - - 306
    III. Acute Sore Throat or Laryngitis, - - 307
    IV. Chronic Sore Throat or Clergyman's Sore Throat, - - - - - 308
    V. Loss of Voice or Aphonia, - - - 309
    VI. Quinsy Sore Throat or Tonsilitis, - - 309

CHAPTER XVIII.

THE TRACHEA OR WINDPIPE, LUNGS AND THEIR DISEASES, - - - - - - 312
    I. The Trachea, - - - - - 312
    II. The Lungs, - - - - - 313
    III. Asthma, - - - - - 314
    IV. Bronchitis, - - - - - 315
    V. Capillary Bronchitis, - - - - 317
    VI. Pleurisy, - - - - - 318
    VII. Pneumonia, - - - - - 320
    VIII. Consumption, - - - - - 322
    IX. The Prevention of Consumption, - - 325

CHAPTER XIX.

THE ŒSOPHAGUS AND STOMACH, - - - 328
    I. The Œsophagus and its Affections, - - 328
    II. Description of the Stomach and Digestion, - 329
    III. Dyspepsia or Indigestion, - - - 331
    IV. Gastritis, Gastric Fever or Inflammation of the Stomach, - - - - - 334
    V. Gastric Ulcer or Ulcer of the Stomach, - 335
    VI. Nausea and Vomiting, - - - 336
    VII. Gastralgia, Stomach Ache or Neuralgia of the Stomach, - - - - - 337
    VIII. Cancer of the Stomach, - - - 338
    IX. Loss of Appetite, - - - - 338
    X. Unnatural Appetite, - - - - 339
    XI. Hiccough. - - - - - 340

CHAPTER XX.

THE LIVER, SPLEEN AND GALL BLADDER, - - 341
    I. Description of the Liver and its Functions, - 341
    II. The Gall Bladder, - - - - 344

		PAGE.
III.	Diseases of the Liver in General,	344
IV.	Congestion of the Liver,	345
V.	Jaundice or Icterus,	346
VI.	Cirrhosis or Hardening of the Liver,	348
VII.	Gall Stones and Bilious Colic,	349
VIII.	Other Affections of the Liver. 1. Abscess of the Liver. 2. Cancer of the Liver. 3. Fatty Degeneration of the Liver. 4. Amyloid Degeneration of the Liver. 5. Acute Yellow Atrophy. 6. Hydatid Disease of the Liver.	350
IX.	The Spleen and its Diseases. 1. Inflammation. 2. Enlargement.	352

CHAPTER XXI.

THE HEART, CIRCULATION, PERICARDIUM, BLOOD VESSELS AND THEIR DISEASES, — 354

I.	Description of the Heart and its Valves,	354
II.	The Circulation,	357
III.	Overwork of the Heart or Heart Strain,	359
IV.	The Pericardium or Heart Sac,	359
V.	Inflammation of the Heart Sac or Pericarditis,	360
VI.	Valvular Disease of the Heart or Endocarditis,	361
VII.	Angina Pectoris or Neuralgia of the Heart,	363
VIII.	Palpitation.	364
IX.	Various other Diseases of the Heart. 1. Hypertrophy or Enlargement of the Heart. 2. Fatty Degeneration,	365
X.	The Blood Vessels and their Diseases. 1. Aneurism. 2. Varicose Veins,	366–367

CHAPTER XXII.

THE INTESTINES, RECTUM AND THEIR DISEASES, — 368

I.	The Small Intestine,	368
II.	The Large Intestine,	370
III.	Diseases of the Rectum. 1. Congenital Deformity. 2. Injuries of the Rectum. 3. Fissure and Ulcer. 4. Rectal Abscesses and Fistula. 5. Itching about the Anus or Pruritus. 6. Piles or Hemorrhoids. 7. Prolapse of the Rectum. 8. Polypi,	371–375
IV.	Other Rectal Affections. 1. Stricture. 2. Cancer,	375
V.	Rectal Alimentation.	376

		PAGE
VI.	Intestinal Catarrh,	376
VII.	Dysentery,	378
VIII.	Cholera Morbus,	379
IX.	Cholera, Asiatic,	381
X.	Inflammation of the Bowels, Obstruction and Appendicitis,	383–385
XI.	Hernia, Breech or Rupture,	385
XII.	Peritonitis,	387
XIII.	Colic,	388
XIV.	Constipation,	389
XV.	Worms,	391–395

CHAPTER XXIII.

THE KIDNEYS AND THEIR DISEASES, - - - 396
   I. Description of the Kidneys, - - - 396
   II. The Secretions of the Kidneys, - - 398
   III. Diseases of the Kidneys. 1. Gravel. 2. Renal Colic. 3. Pyelitis. 4. Abscess. 5. Cancer. 6. Hydatid Disease, - - 399
   IV. Bright's Disease, - - - - 400
   V. Diabetes, - - - - - 403
   VI. The Supra-renal Capsules, - - - 405
   VII. How to Preserve the Health of the Kidneys, - 405

CHAPTER XXIV.

THE BLADDER AND THE URINARY APPENDAGES, - 407
   I. Description of the Bladder and Neighboring Tissues. 1. The Ureters. 2. The Urethra. 3. The Prostate Gland. 4. Cowper's Glands, - - - - - 407
   II. Acute and Chronic Cystitis or Catarrhal Inflammation of the Bladder, - - - 408
   III. Retention of Urine, - - - - 410
   IV. Suppression of the Urine, - - - 411
   V. Enuresis or Incontinence of Urine, - - 412
   VI. Stone in the Bladder or Vesical Calculus, - 413
   VII. Enlarged Prostate, - - - - 414
   VIII. Other Obscure Affections, - - - 416

CHAPTER XXV.

THE MALE GENITAL ORGANS AND VENEREAL DISEASES, - - - - - 417
   I. Description of the Male Genital Organs, - 417

xiv   CONTENTS.

                                                                              PAGE.

  II. Affections of the Male Genital Organs. 1. Phimosis. 2. Para Phimosis. 3. Congenital Malformation. 4. Warts. 5. Cancer of the Penis. 6. The Testicles. 7. Varicocele. 8. Hydrocele. 9. Hæmatocele. 10. Orchitis. 11. Other Minor Affections,   418–421
 III. Chancre and Chancroid or Venereal Diseases,   421
 IV. Acquired Syphilis, -   -   -   -   422
  V. Hereditary Syphilis, -   -   -   -   424
 VI. Gonorrhœa, Urethritis or Clap and its Complications. 1. Orchitis. 2. Bubo. 3. Chordee. 4. Gleet. 5. Stricture. 6. Gonorrhœal Rheumatism. 7. Purulent Ophthalmia. -   -   -   -   425–429

CHAPTER XXVI.

THE FEMALE GENITAL ORGANS, -   -   -   430
   I. Description of the Female Genital Organs. 1. The Female Pelvis. 2. The Ovaries and their Functions. 3. The Fallopian Tubes. 4. The Uterus or Womb. -   430
  II. Menstruation and its Disorders. 1. Menstruation. 2. Delayed Menstruation. 3. Profuse Menstruation. 4. Cessation of Menstruation. 5. Care of Menstruation,   433–435
 III. Affections of the Female Genital Organs. 1. Pruritus or Troublesome Itching. 2. Leucorrhœa, Whites or Female Weakness. 3. Gonorrhœa in the Female. -   -   436–438

CHAPTER XXVII.

CHILDREN'S DISEASES, -   -   -   -   -   440
    I. Chicken Pox or Varicella, -   -   -   440
   II. Croup, True or Membranous, -   441
  III. Croup, False or Laryngismus, -   -   443
  IV. Cholera Infantum or Summer Complaint, -   444
   V. Diphtheria, -   -   -   -   -   448
  VI. Measles or Rubeola, -   -   -   -   451
 VII. Measles, German or Roseola, -   -   -   453
VIII. Mumps or Parotiditis, -   -   -   454
  IX. Scarlet Fever or Scarlatina, -   -   -   456
   X. Whooping Cough or Pertussis, -   -   459
  XI. Disinfection During and after Diphtheria and Scarlet Fever, -   -   -   -   461

CHAPTER XXVIII.

		Page
Fevers,		464
I.	Bilious or Remittent Fever,	464
II.	Malarial or Intermittent Fever,	465
III.	Catarrhal Fever, Influenza or La Grippe,	468
IV.	Neuralgic Fever or Dengue,	470
V.	Typhoid Fever,	471
VI.	Typhus Fever,	474
VII.	Yellow Fever,	476
VIII.	Puerperal Fever,	477

CHAPTER XXIX.

Nervous Diseases,		479
I.	Epilepsy.	479
II.	Hysteria,	480
III.	Catalepsy,	482
IV.	Ecstacy,	483
V.	Chorea or St. Vitus Dance,	484
VI.	Convulsions, Fits or Spasms,	486

CHAPTER XXX.

General or Unclassified Diseases,		488
I.	Rickets or Rachitis,	488
II.	Erysipelas,	490
III.	Rheumatism,	491
IV.	Gout,	494
V.	Obesity,	496
VI.	Small Pox or Variola,	497
VII.	Varioloid,	499
VIII.	The Prevention of Small Pox or Vaccination,	500

CHAPTER XXXI.

Various Inflammatory Affections,		502
I.	Inflammations,	502
II.	Abscesses,	504
III.	Felon or Whitlow,	505
IV.	Onychia or Suppuration of the Matrix,	506
V.	Ingrowing Nail or Onyxis,	507
VI.	Chilblains,	508
VII.	Boils and Furuncles,	509
VIII.	Carbuncles,	511

		PAGE
IX.	Malignant Pustule or Anthrax,	512
X.	Glanders,	513
XI.	Hydrophobia or Rabies,	514
XII.	Tumors.	516

CHAPTER XXXII.

MARRIAGE AND MATERNITY,		519
I.	Marriage,	519
II.	Reproduction,	523
III.	Symptoms of Pregnancy,	525
IV.	Diseases of Pregnancy,	526
V.	Advice to the Pregnant,	529
VI.	Miscarriage,	530
VII.	Labor, Stages and Management,	531
VIII.	Management of Infants,	536
IX.	Care and Education of Children,	542

CHAPTER XXXIII.

NURSING. DIET FOR THE SICK AND HOW TO PREPARE IT,	546
I.	Nursing,	546
II.	Diet for the Sick and its Preparation,	549

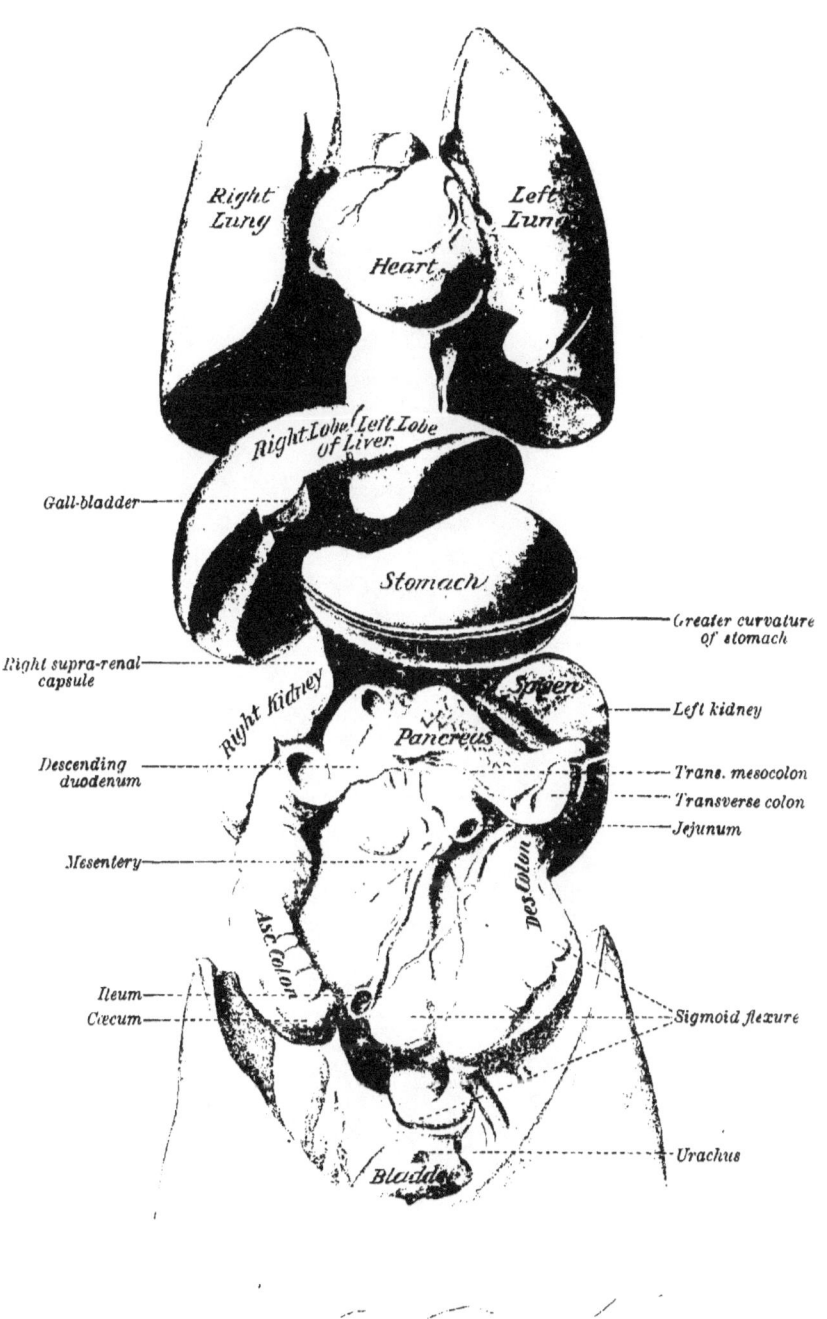

Relations of internal organs. Anterior view.

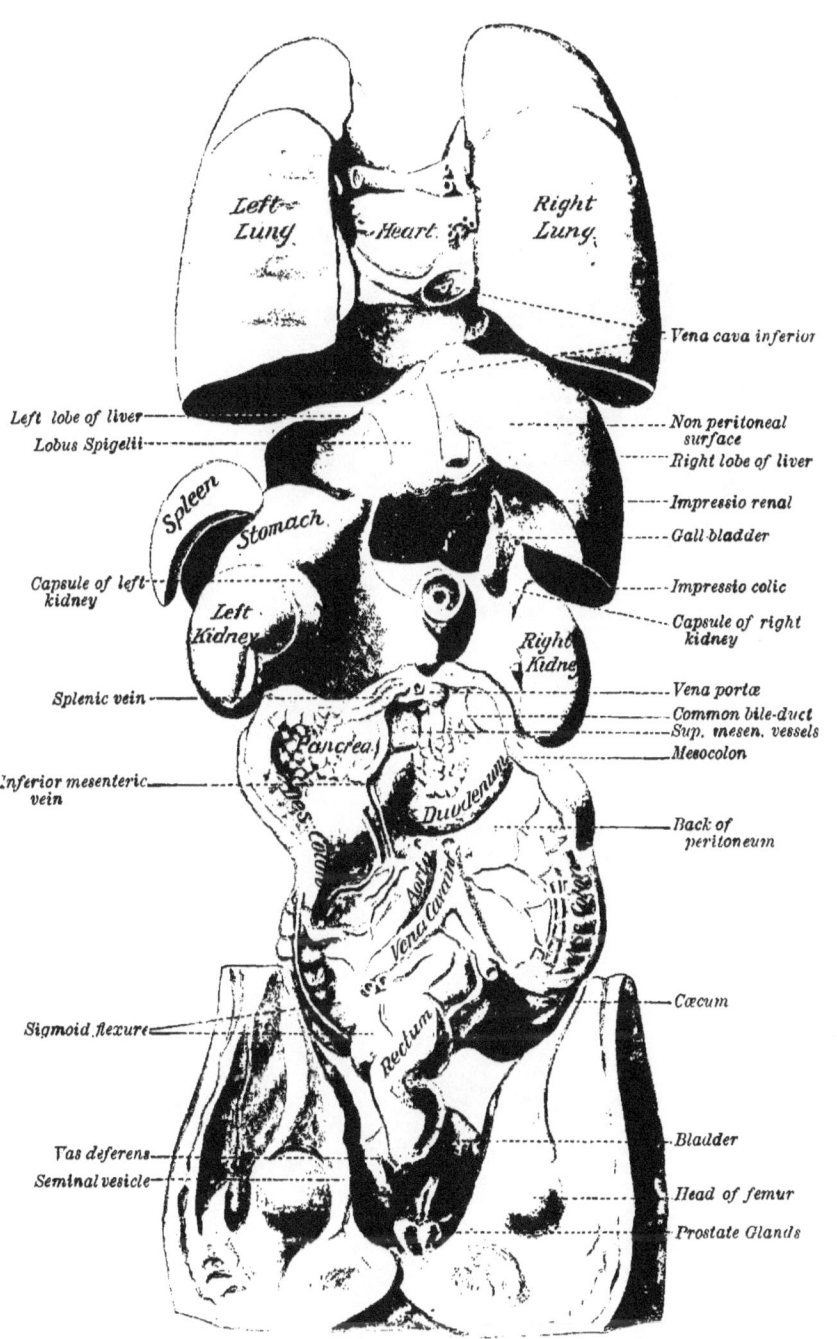

Relations of internal organs. Posterior view.

CHAPTER I.

INTRODUCTORY ARTICLES.

I. MEDICAL PROGRESS. X RAYS.—II. MEDICAL STUDY FASCINATING.—III. MEDICINE A POPULAR SCIENCE.—IV. MEDICAL COMMON SENSE.—V. GENERAL CAUSES OF DISEASE.—VI. SPECIAL CAUSES OF DISEASE.—VII. BACTERIA, OR GERMS IN DISEASE.

I.—MEDICAL PROGRESS.

MEDICINES must have been used at quite an early period in human history, the conditions of life being such that disease is inevitable. Only in jest can one habitually cast out the doctor and "throw physic to the dogs."

To trace the history of medicine for a thousand, or even a hundred years, however interesting the process, becomes too tedious. In the past, many strange agents have been employed medicinally, which seem to us ridiculous, as for instance the hag-stone, which was supposed to keep the troublesome witches from sitting upon the sleeper's stomach, and thus prevent the nightmare

The history of medicine has been associated to no little extent, with charlatans and pretenders; notwithstanding, we flatter ourselves that medical science has been making remarkable progress during the last half century.

The medical men of to-day are trying faithfully to answer these questions:

What ails the sick? What is the best method of treating disease? How can disease be prevented?

Notice what recent medical science has done to answer this question: What ails the sick?

It produces the microscope, to examine diseased tissues, and announce with certainty, the difference between a cancer and a harmless growth.

It is able to disclose disease germs when they exist in the saliva, the sputa, the urine and other excretions, as well as in the food and water which we consume.

It brings forward the fever thermometer, to record the accurate temperature of the body, and is capable of revealing whether pus is forming, or other danger signals.

It has invented the stethoscope, to exaggerate the abnormal sounds in the lungs and heart, so that diseased conditions are readily recognized.

It provides many other delicate instruments to assist in the examination of the eye, the throat and other obscure organs.

By the aid of these modern inventions, we are far better able to obtain a correct answer to the question: What ails the sick?

Great progress has been made in modern times toward answering our second question: What is the best method of treating disease?

Physiologists have made important discoveries with living animals causing them to suffer for the good of man. There is no question but what much definite knowledge concerning the action of medicines upon the blood, the nerve centers, and other important tissues, has been obtained by these experiments upon the lower animals. In this, and in various other ways, medical science has been constantly advancing and the sufferings of mankind correspondingly alleviated.

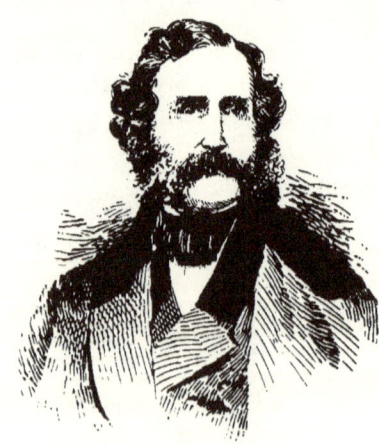

DR. WILLIAM T. G. MORTON.

The discovery of Ether and Chloroform for the relief of pain, marked an important advance in the science of medicine, while words almost fail to portray the benefits which attend their use in surgery. There are many surgical operations made successful by their use, which could not be attempted without them.

Dr. William T. G. Morton, the Boston, Mass., dentist, who discovered anæsthesia, and opened up the way for painless operations in Surgery was born in 1819, and died in 1868. His claim was satisfactorily demonstrated on the 16th of October, 1846, at the Massachusetts General Hospital. Before that time whenever misfortune rendered the surgeon's knife a necessity, the patient experienced an extreme sense of suffering and untold agony. Since then and for all future time the agony of the operating room has been and will forever be "steeped in the waters of forgetfulness."

The injection of medicine under the skin, a comparatively recent method, antidotes and relieves the most agonizing pain. The hypodermic use of medicine, while it should be employed exclusively by physicians, has much in its favor. The medicine enters the circulation immediately, and is not altered and changed by the slow process of digestion, as it is when administered by the mouth, and it is able to relieve the severest pain in a very brief space of time, and thus beginning inflammations are conquered at the very threshold. There are many medicines which could be administered in this way to great advantage, and are likely to be so employed more frequently in time to come.

Electricity is an agent that has come somewhat to the front in medical practice, and is sometimes curative when other remedies have failed. It is used to improve the nutrition of wasting muscles, by stimulating and strengthening their nerve control; hence it arrests atrophy or wasting, and restores power to limbs that are partially paralyzed. It is also used to remove superfluous hairs from fair faces, to destroy moles, birthmarks, and for various other purposes.

Anyone can observe that great progress has been made in the management of acute diseases, in recent times; instead of depletion, blisters, blood-letting, setons, issues, heroic doses of mercury and other powerful drugs, we present a method which we are certain yields better results. We sustain the strength of the patient and make use of good nursing and hygienic measures with increased success.

The working of nature is at present more fully recognized in treating the sick; it is found that with timely and simple assistance, she is often able to work the miracle of healing, with the aid of but very little medicine.

Still more important than the questions already answered is this last one: How can disease be prevented?

Anxiety to answer this, has led to the vigorous study of hygiene and sanitary science. Such study is comparatively recent. Much attention is now being properly given to our water, ice, milk and other food supplies. The infectious germs, only recently recognized, producing typhoid and scarlet fever, diphtheria, consumption, and an exceedingly large list of other diseases, have been investigated with untiring diligence, and with the avowed aim of preventing the spread of these undesirable, and often fatal infections or contagious diseases. The habitat of these germs is sought out to find where they originate and multiply, and what are the conditions favorable to their spread and multiplication. To this end, defective sewerage is inspected and remedied, well water suspected of contamination is analyzed, and a thousand matters are awakening general attention which relate to the prevention of disease, and hence the germs of disease are often destroyed and its spread prevented.

We have learned that it is easier, safer, and less expensive to prevent disease, than to restore health after weeks of prostration and suffering.

There were never more agencies at work to prevent the spread of disease than at present, and as for medical men, they were never more intelligent, or better able to cope with it and baffle its ravages. In respect to these matters, the day which has dawned upon us knows no sunset. Eminent men may die, but progress in the healing art is destined to a perpetuity as lasting as the race. Facts are constantly accumulating, discoveries are being multiplied for curtailing human maladies, relieving human suffering, and checking the spread of infectious and contagious diseases.

The present is often spoken of as the age of invention, the age of rapid transit, rapid transmission of speech, wonderful machinery and a thousand inventions, which, in the light of the past are marvelous; but at the same time thoughtless persons are prone to intimate that medicine is now and has forever been at a standstill, that so far as the medical profession is concerned, there has been no progress. Such imputations are utterly without foundation. There is no body of men more keenly alive to every scientific improvement in the sphere of their labors than the large and educated body of physicians practicing medicine throughout our broad land.

THE X RAYS.

The discovery of the X rays by Professor Röntgen of Wurtzburg was announced during the preparation of this work. It has proved to be of unusual interest to the scientific world, and has stimulated experimentation in the field of electrical research enormously.

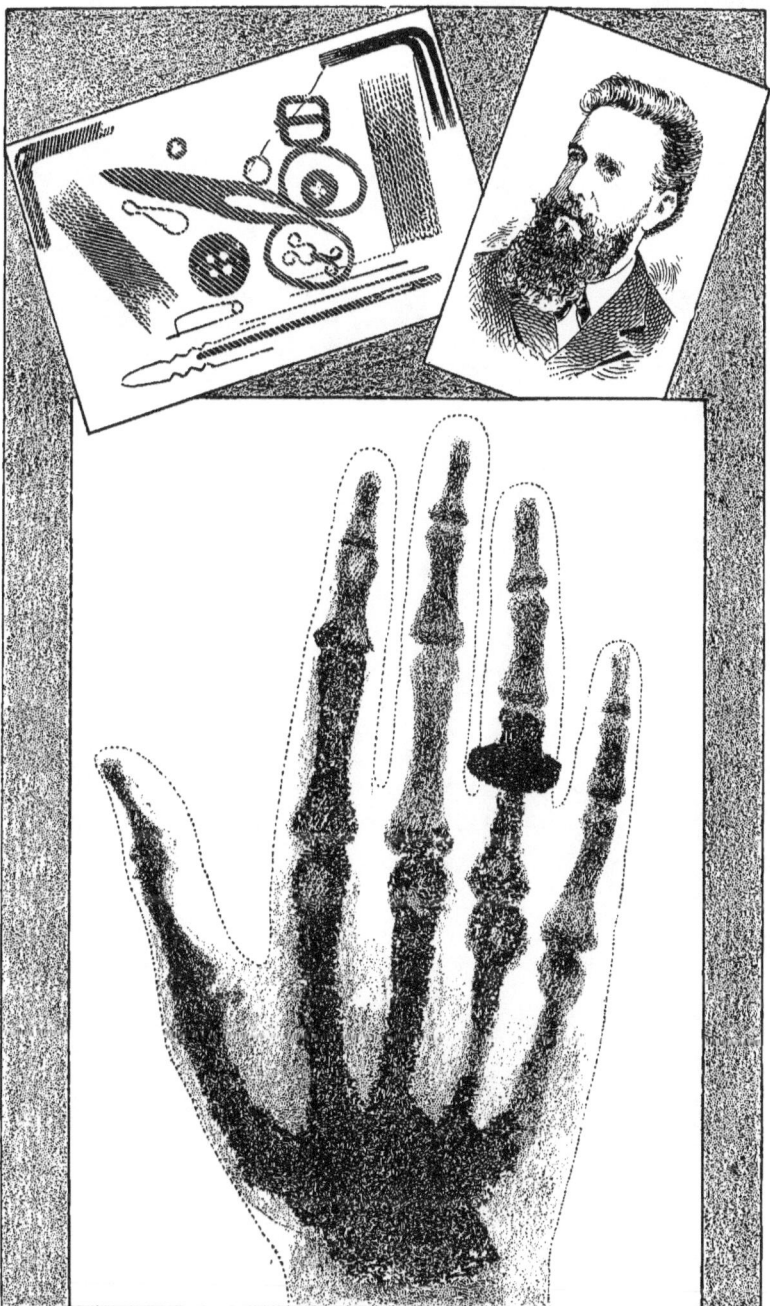

1.—Photographs of scissors, needles, pins, etc., enclosed in a leather case with metal cornerpieces. 2.—Dr. William Konrad Röntgen, discoverer of the X Rays, Professor of Physics at the Royal University of Würzburg. He had only a local reputation before the announcement of the discovery of the X Rays but on account of this he has suddenly become famous 3.—Photograph of a lady's hand, showing the bones, and a ring on the third finger, with faint outlines of the flesh.

The previous employment of electricity for the larger development of light and force is phenomenal, for during the past ten years our methods of street travel and lighting have been revolutionized. Thus the world had been prepared by the rapid progress of the recent past to give this new discovery fitting attention and widespread notoriety.

It was at once perceived that the Röntgen discovery would be of extraordinary interest to medical men, as its practical side has a special bearing upon the further and more complete examination of the living tissues of the human body.

It has been known for many (40) years, that the negative or cathode current, when passed through a glass vacuum tube, produces a vivid fluorescence. Professor Röntgen discovered that when passing a rapidly interrupted current of these cathode rays through a glass vacuum tube, some of the rays penetrate more or less certain substances and cast a shadow picture upon a photographic plate, the distinctness of which depends upon the character of the substance exposed. In brief the whole process is carried on by means of a Ruhmkorph coil connected with a Crookes tube. The portion of the body to be examined is placed between an opening in a disk of the tube and a sensitive photographic plate. The rays which penetrate and cause the shadow on the plate may be cathode rays, ultra-violet rays, or others associated with them. Just what rays produce the picture is as yet not definitely known, and hence the discoverer called them X rays, because X is used to denote an unknown quantity or factor.

The picture made by the employment of the X rays has received a variety of names, but as yet no scientific term suggested seems more appropriate than Skiagraph, which literally means a shadow writing.

The X rays, though imperceptible, readily pass through flesh, leather, clothing and other similar substances. They pass less readily through bone or metal, except aluminum. Glass through which ordinary rays of light pass with much readiness almost completely obstructs the passage of the X rays.

When the human hand or foot is exposed in the manner already indicated, a shadow picture is formed upon the photographic plate which reveals the outline of the hand, foot or other part exposed. In this shadow picture the muscles and soft tissues show only a little in their outline, the bones themselves show much plainer, so that it is possible by this process for one to see a picture of his own framework; as though a living person could look upon his own skeleton.

Any foreign body, as a piece of glass, needle, bullet, or other piece of metal, is readily detected and located, also any deformity such as results from a fracture or dislocation, or an abnormal growth or bone enlargement may be discovered so that it may be remedied.

Up to the present time the hands, feet, forearm, and such portions of the body, are more successfully penetrated by the X rays than the head, which is surrounded by thick plates of bone on all sides.

The trunk and pelvis for similar reasons are as yet difficult to penetrate, and thus reproduction upon a sensitive plate by this interesting process awaits other discoveries to perfect the methods employed.

Many improvements for producing these shadow pictures have been suggested and attempted with more or less success in nearly every electrical laboratory.

As the matter now stands the discovery of the X rays is a great aid in certain diagnoses and promises to render the surgeon especially valuable assistance in the performance of his delicate and often difficult work.

II.—MEDICAL STUDY FASCINATING.

Medical study possesses a peculiar and remarkable fascination! Who does not wish to know more about the mechanism of the human body, and the laws which govern it, whose keeping bring health and delight, and whose violation entails sickness, distress and death?

What can be of more practical service than to know how to keep well and strong, and perpetually young?

The owner of a valuable horse is particular about his care, his food, grooming, shoeing, the fit of the harness, in fact, whatever conduces to the good looks and lofty bearing of this noble animal. Inasmuch as man is better than the horse, ought he not to receive greater attention? It is a part of our mission to devote such care to ourselves and the race as will conduce to the health, happiness and longevity of all. In order to do this, we must devote an intelligent interest to a large variety of subjects. Attention must be given to cleanliness, for frequent baths are necessary to keep the skin in a healthy condition. The eyes, the ears, the teeth, the hands, the feet, all require especial care. Exercise, rest, clothing, proper food for the body and mind, are important. How fascinating ought to be the consideration of all these subjects, so intimately are they related to the important question of our health! We do not exaggerate when we say that there are no more interesting subjects than these which relate to medical study, in its bearing upon healthy men, women and children; subjects which are thoroughly treated in this household work.

III.—MEDICINE A POPULAR SCIENCE.

Formerly the physician appeared to have a monopoly of medical knowledge, and was regarded with profound veneration. He was considered the wisest among men, whether he spoke or remained silent. Even the movement of his head in the sick room was ominous. This old time veneration for professional men belongs to the past. Medical subjects are no longer shrouded in mystery, which only the physician cares to penetrate.

The human body is not, as formerly, but little understood and studied by the masses. Even the school children are now taught the rudiments of anatomy and physiology, and many besides professional persons know considerable about one or more of the several branches of medicine.

Intelligent people are everywhere discussing hygienic measures, the prevention of sickness, the quarantine of contagious diseases, the causes of disease, the latest theories, especially the germ theory and other kindred topics. Nearly every household magazine, at the present time, has its medical department for answering the many questions proposed by its readers, and various medical subjects are studied and written up, so that medicine to-day, may be especially regarded as a popular science.

This increased interest in medical subjects is to be hailed with delight, for the more intelligent the people are concerning these matters, the more satisfaction can be derived, and the greater the success which will attend treating their ailments.

A smattering of medical knowledge is likely to make people fussy, superstitious, and the easy victims of prejudice or incompetency. A general and cultivated understanding of these subjects renders a person sensible, self-reliant, and better fitted to act deliberately and wisely in times of emergency and danger. Such persons, instead of being frightened, and ready to faint at the sight of a drop of blood, render timely and valuable assistance to the injured.

The more generally medical knowledge can be disseminated, the better it will be for the physician, for he is liable to have his best suggestions hindered, and his anxious hopes blighted, by the want of intelligent co-operation. The physician is sure to experience far greater pleasure in his earnest and difficult work, when his suggestions are helped to the utmost, by intelligent co-operation, and his patient is correspondingly benefited.

Medical subjects, too, of all others, broaden the mind, enlighten the understanding, and fit men and women everywhere to better fill their places in a world of suffering and misfortune.

IV.—MEDICAL COMMON SENSE.

There are usually thought to be several schools of medicine. In reality there ought to be only one, and that one broad and liberal enough to embrace every method and remedy of positive value. Prejudice has done much in the past to prevent the best results of medical science. It has been fostered by selfishness, and encouraged by ignorance. The age of prejudice fortunately is slowly passing away, and yet how few, even at the present time, know that apart from pretensions, there is but one field of medical science. The field, it must be remembered, is a very broad one, for there is no patent upon medical books, or medical knowledge, and no monopoly of these can be created.

The first requisite of a medical student, as of every other, should be a teachable spirit, and he should resolve to receive the truth, from whatever source it originates. The untaught mind is like a dark room, and we must throw open the shutters and let in the light unhindered. It is fortunate indeed that many a mind is broader than its professed creed, and it is to be hoped that every one who practices the healing art, is progressive enough to lay aside prejudice, and make use of the very best known remedies, in the very best manner possible.

There is no question but what medicines have sometimes hindered the process of recovery, and in such cases better results would have been obtained without them. It is as important to know when to withhold, as when to prescribe. When medicinal agents are necessary they should be used in such doses as will assist nature to reach the desired result. The law of cause and effect should not be ignored; for it should operate constantly when we attempt to work any preceptible changes upon diseased conditions. We must apply the same good judgment to medicine which is successfully applied to farming or shop-keeping.

For the reasons given above this book contains no sections upon homeopathic, eclectic nor other *special* methods of treatment.

It proposes to recognize truth from all reliable sources and any remedy sufficiently important to be embodied into this work has not been intentionally withheld nor obscured on account of its origin or advocates; the same is true with respect to the medical doses recommended; for in all cases where admissible the medium dose rather than the maximum has been given the preference.

The design has been toward a broad, liberal and modern system of medical belief and practice. There has been no intention of narrowing the broad circle of medical knowledge nor of fostering prejudice.

V.—GENERAL CAUSES OF DISEASE.

Medical study trenches upon a much wider field than the curing of disease. It embraces a large variety of subjects of vital importance to the health and well being of the family and community. A consideration of these topics, so closely allied to medicine proper, cannot be omitted without failure to understand the obscure causes of many important affections. In order to treat the sick intelligently, one must consider the question of diet, exercise, ventilation, clothing, climate, proper nursing, and many other subjects related to the welfare of those suffering from acute or chronic affections.

It is necessary to study the causes of diseases, in order to learn how to bring about their removal. We must understand how contagious diseases spread, in order to check, successfully, their onward march. It is usually necessary to know the cause of a patient's suffering, in order to administer the proper remedy.

When sickness invades a family or breaks out suddenly in some particular locality, the foremost question is,—What caused the outbreak? The physician is not the only person interested in the origin of disease. It is a matter of vital interest to the general public. Hence, at the present time, others beside the family doctor, are asking the following questions: Is the location of this house a healthy one? Is the cellar clean, dry, light and well ventilated? Is the plumbing modern and worthy? Is there anything about the house or its location that can favor the introduction or assist in developing disease? If there is any defect about the sanitary condition of this dwelling, can it be successfully remedied? Has it been thoroughly disinfected since it gave shelter to contagious disease?

As population multiplies and becomes more crowded in the large cities a knowledge of the causes and the methods of prevention, especially of the infectious and contagious diseases, becomes more essential to all classes, the rich and the poor alike.

Questions of no less importance about the water supply, concern us all. When we consider that the many outbreaks of typhoid fever, entailing upon communities vast cost and large mortality, are, or can be traced in nearly ever instance to water polluted by infectious germs, an abundant supply of pure water cannot be regarded with indifference.

Many diseases are also caused by unhealthy occupations. It is essential that those inheriting a debilitated condition of the system or who are otherwise unfitted for the dangers and hardships of certain callings or occupations should avoid them.

Mental worry and anxiety exert a depressing influence upon all the processes of life. So well is this recognized, that the saying has passed into a proverb, that "worry kills more people than hard work." It is probable that this well-known fact accounts for the many frequent deaths among public men, in the prime of life. Men of business, men at the head of great enterprises, politicians and statesmen are no doubt often heavily laded with vexatious care and exposed to a fatiguing mental strain, which weakens digestion, induces insomnia, and causes the prostration of the whole nervous system. Many sensitive men, who occupy positions of great responsibility, are fearfully fretted and annoyed by needlessly harsh and cruel criticisms. Is it a matter of wonder, when they envy the health of the daily toiler, whose food, though coarse, is sweet, and whose sleep is refreshing? We shall never know how large the list is, of this vast number, cut off in the prime of life, in the midst of their activities, disappointed, grieved, wounded and broken-hearted. Only physicians are able to perceive how widespread are the nervous troubles which grow out of our intense activities, our struggles to get ahead in the world, the constant worry and perplexity which in the heat of the strife is so exhausting.

Our variable and ever changing climate often exerts a deleterious effect upon infants, old people and those otherwise debilitated.

A large number of acute and chronic affections are supposed to have their origin in that almost indescribable process which is denominated *taking cold*.

Intemperance, and other reprehensible habits, should not be lost sight of in this enumeration.

From the intimations of this brief article you will observe that the causes of disease form a very complex and exhaustive subject, which must receive detailed attention elsewhere, for here we have only touched upon them in the most general manner.

VI.—SPECIAL CAUSES OF DISEASE.

The number of defined diseases is put down as two hundred and fifty. Of these, about one hundred are more or less fatal, and add to the death rate. In a comparatively few instances, accidents and unavoidable calamities, such as storms, floods, earthquakes and lightning, increase slightly, the rate of fatalities.

But for the fatal diseases, man would, with the few exceptions noticed, live a natural life, and die a natural death.

In old age, death is a natural process, for it is simply conformity to nature.

With but few exceptions, disease comes from without, and like a foreign foe attacks the system. This is readily seen in contagious diseases, while hereditary diseases, like scrofula and syphilis, appear to be exceptions.

It has been discovered quite recently that contagious diseases are due to organic poisons, which enter the system in the form of microscopical disease germs from the air or water consumed by the individual. These germs find in the human body favorable soil for their development, and begin to multiply and so affect the blood and other tissues as to cause sickness, prostration, and often death.

Atmospheric conditions are prominent factors in the causation of such diseases as bronchitis, croup and catarrh, and the heat of summer and autumn is prominent in causing diarrhœal diseases.

Some diseases extend everywhere, while others are found only in certain sections. Yellow fever requires a high temperature, while consumption is limited by excessive cold.

A very large number of the well-known diseases are preventable, their progress can be checked, and their spread limited. In other words they can be controlled.

Diseases resulting from over work can be prevented, because they are self induced. Other diseases which result from the habitual use of debilitating agents, as alcohol, tobacco, narcotics and poisons are preventable.

Contact with those dreadful diseases which work through human passions, as syphilis, can be prevented. This is a foul and dreadful disease, for it pollutes all life which it touches and travels down to blight the innocent ones of future generations.

Among the old medical writers the predisposing and exciting causes of disease were much dwelt upon. When insanity appeared in a family through several generations, they said such a family was predisposed to mental disease. Other families were predisposed to scrofula, others to gout or rheumatism, to epilepsy, to cancer and other diseases. The second term, exciting causes, was much in vogue.

Sedentary habits are regarded as the exciting cause of constipation. Want of cleanliness is considered to be the exciting cause of certain affections of the skin. Poor ventilation causes diseases of the blood and respiratory organs, loss of sleep, mental disturbances, and improper food taken into the stomach, dyspepsia. Colds are generally considered as an exciting cause of many diseases, as croup, bronchitis, catarrh, etc.

The diseases which result from old age should be regarded as natural. They are especially heart failure and stomach failure. The digestive apparatus is worn out and is no longer able to perform its task. In old age congestion of the lungs is common, owing to a weak condition of the circulation.

Heat produces burns, and excessive heat of the sun, sunstroke. Cold causes frostbite, lack of food, starvation. Intemperance produces a long train of bodily disturbances. Tobacco and opium produce typical diseases, and you are referred to the articles upon those topics.

VII.—BACTERIA OR GERMS IN DISEASE.

Reference has been made so frequently to the influence of germs or bacteria in causing disease, that a brief review of a few things known about them will help us to a more intelligent understanding of this interesting subject. The microscope has revealed a vast army of life which is invisible to the naked eye, and because the bacteria are visible only by means of its power, they are often called micro-organisms. So minute are these germs that it has been difficult to decide whether they belong to the realm of animals or plants. They are so small that several hundred of them would scarcely stretch across the head of a pin.

It is only within the last half century that these germs have been recognized and studied. In fact such recognition and study was impossible previous to the perfection of a microscope which would magnify three or four thousand diameters. One of these microscopes reveals a drop of water as an animated skating rink, containing many millions of these micro-organisms.

They vary in shape. Some are spherical or egg-shaped, and these are known as micrococci; others are rod-shaped, like a match or pencil, these are bacilli; still others are spiral, like a corkscrew, these are spirilla. The rod-shaped are the most common variety. They are composed of a cell and enveloping material. It is usual to stain them red, blue or violet, in order to trace their outlines more perfectly.

Their movements are accomplished by means of hair-like projections or cilia, which have been successfully photographed.

When the conditions are favorable for these germs they multiply rapidly; these conditions are warmth, moisture, oxygen and organic matter. The estimate of their multiplying ability is marvelous if they encounter no obstructions.

Fortunately the struggle for life is especially severe among these lower orders of microbes, and the weak go continually to the wall. One variety may feed upon and destroy another, or one variety may become extinct for lack of material to provide nourishment. Some are poisonous, and poison each other. Some species are enemies and cannot thrive together; some cannot live without other varieties, and if separated, die.

Many of these germs are harmless, so far as the human race is concerned, while others are beneficial, and absolutely essential. The latter are our invisible friends, and indispensable to human existence. Only a few are capable of producing disease, and find favorable conditions for their development in the human body.

They may be cultivated like plants and flowers. Some thrive

in this, others in that medium; some kinds will grow on a piece of cooked potato; some in beef broth; some thrive by means of heat; others can endure a great amount of cold and survive freezing.

Germs are the agents of putrefaction; they reduce all animal matter after death, to dust, and set free all kinds of odors, good and bad, sweet and sour. They are found everywhere, but are more abundant where putrefaction is going on. They exist in the water, in the soil and on all plants, vegetables and fruits.

It may be remarked that the canning of fruit is simply a process to keep out the germs which produce fermentation; boiling destroys them and sealing the can keeps out those that pervade the atmosphere.

In this connection, it will help our understanding of this whole subject to define what is meant by a spore. A bacterium that is unable, for the time being, to reproduce itself, becomes a spore. Spores become dry and lie dormant, like the seeds of a plant, till they are brought into favorable conditions for their development. These spores are carried about in the air, and float about our rooms like particles of dust, as if searching for moisture and a foothold. When such opportunity is found, they develop like the seeds of plants, and produce a progeny. The dried yeast germs are examples of these spores; they lie dormant until they are introduced into the moistened flour, when they begin to multiply with marvelous rapidity.

We have already hinted that there are certain varieties of germs which, in the human body, produce disease. Their activity liberates poisons called ptomaines, which produce fever, sickness and a train of systemic disturbances. We shall endeavor to give, in condensed form, a few of the leading facts which have been learned about these disease producing germs or bacteria.

The causes of disease have baffled all former ages. When the germ theory was first proposed to account for the mysterious origin of certain diseases, it had only a few believers, but the more carefully and thoughtfully intelligent persons investigated the subject, the more converts to this teaching were multiplied, till at the present time all scientists have adopted the germ origin of infectious diseases.

The revelations of the microscope have banished ancient superstitions, and brought to light millions of agents which swarm in the air and water about us, most of which are not only harmless to the human body, but are absolutely essential to its well being. Some of these germs, however, are found to be always present in certain forms of disease, and it is believed that they cause its outbreak. There are certain diseases which when introduced into a family or community, spread more or less rapidly. A small quantity of the disease poison, no matter whether introduced into the system in the act of respiration or with the food and drink, reaches the circulation, and creates a marked disturbance, especially rise of temperature, due to the rapid multiplication of this poison, or septic material. The multiplication of this septic material resembles the action of yeast, a little of which soon permeates the whole mass. It multiplies with marvelous rapidity, and produces fermentative changes. One sort of germs produces measles; another, typhoid fever; another, consumption; still another, small pox; another, chicken pox; and so on through the large list of contagious diseases.

These varieties of germs always reproduce themselves, and are always true to their kind. The yeast germ always produces the same kind of fermentation, the measles germ always produces measles, and never small pox. The small pox germ never begets cholera, and so on, to the end of the chapter.

Each variety of germ works under its own special law, but in all some general methods are observed. Upon exposure to the disease contagia or germs, a certain time is necessary for their development, this period is known as the incubation; during which time the disease lies dormant in the body. The period of incubation varies from a few hours, as in scarlet fever, to several weeks or months, as in hydrophobia.

Having had a germ disease once, we are not likely to have that same disease again. The yeast germ will not work the second time upon the same mass. It consumes all the material favorable to its growth and development the first time, so that there is nothing left for it to feed itself upon in the future. Introduced the second time, the germ is most likely to die of starvation, unless new material has been elaborated upon which it can subsist.

In some of these germ diseases the poison or infectious germ, can be approached nearer than others, without danger of contagion. In small pox or measles it is either necessary to come near the infected person, or else in contact with some object, as clothing, that has been about or near the sick person, or the dried spores which are capable of communicating the contagion. In diseases like cholera and yellow fever, the poison is wafted through the air for some distance. It is perfectly safe to pass by a house where small pox exists, and there is little danger of contracting the disease, but the district even, where cholera or yellow fever exists cannot be visited without peril.

In some diseases, the poison is introduced by means of infected drinking water, or the emanations of infected water carried into the house by means of sewer gas. Other disease germs must be brought into actual contact with the mucous membrane, of which gonorrhœa and syphilis are examples.

Each year the character of these disease germs is becoming better understood. The enthusiastic labor of Louis Pasteur has done much to bring about an understanding of the character of bacteria. Such infinite painstaking as he has manifested has not been too highly rewarded by the eminence he has attained, and the unusual honor he has received. Sir Joseph Lister applied the principle enunciated by Louis Pasteur to the dressing of wounds. By keeping disease germs out of wounds, they heal without the development of erysipelas, or the formation, in many instances, of a single drop of pus.

A knowledge of the character of these disease producing germs helps us to know what course to pursue in each case, in order to prevent the spread of the contagion. Some are readily destroyed by one agent, and others by another. In general, the sick should be isolated from the well, and when the disease is over, disinfection and thorough destruction of the germs should take place. The fumes of burning sulphur destroy the germs of diphtheria and scarlet fever; boiling destroys the typhoid germ in drinking water, and renders it harmless. Cold destroys the yellow fever germ, and heat the small pox germ.

When proper disinfection is neglected, or when the work is imperfectly done, cases of contagious disease multiply. Disease germs are easily destroyed outside of the human body if we only know how. They are destroyed with great difficulty after they have entered the circulation. It is not wise to imitate the man who swallowed a potato bug and then Paris green to kill it. All germicides are poisons, and can be used to much better advantage outside than within the human body.

CHAPTER II.

SANITARY SUBJECTS.

I. The Choice of a Home.—II. The House Furnishings.—III. Drainage and Sewerage.—IV. The Air and Ventilation.—V. The Water Supply.—VI. Food.—VII. Clothing.—VIII. Climate.—IX. Exercise.—X. Longevity.

I.—THE CHOICE OF A HOME.

"He who has health has hope; and he who has hope, has everything."

THOSE who have abundant means experience but little trouble in the choice of a home. They can select an elevated position, on dry, porous soil, where the surroundings are attractive, and the sunlight makes cheerful and healthful the rooms of the house. They can have the best drainage and sewerage possible, for there is no commodity which money will not buy. They can employ competent and skillful architects, to supervise the work of building, and carry into effect the most advanced knowledge in respect to ventilation, plumbing and other hygienic requisites which conduce to the health and happiness of the family.

There is a large and respectable class, however, who cannot select the situation and build the house they would like; they are compelled to make the best selection possible for a quite limited sum of money.

If laboring men could choose their homes in accord with their intelligence and taste, they would undoubtedly prefer elevated and healthy situations, dry soil, pure air and water, abundance of sunlight, and thorough drainage. Abundant means add greatly to the ability of building homes after the most approved patterns; in fact, it is the indispensable requisite for carrying out advanced health measures to any marked degree.

The truth is, that a laboring man, with a family to support, is obliged to provide such a home as his limited earnings will command. This is the reason he is so often forced into unhealthy and filthy quarters, where the rooms are small and receive but little sunlight, where the alleys and streets are foul and odorous. He has not preferred for his family, mouldy walls, damp cellars, filthy alleys, defective drainage, and a polluted atmosphere, but he has become the creature of necessity, and he has been unable to escape his environment. Between the wealthy and the unfortunate poor alluded to, every grade of necessity intervenes.

Only a portion of the income can be expended for rent; in addition food, fuel, and clothing must be procured, and a margin allowed for incidentals. No family, at the present time, will be satisfied with the bare necessities of life. Clothing must not only be warm and durable, but it must also be tasty in appearance. The wife feels compelled to dress herself and children so as to avoid ridicule, and be admitted, at least, to the privileges of common society. A man who retains his self-respect cannot permit his family to be regarded nor treated as outcasts; it then becomes necessary to conform somewhat to the customs of the times so far as they are harmless, and to be in touch with the people among whom one lives.

The laboring man who has a family to support, unless he receives more than the average wages, must practice a rigid economy. The expenses and wages must be in proportion; for the income must equal or exceed the outgo. In addition to the ordinary expenses the unexpected is always likely to occur, so that where five dollars were planned, ten are often required. Sickness, though undesired and unprepared for, is liable to come, and who can deny a sick child the luxuries which a fevered or abnormal condition demands. If the wife is sick, expenses multiply rapidly, hired service must do the work she so cheerfully performs, and so reluctantly puts aside. These are some of the odds against which the laboring classes are often compelled to struggle in our large cities. The first, most difficult, and most important lesson for them to learn is economy, if they would ever become the independent possessors of a dwelling place.

The problem at first is a hard one. It is not merely to live on the income, but to lay by something each year for the purchase of a home. It is easy for a family of average size to dispose of a large income, when the desires are not restrained, and extravagance prevented. Every man ought to look forward, for many reasons, to the possession of a home. Landlords are often petty tyrants, doing only what they are compelled for the health and convenience of the tenant. The laboring man, aided by his wife, ought to make a heroic effort to escape such tyranny, and become the independent possessor of a home, which will conduce greatly to the health and happiness of his family.

The author of this work, a few years ago, attended three cases of diphtheria in a tenement house, where an examination of the sanitary condition of the premises revealed a desperate condition of affairs. The sink drains were conducted, about twenty feet from the back door to a surface privy vault, which was overflowing from heavy rains and surface water, and the overflow found its way back into the cellar, and stood there, a pool of filth about two feet deep. From such places, unworthy the name of home, the laboring man ought to pray earnestly to be delivered, and so strive to improve his condition by rigid and enforced economy, that he can become the owner of a more suitable and homelike dwelling.

Co-operative banks and building loan associations have accomplished much in helping these worthy and scantily paid laborers out of their difficulties. In making choice of a home avoid damp, unhealthy locations; do not be tempted into a swamp or peat bog by a cheap lot. An elevated position is always preferable for a house; sandy soil or gravel is desirable, sunlight is free, and enters wherever permitted, carrying cheerfulness and good health. It is a destroyer of disease germs, and contributes more than we are aware to cheerfulness, happiness and longevity. Sleeping rooms ought to be large, well ventilated and admit abundant sunlight. Nearly one-third of our time is spent in sleep, and to occupy rooms which are small, damp, and otherwise unsuitable for such a large proportion of time, is to invite rheumatism, malaria and other undesirable diseases. In buying a home already constructed, examine the woodwork in the cellar, this will give you a clue to the desirability of the place or the reverse. If you find dampness, mould and decaying timber, do not negotiate for the premises, no matter how low the figures.

A house is not desirable covered in and about with dense shade. Shade trees are delightful a proper distance away, but if too near, they render a house damp and unhealthy.

II.—THE HOUSE FURNISHINGS.

Dust accumulates and abounds in human habitations; it always contains undesirable properties, and whatever harbors it and prevents its thorough and constant removal is, from the standpoint of health, undesirable in the furnishings of a home.

Managers of hospitals have at length learned the best way to keep out infectious disease germs. You do not find carpets upon the floors, paper upon the walls, draperies, pictures and upholstered furniture as formerly, because it has been learned at last that all these beautiful products of a modern civilization are liable to become a menace to the health of the inmates. What is true of hospitals would be as forcibly true of all our homes, if they were constantly crowded with the sick.

The objection to woolen carpets, upholstered furniture, draperies and such like, is not their convenience, elegance or cost, but it is that they become the receptacles of dust, and when stirred or moved by a footstep, they send into the surrounding atmosphere a cloud of dust and lint which, if destitute of disease germs is, to say the least, irritating to the air passages, and unfavorable to the enjoyment of perfect health. A hard floor, with mats or movable rugs, which are daily shaken, is free from the objections which arise against a carpet fastened to the floor and removed for purposes of cleaning only once or twice a year.

All furniture should be plain, chairs cane-seated and without upholstery. The less furniture put into sleeping rooms the better for health purposes. A matting carpet is cool, is easily cleaned and preferable to tapestry or brussels. Draperies and portieres are undesirable, for they harbor dust, which, upon the slightest agitation, is precipitated into the air, and gives to a person whose air passages are especially sensitive, a stuffy, unpleasant sensation, and in other instances produces such difficulty of breathing, as to render the victim unable to sleep or rest.

It is the over-furnishing of the homes of the wealthy which makes their apartments often more unhealthy than those of the poor, including polluted air and lack of ventilation. When contagious diseases gain a foothold in these costly furnishings they are dislodged with difficulty, and for this reason, consumption, diphtheria and scarlet fever, are often more obstinate and malignant in homes of gorgeous interior, than in the humble abodes of the poor. Many die surrounded by all the elegances and conveniences of civilization, the victims of myriads of disease germs, floating in the respired air, who would have recovered in tents by the seashore, or in the pine woods, with only nature's soft carpet beneath them, and the sweet, pure air and blue sky around and above them. It is quite possible to sacrifice too much for elegance, convenience, and the gratification of our taste for beautiful and costly furnishings.

The health of the wife and her vigorous and rosy children, a thousand times more than compensate for attention to all these details of furniture, whose principal ends ought to be utility and cleanliness. In the homes expensively furnished we often find the husband the only party whose countenance bears upon it the evidence of health, and for the reason that he spends a large part of his time away from home. The wife appears faded and sickly, and the few children, or often lone child, still spared by disease and death, are slender, pallid, irritable and unhappy.

There is no deficiency in what money can buy, but a sad deficiency, perhaps, in the best gifts of nature, rosy cheeks, sparkling eyes, smiling lips and healthy bloom.

III.—DRAINAGE AND SEWERAGE.

These hygienic articles only contemplate the consideration of subjects closely related to health, with a view to the prevention of disease. It is therefore unnecessary, for practical purposes, to follow the usual course, and consider drainage and sewerage as two separate subjects, the former referring to surplus water about a house from rain and damp soils, and the latter to excrementitious matter including the refuse of the kitchen and sink. We will agree at the outset, to understand by drainage, all the surplus of water, and the waste material capable of fermentation and decomposition, which it is necessary to remove beyond the reach of human habitation, in order to prevent dampness and the pollution of the soil and atmosphere. Most of the waste products of human habitations in cities, are conducted away in drain pipes aided by the inflow of water. These conveying pipes ought to be of sound material, with perfect joints.

Defects in drainage are due to a great variety of causes, among which may be mentioned the hasty construction of houses; the soil about them settles, and often disarranges and strains the pipes, and opens their joints. Drains placed in new or made soils, should have the earth packed solidly about them by tamping, in order to prevent the dangers which result from injury to the pipes and the escape of sewer gas into the cellar or surrounding soil.

Cheap plumbing is always dear in the end, and that which is costly may be spoiled by bad workmanship and prove unsatisfactory and unsafe. When doing a job so important as the house plumbing, use only good materials, and employ only reliable workmen. It is poor economy to scrimp here and get a poor job. Have the best plumbing which experience has sanctioned, and have it adequate for the demands made upon it.

Plan for a dry cellar; if necessary, have it cemented, and place tiles below the cellar bottom to drain away moisture, and conduct it outside the walls. Avoid surface sink-drains if possible. When there is a system of adequate sewerage, the refuse from the sink empties into the sewer. Look diligently to see that these pipes do not become loaded inside with grease, and be sure of good trapping to keep gases and odor out of the house. Perfect plumbing is such a rarity that sewer pipes should never be carried into sleeping rooms, nor into the closets which open out of sleeping rooms, for the purpose of having handy washbowls.

The water-closet and bath-room should have an abundant supply of water, the former should have the overhead flush. The elevated cistern should contain several gallons and deliver it with such force as to secure thorough cleansing. The "pan" closet is unsatisfactory, filthy, and ought not to be tolerated. It is flushed by a valve in the supply pipe, which delivers an inadequate amount of water for flushing purposes and often leaks, wetting the woodwork about the seat bowl. In the modern appliances, the cistern or reservoir is elevated and the space about the bowl is left open, which secures cleanliness and ventilation; this is a great improvement on the pan closet with leaky pipes and a space boarded up about the bowl which cannot be easily reached and cleaned.

Whatever the system of sewerage, make sure that the soil about your dwelling does not become polluted with refuse liquids, and become the breeding place of germs; also make sure that sewer gas and unhealthy odors do not gain admittance to your house.

A few things are absolutely essential for the maintenance of health; these are pure air, pure food, and pure water. Pure air is impossible without pure soil. Water must not be contaminated by proximity of the supply to vaults and cesspools, nor must it be permitted to absorb sewer gas.

Proper drainage is of paramount importance to the health of a family. It is not always easy to state the precise relation between ill-health and improper drainage. It has been proved, however, that diphtheria is much more prevalent in damp localities. Dampness and filth, while they do not of themselves cause diphtheria, seem to furnish the essential conditions by which this disease thrives and becomes malignant. Human beings naturally pollute their surroundings, both the atmosphere and soil; as population becomes more dense the danger multiplies. The unpolluted country with its pure air and water possesses the ideal requisites for perfect health, while the crowded city where poverty and filth abound, offers all the favoring conditions for the development and spread of disease. Hence the saying that "God made the country and man the town" has long since passed into a proverb. It is well known that typhoid fever germs may gain an entrance into houses and prostrate the inmates with tedious and expensive disease by means of imperfectly trapped sewer connections.

The nations of the old world have been slow in learning that cleanliness is an important factor in staying the march of devastating diseases; they have manifested great carelessness in polluting with filth the soil and atmosphere about their habitations, and hence the plague and other frightful epidemics have swept over Europe repeatedly, leaving in some rare cases not more than one-tenth of the population alive, and in other still rarer cases whole districts were abandoned to the wild beasts, the entire population dying leaving only a desert and desolation behind. During four years in the fourth century we learn that the plague or black death, resulting from the filthy conditions of life, destroyed forty millions of people. The cholera of India is attributed by modern writers to the filthy habits of the pilgrims. These diseases together with scurvy and typhus fever, are now almost unknown among civilized nations, abolished by better health measures and attention to the removal of filth and decomposing vegetable and animal substances. It is only quite recently that people are beginning to comprehend the causes of disease and manifest an interest in those conditions which render the existence and spread of disease possible, and it is still more recently that they are earnestly trying to master the knowledge which will altogether banish many of the contagious and infectious diseases.

A few practical thoughts should be thoroughly impressed upon the minds of everyone. The removal of all filth from the habitations of man to some place where it cannot vitiate the atmosphere, pollute the water, nor breed disease should be speedily accomplished. The drain pipes which carry off the kitchen slops should be securely trapped, and in hot weather proper disinfectants should be dissolved in hot water and poured into the sink; copperas is excellent for this purpose. Garbage should be removed before decomposition takes place and foul odors arise therefrom. Where there are no sewers in the country the slops from the sink should be carried away from the house where they may be used for fertilizing fruit trees and the garden. In the country all drains should be carried far away from the well if it is used to supply water, neither should surface water, the result of heavy rains, be permitted to reach it.

The water-closet in the country should be abundantly supplied with dry earth, charcoal or ashes, and these should be freely used so as to absorb the liquids and prevent odors. A solution of copperas should be used occasionally and no neglect in emptying the contents of the receiving box should be permitted.

People living in the country should remember that typhoid fever is more prevalent in small places than in the city, and the contagious germs usually enter the system by means of polluted water. Wherever odors are noticed they should be regarded as signals of danger, and receive prompt and efficient attention. It is likely that the best methods of drainage have not yet been devised. Some method, unprejudicial to health, is needed which will prevent the pollution of our rivers and streams and which will enrich our soil by using it for fertilizing purposes.

IV.—THE AIR AND VENTILATION.

The air performs a very important service in the animal economy. It is a mixture composed of nitrogen, oxygen, carbonic acid, moisture and small amounts of organic matter. Nearly four-fifths of this mixture is nitrogen, which has only the one known office of diluting the oxygen sufficiently to render it suitable for the requirements of respiration. The most important constituent of the air is oxygen, and without this vital element no animal life could be maintained. Neither could animal life exist in an atmosphere of pure oxygen, for it is too stimulating and it has to be diluted very much to adapt it to the requirements of respiration.

Combustible substances burn with a greatly increased brilliancy in an atmosphere of pure oxygen, and many which are not combustible under ordinary circumstances will burn freely in such an atmosphere.

The oxygen which we breathe is the great source of animal heat. It gives health and bright, red color to the blood. It acts as a stimulant to the brain, the muscles and all the functions of organized life.

Air contains a small quantity of carbonic acid, a varying amount of moisture which renders the act of respiration more easy and some other substances in small amounts which are quite unimportant. Air like water is a solvent of other substances, and for this reason is often very impure. The act of respiration adds to the impurity of the air about us and soon renders it unfit for use, unless there is constant renewal and ventilation. In the act of breathing oxygen is taken from the air and carbonic acid is added. A person breathes about twenty times a minute, using on an average sixteen cubic inches of air each respiration, or nineteen thousand cubic inches each hour. Every person may therefore be said to vitiate about one cubic foot of air each minute. The combustion of every pound of coal consumes the oxygen out of one hundred and twenty cubic feet of air. A single candle consumes the oxygen of ten cubic feet of air each hour and an oil lamp about twenty cubic feet. A person's sleeping room ought to contain one thousand cubic feet of air to provide sufficient amount for respiration during a single night. It is the oxygen of the air which sustains life, and by maintaining a condition of slow combustion in the body maintains the animal heat. It also comes in contact with the carbon in our stoves and furnaces, and thus the process of combustion is carried on and heat is evolved. For breathing purposes the purity of the air is of no little consequence. Some of the diseases which result from breathing impure air are those of the respiratory organs, as catarrh, bronchitis, asthma, broncho-pneumonia, etc.

Wall paper colored by arsenical pigments may give rise to poison vapors sufficient to produce symptoms of that particular poison upon the occupants of a room. In paint shops the vapors and particles of lead may escape into the air in sufficient quantity to produce after a long time symptoms of lead poisoning. Those working in quicksilver mines often absorb mercurial vapors sufficient to produce the symptoms of poisoning. The impurities of the air also produce disorders of the digestive functions. The air may contain, and transport disease germs, it may be loaded with impurities arising from the soil or from decaying vegetable and putrefying animal matter, or pollution arising from human habitations. It is on account of this tendency of the air to absorb impurities and transport them, and to carry disease germs, that we cannot be indifferent to the squalor and disease of the slums of a city. The health and cleanliness of one home concerns every other home in the vicinity, and from a hygienic standpoint every man becomes his "brother's keeper."

VENTILATION.

As human beings rapidly pollute the air about them, the subject of ventilation is of prime importance. The act of respiration removes oxygen from the air and in its place is found carbonic acid, ammonia, sulphureted hydrogen and decomposing organic matter. It is maintained that from the moisture in the expired air a very poisonous liquid can be distilled capable of producing almost instant death. The process of ventilation is to let out the polluted air, and admit pure air in its place. In a work of this kind we must consider ventilation in a practical manner; for we cannot enter into the theoretical, scientific or chemical study of the subject. This must be left to the domain of special works. The dangers from polluted air demand our notice because they come under the head of the prevention of disease. Some of the more immediate and noticeable results of impure air are headache, languor, loss of appetite, faintness, vomiting and diarrhœa. It is well known that some persons are more susceptible to the effects of impure air than others, usually the weak, the debilitated, infants and children showing the first and clearest signs of suffering, while the middle aged, the vigorous and strong are affected the least.

Where the blood is thin and deficient and the lung capacity is small the results are most marked and disastrous. A skilled person can judge much concerning the efficiency of ventilation from the appearance of the inmates of the house. Those habitually subjected to the influences of impure air reveal a pallid, anæmic condition, a want of color in the face, a peculiar lack of vitality.

Special attention ought to be given to the ventilation of public halls, theatres, churches, and above all in the order of importance, schoolrooms. The crowded condition especially of city schoolrooms and the tendencies and lack of vitality on the part of the younger children, make them the easy victims of a vitiated atmosphere. It would be better for children to remain partially uneducated, than to be poisoned, dwarfed and ruined by the pollution of schoolroom atmosphere.

An item which interferes with ventilation in cold climates is the expense. The changing of the air means the loss of heated air and the incoming of cooler currents to take its place. Heat is expensive, school boards and other authorities usually vote cautiously and too exclusively on the side of economy, rather than on the side of pure air, health and incidental expenses. With the poor who live in small, overcrowded rooms heated by the cook stove, the question of ventilation is often entirely overlooked in the efforts put forth to keep from freezing.

Floating dust is the housekeeper's nuisance. In order to remove it from a house spread a line of damp sawdust across the room and sweep it before you, or if woolen carpets are to be cleaned, dampen the sawdust with a carbolic acid solution. In this way cleanliness and disinfection can be combined. After sweeping, damp cloths should be used to remove the remaining dust from furniture and woodwork. It aids very much in removing the dust to open the outside doors and windows while sweeping, as the air loaded with dust and lint, is driven out by the incoming currents. The dust of rooms is composed of a great variety of pulverized substances including filth and lint, and is to say the least, irritating to the air passages. It may become quite an important factor in chronic diseases of the nose, throat, bronchial tubes and lungs. It is important to drive it out of the house.

In considering the dangers which threaten human abodes, almost a monopoly of attention and interest have been given to sewers and the drinking of polluted water. Contagious diseases, however, are not transmitted by odors nor by air contaminated by the decomposition of vegetable or animal matter in sewers or elsewhere, unless the specific germs of contagion are present. Decaying cabbages or potatoes are unhealthy and render the air unsuitable for respiration, but they cannot convey diphtheria nor other infectious and contagious diseases, unless in addition the germs are present which produce the infection or contagion; as, however, they furnish an excellent hiding-place for disease germs, ventilation demands the removal of all decaying substances from the cellar and all the filth and mouldy articles which are so prone to accumulate even in the best regulated homes, in cellars, pantries, dark passages and out of sight places.

The air of the cellar constantly penetrates the other rooms of the house and it should be made sweet and wholesome at all times by ventilation. It is unkind to charge Providence with the results of our filth, impure air and laziness. Mould and mustiness in the cellar are danger signals and should be driven out by persistent ventilation and an abundant use of whitewash.

Anything which vitiates the atmosphere rendering it unfit for respiration, must be considered as an indirect cause of disease, and hence there are many apparently insignificant matters often overlooked in the sanitary inspection of health boards, which are of vital importance practically. There are many people who possess a bad breath, the result of decayed teeth or an untreated catarrh. All these causes of polluted atmosphere are easily remedied, but require attention to additional matters aside from thorough ventilation. Some one has properly said that "the price of a healthy, clean breath is eternal vigilance and a toothbrush." Five minutes devoted to cleaning the mouth and teeth after eating would add much to the sweetness and cleanness of many a home, and those who cannot spend that amount of time in the interest of sweetness must be sadly overworked. A few pennies spent for one of the remedies recommended for nasal catarrh will remove the disagreeable odor from that filthy disorder, and those who cannot afford the amount of money required in the interest of a sweet breath must be poor indeed.

If a person's teeth, mouth, nose and skin are in such a condition as to perceptibly scent the air, the effect must be injurious to the person himself. As the odor does not come from the lungs, the foul-mouthed not only breathe out but also breathe in polluted air into their own lungs; hence they poison themselves and become a nuisance to others.

Many workingmen smoke old, filthy pipes. Wherever they go they taint the air with sickening odors. If they enter your home for only a few minutes you are obliged to open the doors and windows to drive out the intolerable and indescribable stench left behind them. They pollute the cramped apartments of their own home and render it unfit for a human being. In the winter when fuel is expensive and pure air is shut out as much as possible, and ventilation is disregarded, think of crowding a family of four or five persons into such a stifling place to live and obtain the oxygen needed from such an atmosphere. Add to these quarters the smoke and odors of cooking and you have a condition of affairs that is truly loathsome.

Just think what a struggle an infant must have, introduced into such an atmosphere at the sensitive period of birth. No wonder the inmates look yellow as if cured by the smoking process. Imagine the germs of contagious diseases introduced into such polluted quarters, and fancy if you can, what the doctor has to contend with. Is it any wonder that the disease is often superior to his drugs? It is fortunate if he has positive views in regard to sanitary conditions, and smashes out a pane of glass or opens a window and drives out the vile air by the incoming of some that is fit for respiration. This will be of nearly as much service as any medicine he can prescribe, and will probably aid the working of his prescription so as to give a fighting chance for victory.

Some of these matters affect more intimately the welfare of the homes of the laboring classes than anything ever touched upon by health boards. There are no subjects of more vital importance to the homes of the poor than cleanliness and ventilation. In Iceland where the houses are destitute of all devices for ventilation, we are told that the odor which arises from the herding together of human beings and animals, the refuse of fish and the filthy habits, is beyond description, and the infant mortality terrible. Births equal the averages in other places, yet population is decreasing, for the majority of children born die within twelve days of an endemic disease generated in the foul atmosphere. It is said that a similar condition of affairs exists in the Hebrides Islands.

The remedy for foul cellars, house odors and musty parlors is ventilation. Bedrooms and bedding should be exposed to the sunlight and air. Faded carpets are more desirable than faded children. Fresh air and sunlight are not only the best disinfectants known, but are the cheapest; for they will save the doctor's call and may prevent the Angel of Death from spreading his dark wings over the household.

V.—THE WATER SUPPLY.

The estimated amount of water required for the use of each person daily, including the bath and closet, averages twenty-five gallons. This estimate is, as it should be, abundant. In all large cities the water from wells except artesian should be avoided; for it is usually polluted by surface drainage and in very deep wells the water is warm and dissolves impurities. In small communities even, the water is liable to become contaminated and produce sickness. Wells should be removed away from all dangers of pollution by barn-yards, privies, cesspools and sink drains. Water absorbs ammonia gas, phosphureted gas, sulphureted hydrogen, and other impurities. Chemically considered all water is impure, but not sufficiently so to prevent its healthful use for drinking purposes.

Great care must be taken in cities to prevent water from absorbing sewer gas. Water which contains decomposing nitrogenous matter is polluted by sewerage and unsuitable for use.

Lead pipes are unhealthy conductors of water, especially if it contains as an impurity lime in solution. Rain water dissolves lead to some extent. A larger amount than one one-hundred and fortieth of a grain of lead in a gallon of water renders it unsuitable for drinking purposes, and if the use of such water is continued for a long time, symptoms of lead poisoning are liable to intervene.

The analysis of water is not as usually supposed a very simple process. There are a variety of methods of purifying water. When mixed with clay and vegetable matter it may be allowed to stand till the foreign matters settle, when the upper portion can be removed. A lump of alum dissolved in a bowl of water curdles the vegetable substances and carries the impurities to the bottom. The amount of alum must be so small as not to be tasted. This method on a small scale is made use of in purifying the water supplies of many cities and large towns at the present time.

It is claimed that when water to which the proper amount of alum, one-third of a grain to each gallon has been added, has passed through a filter every trace of it disappears, the alum uniting according to this theory, with the organic matters in solution forming a coagulum which the process of filtering removes.

A small amount of permanganate of potash may be added to water just sufficient to give it a pink tinge. If the water does not change the color of this addition there is no organic impurity contained in it to occasion fear, and it may be safely used for drinking purposes.

Pure water may be obtained by the process of distillation, and this method is employed by the druggist.

Freezing water into ice purifies it only in theory, and hence ice taken from rivers polluted by sewerage is unfit for household purposes.

Water is sterilized by boiling, as there are no germs that can survive the process of boiling water for ten minutes. This is the most important of all methods for domestic use. Water raised to the boiling point for a short time and then cooled is safe for sick or well persons to drink as freely as needed.

The filtering of water through charcoal and sand removes the solid matters. This is a valuable method and much employed. It will not, however, remove every element of danger in waters contaminated by sewerage, and for this reason the boiling of water is a means of great safety.

Rain water collected in cisterns and filtered through charcoal and sand is in many sections abounding in minerals the most healthy water that can be obtained. A good filter can be extemporized by a little ingenuity which will serve an admirable purpose. Take a barrel, fix in a faucet near the bottom; a few inches above the bottom put in a false bottom full of holes and over this stretch a layer of flannel. Then put in a two-inch layer of clean gravel, and above this a layer of pounded charcoal. Repeat this process, adding a layer of clean, small gravel and then a layer of charcoal, till within one foot of the top of the barrel. The last layer should be gravel covered with another layer of flannel held in position by half a dozen clean stones, so as to hold all in place when a bucket of water is turned in. Draw off the filtered water from the faucet.

Spring water, which is not too heavily charged with minerals, and coming from elevated regions above and beyond human habitations, is healthful. Water is decomposed into hydrogen and oxygen by means of electricity, for the purposes of experimentation; there being just twice as much hydrogen as oxygen by measure.

Pure water is destitute of smell and taste and is colorless except in large quantities, when it has a bluish tinge. Water is constantly evaporating from the surface of the earth and passing into the air as an invisible vapor, so that the air is always more or less charged with moisture. This vapor is condensed in the higher and cooler currents of the atmosphere, and descends to the earth again in the form of rain.

Water unlike most other substances is expanded by cold, and this fact is of very great consequence, as otherwise ice would settle to the bottom of rivers and lakes where the rays of the sun could never melt it.

Impure water, especially that contaminated by sewerage, causes no little disturbance to health, such as loss of appetite, dyspepsia, gastritis and diarrhœal diseases. The breaking out of diarrhœal affections in any community ought at once to direct attention to the water supply. It has already been noted that the germs of typhoid fever and cholera may be introduced into the system through the pollution of our water supply with human dejections. Stomach worms also gain an entrance into the system through unsuitable drinking water. How important then to the health and well being of every family is the consideration of this subject.

VI.—FOOD.

Waste and repair are the phenomena which characterize all animal life. Every process of thought or motion, whether voluntary or involuntary, involves destruction of tissue. The more vigorous the thought or muscular activity, the more rapid the process of waste. The activities of the student's brain, the anxieties of the man of business, the sedentary occupations of the professional man, consume force and produce bodily waste as well as the muscular efforts put forth by laborers in swinging the scythe, lifting the sledge or following the plow. The involuntary movements of the lungs in breathing or the heart in maintaining the circulation consume a certain measure of force, and this force is produced by the combustion and destruction of tissue.

Nature is constantly demanding fuel for her fire. The lungs bring fresh oxygen to the blood nearly twenty times each minute; for oxygen being essential to combustion, a constant and never-failing supply must be provided. It would be inconvenient, however, to eat food as constantly as we breathe, and so a stomach or receptacle for food is provided, and by eating at intervals, usually about three times a day, enough for nutrition is stored up to meet the requirements of the body in repairing its wastes, and hence an equilibrium is maintained both of nutrition and animal heat. When the store of food in the stomach is exhausted, nature admonishes us by a feeling of hunger and thirst, a desire for food and a relish for it, which makes the gratification of the appetite in health one of the most common pleasures of living.

When we consider what a complex piece of machinery the human body is and that whatever enters into its composition must be supplied from our food, it seems as though it would be essential to employ a chemist to preside over the culinary department of the household, and instruct the cook in order that our food may contain lime, sulphur, magnesia, soda and potash for the muscles and bones, phosphorous for the brain, iron for the blood, together with other mineral salts and acids which unite to build up a human body. The chemist, however, can be dispensed with because nature has anticipated all the requirements of the body, in the great variety of foods placed at our disposal and if the appetite is normal and the food supply is not too scanty and too limited in variety, she can develop and maintain a healthy body, but if some abnormal development of the appetite exists so that the food demanded by nature is loathed, or there is poverty in the amount and variety of food, then diseases of nutrition may develop, as rickets, a crooked spine, anæmia, gout and scurvy, while under such conditions the course of scrofula and consumption is greatly accelerated.

Where the food supply is abundant, very little attention has to be given by the individual to the consideration of its constituents or as to whether it contains the essential elements required by the body. For the appetite will be a safe guide, unless it has been pampered and spoiled like some only child by too much indulgence. The appetite is not an infallible guide, since it must be controlled, especially in children, by persons of reason, good judgment and experience. It is safe to gratify the appetite to a reasonable extent by good wholesome food of which persons rarely over eat.

The danger of over eating is not from the appetite, but from the arts of the cook by which foods are made too rich, too highly seasoned or too concentrated for the stomach. As a rule the plainer and more simple the preparation of food, the more wholesome it is, and the less danger there will be of over feeding. We can already see why suitable, nutritious and wholesome food is such an important factor in preserving the health of individuals and families. A thorough study of nutritious and wholesome food involves a consideration of the chemical composition of the various articles of diet; but this cannot be entered upon in a work like this, which covers so great a variety of subjects in a single volume. It will be sufficient to give a few practical hints, and direct those who wish to study the subject further to special works on physiology.

As to the disputed question in regard to animal foods, the vegetarian contends that vegetable foods only are intended for use, that the slaughter of animals is cruel, repulsive and wicked. He does not, however, hesitate to partake freely of milk, eggs, cheese and butter. As these belong to the list of animal foods, even those who profess to be vegetarians are so only in name. Experience teaches that a mixed diet of meat and vegetables is the most natural and wholesome. Too large an amount of animal food causes congestion of the liver, and probably enlargement of that organ. Sedentary persons and the aged, who use too much meat, develop a tendency to gout, disorders of the blood, degeneration of the arteries and apoplexy. An excess of foods containing fat, produces bilious troubles and obesity; while a diet of rice and starchy foods requires the consumption of too large an amount in quantity to satisfy the bodily requirements; and the development of body and mind in nations too exclusively confined to their use, is notably inferior. Good milk contains all the elements of nutrition and is an excellent and nutritious article of food. Of all foods it is the most suitable for infants prior to dentition.

The two great classes of foods required by nature are the nitrogenous foods, so called because nitrogen enters largely into their composition, and the carbo-hydrates or non-nitrogenous. A human being could not thrive on an exclusive diet of either. The nitrogenous foods are represented by muscle or lean meat, fish, the caseine of milk, the gluten in bread, the albumen of the egg, beans, peas and other vegetables. These also contribute to the formation of muscle or flesh, while the carbo-hydrates are represented by starch, sugar, oils and fats. These latter are the heat and fat producing articles of food. They unite with oxygen in the body and produce a slow combustion, by which heat is evolved. The heat of the body is maintained during summer and winter at an even temperature of $98\frac{3}{4}$ degrees.

It must be remembered that many articles of food contain both the muscle or flesh forming and fat producing elements, as well as small amounts of minerals required by the body. The cereals also contain phosphates; potatoes, cabbage and other vegetables contain the salts of potash; beets and other vegetables contain iron; the yolk of an egg, sulphur; meat contains, in concentrated form, food for the muscles and brain and the same mineral constituents as are required by the human body. The most substantial, nutritious and easily digested meats are beef and mutton, and none are more healthy. Water and common salt are among the important articles which are required for the nutrition of the body, a large proportion of which is water. Water assists in the digestion and assimilation of food; for it is nature's solvent. It keeps the blood in the proper fluid condition, so that new material can be carried to build up the tissues, and it dissolves the waste products and holds them in solution so that they can be removed by the kidneys, bowels, sweat glands and the lungs.

The art of cooking has much to do with the digestibility and appropriateness of the diet. Many foods would be unsuited to our use unless cooked. It is to be remembered that foods may be injured and made indigestible by improper cooking. Fried foods and articles permeated by grease are difficult to digest, and are certain to overtax and distress the stomach of the student and others of sedentary habits. Heavy bread, strong tea and coffee, alcoholic stimulants, and many other things which could be mentioned are injurious to the stomach and detrimental to the health.

It is not necessary to purchase the highest priced pieces of meat in order to obtain healthy food. The cheaper pieces are toothsome and nourishing when properly cooked. The succulent vegetables should be sound and fresh, and in such condition are healthy and desirable. Meats should be used before becoming tainted; and stale eggs are very undesirable for food. The foods prepared for our use, of whatever kind, should be sound and wholesome, properly cooked and deliberately eaten. The variety should be sufficient and the amount abundant in order to supply all the elements which nature requires to produce cartilage, bone, muscle, brain and nerve, and to supply the force which our activities of body and mind constantly expend. Muscular force and nerve force we consume more rapidly and lavishly than less civilized nations. When the food supply is just sufficient to repair the wastes of the body and maintain the tissues, the bodily weight remains constant, if the food supply is inadequate, the weight diminishes; and when the food supply is taken in excess, the weight is liable to increase. When this latter process is going on too rapidly, the amount of food should be diminished, and exercise increased. Nature makes considerable provision for the removal of the surplus food material which she does not require, and rigorous exercise favors the process.

Persons who are accumulating flesh or fat too rapidly, ought to diminish the luxuries of the table and increase their out-door activities. The danger of taking too little exercise is greater than of taking too much food.

The amount and quality of food required is influenced considerably by the occupation and climate. Those who perform severe manual labor require a substantial diet of both the muscle and fat producing foods. In cold climates more food is consumed, especially the fats and oils; for nature demands these in order to maintain the animal heat. In temperate climates more of the fat producing foods are used in the winter to supply the demands of nature, while in the summer, fruits, berries and vegetables are more plentiful and their increased use more appropriate than fat meats. Every person requires some fat at all seasons, but as scarcely anyone eats bread without butter, or potatoes without gravies, this demand is supplied in our ordinary diet.

The action of the saliva, the secretions of the stomach, the pancreas, the bile and the intestinal juices upon the food belongs to the subject of digestion, and is mentioned in its appropriate place.

Tea and coffee are largely used throughout the civilized world. They are somewhat stimulating in their effects and prevent waste of muscular and nerve tissue. It is a well-known fact that those using tea and coffee consume less solid foods. When used, the amount should be moderate and if nervous troubles are developed or augmented, their use should be restricted, or even discontinued if necessary. Coffee, as well as tea, is a quiet stimulant to the nervous forces. It quickens the intellectual faculties, aids digestion, invigorates not only the brain but also the body and increases mental and physical endurance. The drinking of coffee at night usually produces wakefulness. Good coffee can be obtained only by buying it in the kernel. It should not be too coarsely nor too finely ground. It is best made by adding boiling water and should be prepared as wanted, for if boiled too much the delicate aroma is dissipated and restaurant or boarding house coffee is the result. Both tea and coffee contain tannin, and too much boiling extracts this undesirable astringent, which produces constipation. Cocoa makes a nutritious and healthy drink when properly prepared.

Children should not be allowed to drink tea and coffee. In their stead they should be supplied with milk, which is not stimulating, more nutritious and much better adapted to their needs. Feeding the sick is treated elsewhere, as it forms an important part in their recovery and restoration.

VII.—CLOTHING.

If this subject had no bearing upon the prevention of disease it could be dismissed with few words. The relation however between clothing and health is so intimate and important as to demand recognition. The uses of clothing are so numerous and the services it performs so manifold, that it ought to awaken the interest of all who are solicitous about the preservation of their health.

As made use of in civilized countries its principal office is to cover and conceal the person, except the hands and face and a portion of the head. In a narrow and heated belt of the tropical world, savage tribes almost wholly dispense with clothing and in consequence are but little burdened with what in civilized countries constitutes a considerable item in the column of expense.

Many of the animals have a covering of hair which protects them from the changes of climate, adapting them to the heat of summer and the cold of winter. In the early fall winter's approach is anticipated by a luxuriant growth of the fur which becomes thick and heavy. Near the approach of spring the shedding process occurs and the hair falls rapidly and thus the heat and cold are anticipated and provided against yearly. Man has a similar protection for his head but the wearing of fashionable hats and other effects of modern civilization have an unfavorable influence upon the hair, the bulbs are injured and the hair often falls from the crown and dome of the cranium by or before middle life.

Civilization appears to be especially destructive to the teeth and hair.

Another use of clothing is protection from external injuries, but especially from the effects of heat and cold. In the temperate and frigid zones protection from the rigor and changes of the climate is a necessity. It is doubtful whether human beings could be sufficiently toughened to endure the variations of the climatic changes of the temperate zone even, without clothing. The colder and more changeable the climate the more apparent and forcible is the necessity for suitable clothing. It is a well-known fact that the body becomes heated by exercise and in this condition the pores of the skin gradually open wider, the sudorific glands are stimulated by warmth to increased activity and a large amount of moisture is carried to the surface of the body, where evaporation takes place rapidly in order to lower the temperature and establish an equilibrium.

In this relaxed condition clothing prevents cold currents of air from coming in direct contact with the skin, the results of which would be a shock of the cutaneous nerves, a rapid flow of blood to the internal organs with congestion of the same, chilling of the surface and the taking of a cold which so often proves disastrous.

Another important use of clothing is to prevent a rapid escape of the animal heat. This is lost in two ways, by evaporation and radiation. When evaporation is too rapid the surface is cooled too quickly, the body is chilled and often with serious consequences. Clothing then has its most important use in retarding the cooling process. Those fabrics are most suitable for clothing which are the poorest conductors of heat, as they most retard evaporation and radiation.

Among the poor conductors of heat are silk and woolen, while cotton and linen represent the opposite quality. Owing in part to the expensiveness of silk, woolen may be regarded as the best known material for many articles of wearing apparel. It has great affinity for that moisture and retains it in large amount. It is owing to the fact evaporation goes on so slowly from its meshes that one does not feel cold and clammy after sweating, as is the case with muslin or linen.

It is the slow evaporation of moisture from woolen which renders flannel so comfortable for summer wear. Clothing itself is neither warm nor cold. Its serviceable use in winter depends upon its ability to retain the bodily heat and in summer to prevent rapid evaporation of moisture. Woolen clothing meets both these requirements, for it is porous, containing air in its meshes and hence does not permit heat to escape like cotton or linen.

Another use of clothing is adornment. This in civilized countries occupies much thought and attention, and often overthrows the best teachings respecting its sanitary use. Fashion is often averse to the more legitimate use of clothing, but so much has been said in this line as to render its repetition uncalled for and hackneyed.

The essential requisites of clothing are comfort and warmth. Men are more apt to dress comfortable than women; for they ordinarily pay less attention to the dictates of fashion and would not hesitate to violate her mandates if she ventured to interfere too perceptibly with male attire. Men do not gracefully submit to discomfort and violate the laws of health, since they are not as patient and resigned in tribulation and suffering as their less complaining sisters.

The appearance of women at receptions in winter with the fashionably low cut dresses which expose the throat, chest and arms, if in good taste, sadly conflicts with every requirement of health. Whatever violates the sanitary demands of clothing should be abandoned as unbecoming and unsuitable no matter what other advantages may be claimed.

Clothing should be worn sufficiently loose to permit full play and natural movement of all the muscles of the body. To dress otherwise or to constrict the waist and change the form which nature has chosen as most fitting is foolish indeed, and entails a large amount of suffering in the aggregate. Intelligent persons at least ought to know that a slight waist detracts from the graceful appearance of the human form. Nature needs no remodeling and reshaping with ribs of bone and steel. Life at the best is full of suffering; why multiply our sorrows or shorten our days? Tight lacing produces, by unnatural pressure, injurious effects upon the delicate abdominal organs which cannot escape displacement. It limits the expansion of the thorax, interferes with the play of the diaphragm, the great muscle of respiration, which ought to be free to rise and fall with every breath. Digestion, circulation and respiration, the three great and essential functions of animal life, all suffer evil consequences.

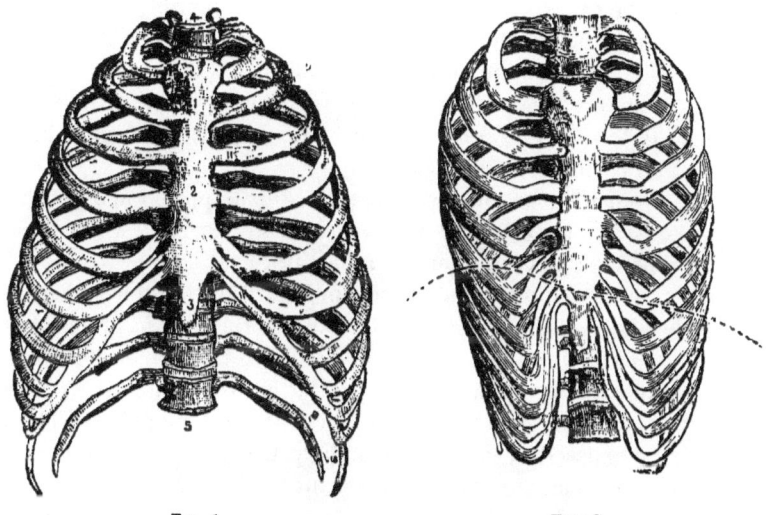

FIG. 1.   FIG. 2.

FIGURE 1.—Bones of the chest in their natural relations.
FIGURE 2.—Bones of the chest which have been distorted by tight lacing

Whatever impedes the circulation though it be only a tight garter, a close-fitting glove or shoe works mischief and obstructs the return circulation of the venous blood. A thing so apparently trifling as a snug garter easily works injury to the valves of the veins in the lower extremities and causes varicose veins and ulcers. One thing leads to another and it is easy for those who understand the delicate structure of the animal tissues to trace the connection between impeded circulation and a reduced vitality, and to trace the relation between tight clothing and pneumonia, consumption, palpitation, dyspepsia, biliousness and the derangement of other delicate organs.

We do not maintain that the errors in clothing are always the cause of the diseases mentioned and many others, but in so far as the vigor and vitality of the bodily forces are depressed by clothing, it becomes a recognizable and important factor in the development of many diseases which could be avoided by a judicious obedience to the teachings of physiology.

Young persons often fail to appreciate the value of good health and stand ready to sacrifice it for what they believe to be an improvement in external appearance. This is often the result of thoughtlessness or a lack of right knowledge. Experience teaches that health may be easily sacrificed, vital force may be lavishly squandered and life cut off before the noontide hour. The teachings of experience usually come too late to rectify the mistake. There are but few persons who are ready to profit by such suggestions. Many are more ready to take pills, powders and potions of bitter drugs than to receive and profit by good advice.

It is astonishing to observe the low estimate placed upon health until, like Esau's birthright, it has been foolishly bartered away when it cannot be bought back at an enormous price.

There are a few other general facts in regard to clothing which are usually well understood. Dark colors absorb the heat from the sun's rays more perfectly than light colors and hence the former colors are more suitable for winter wear and the latter for summer. As the exhalations from the body permeate the clothing it should, as well as bedding, be exposed to the air and sunlight frequently or cleansed by washing. Clothing is sometimes irritating to the skin and if the irritation is continued produces diseases peculiar to that organ. Such defects, as soon as observed, should be remedied.

VIII.—CLIMATE.

The subject of climate cannot be treated exhaustively here, neither is it necessary. There are special works on climatology which go into thousands of details that only interest those making a special study of the subject. There are also many articles in all the encyclopedias on this and kindred topics. Climate is of interest to us from a medical standpoint and we shall briefly consider it in its relation to health and disease.

Man has the faculty of adapting himself to a great variety of climates. He is able to live in the frozen north amid snow and ice, where his clothing must be the skins of animals and such material as will prevent as much as possible the radiation of heat. He is on the other hand able to live in tropical regions where the heat makes clothing almost intolerable.

The two extremes of heat and cold are not as favorable for the best race developments as the temperate climates. In the northern or arctic regions the struggle for life is too severe, the products of the earth are scanty, the races are stunted, dwarfed not only physically but also intellectually. In the tropical regions vegetation is luxuriant, nutritious fruits are produced in abundance with the minimum of labor, man has to put forth but little effort to secure a living and he does not have to store up fuel and provisions and so the tendency is toward indolence and laziness.

The two extremes, distressing poverty or abundant luxury, are also inimical to the best interests of a race. Climate has its bearing on these conditions and is a very significant factor in the welfare and happiness of the human family.

Man is effected physically, mentally and morally by his environment. This he cannot escape except by change of habitation. It determines largely the diseases from which he must suffer.

High altitudes have a well-known immunity from consumption and malarial diseases. Climate is the most important factor in diseases of the air passages. Catarrh, so troublesome in the New England states, especially in winter, is almost unknown in a climate such as Southern California.

Sudden and extreme changes in the temperature work injuriously upon many constitutions. The debilitated are the greatest sufferers from a variable climate.

The northern portion of the United States is subject to these trying variations in a marked degree against which no foresight can always provide. There are periods when the climate is that of a region far to the south; the air is mild, the sky soft and southern, while south winds blow; in an hour the wind changes and cold currents come sweeping down upon our habitations "from Greenland's icy mountains." The robust brave these sudden variations without injury, but persons suffering from diseases of the air passages or lungs are greatly depressed, and sometimes the decision between life and death is made by such climatic changes.

The best climate for consumptives, or those suffering from chronic bronchitis, and other kindred diseases is in those regions where the greater portion of time can be spent daily in the open air the whole year around. This requisite demands pure sky, pure air, dry atmosphere, warm, even temperature and freedom from sudden and violent changes.

Some who are not too far advanced in sickness and who possess a large amount of vigor and endurance improve in cold, salubrious climates like that of Minnesota, while others have better chances for improvement in Florida, Arizona or Southern California. Colorado enjoys considerable reputation at the present time for consumptive patients. It must not be forgotten that change of scene, better health regulations and other minor matters often combine to bring about the improvement which follows a change of climate.

A change of climate often aids indirectly in producing the desired improvement; for it may help to increase the appetite, improve the digestion, increase muscular exercise, which means increased respiration and circulation and consequent gain in bodily weight. It is impossible to give rules in regard to change of climate or to specify the places suitable for different diseases and persons. No one climate is adapted to the requirements of all. Some are benefited by the sea air, while others are made worse. The best method to pursue in regard to change of climate is for each case to seek advice from competent authority. Our own country contains almost every variety of climate modified by altitude, heat, moisture, the ocean currents and many other factors.

Some people prefer other lands and for such there are suitable places in Switzerland, France, Italy and the islands of the sea. Nassau, on one of the Bahama Islands, has the reputation of a mild and even climate throughout the entire year.

Having decided that a change of climate is essential, one should give the new locality a thorough trial and not leave before noticeable improvement can have time to take place. Winter in a southern clime and summer in the Adirondacks would afford variety and diversion for those who are fond of changes and can afford the expense.

IX.—EXERCISE.

There is close relation between exercise and good health. It is not merely important but it is essential to the functions of all the organs and to a normal and healthy condition of the nerves and muscles.

The beneficial effects of exercise upon the nerves will be seen from their relation to all functional activity and every bodily and muscular movement. There are two sets of nerves, known as nerves of sensation and nerves of motion; the former receive the outward impressions and carry them to the brain, the latter transmit the impressions to the place where motion or action is essential. The brain is the capital center of all nerve force and the numerous nerves running to every portion of the body and from every portion back to the brain are like telegraph wires carrying messages to and from the central office.

Back of every movement whether voluntary or involuntary is the controlling nerve influence; when this is disarranged there is a corresponding disarrangement of this or that organ or function, as the heart, stomach or muscular system. Such disarrangement produces dyspepsia, lack of nutrition, constipation, irregular heart action, weakness, prostration and a host of diseases depending upon the character and degree of nerve trouble. This is sometimes so pronounced that the whole mental or physical system is shattered and not infrequently the whole man becomes a mental wreck. We can do little more than suggest here how the nerve force acts and reacts upon every tissue and fiber of the body.

It is well known that motion is produced by the action of the nerves upon the muscular fibers, causing them to relax or contract as necessary. Exercise could not improve the muscular force if it did not equally increase and develop the ability of the nerve force. It is always the trained nerve which controls the action of the muscle fiber. This training of the nerves is the most important result of physical exercise.

Men of powerful muscular development cannot write out their thoughts upon paper unless they have learned the process of writing, unless the nerves and muscles of the hand have been trained to do this work conjointly. Any common handicraft is easy to the trained nerve and muscle, but otherwise difficult or impossible no matter how great the muscular power.

Exercise is just as much a tonic for the nervous system as it is for the muscular system and just as essential, but this fact is usually lost sight of. Exercise is usually considered as having reference simply to muscular development, but let us remember that its relations are as close to the mind as to matter; for no process of the mind or body, no tissue, nothing, can be separated from the nervous system. It is omnipresent in the human organism. Hence all exercise affects primarily the nervous system and through it secondarily the tissues and functions under its control.

Exercise affects the process of respiration favorably; but think for a moment how far reaching such a proposition is. Increased and improved respiration means that more oxygen is taken into the lungs, that the carbonic acid and other waste and poisonous products of the system are more successfully eliminated. This implies purer blood and the remotest tissue and fiber of the body feels the exhilaration almost immediately. It is not essential for your well being to follow up the newspaper advertisements of the dispensers of oxygen for there is oxygen all about you, oceans of it, abundant and to spare, and you may breathe it in freely and become more vigorous and healthy. The Creator who made man and who knows what is necessary for his well being has put as much oxygen in the air as the human body requires, if you will only use it and inflate your lungs with it daily to their utmost capacity.

Exercise increases and improves the heart's action. This, if not excessive, sends the improved blood with greater energy and force to the extremities, and relieves cold feet and hands far more satisfactorily than sitting over a register to get the hot air from a furnace. It is better than medicine in most instances to aid the circulation. There is no more satisfactory tonic for a weak heart, purple veins, cold extremities and pale cheeks than exercise judiciously taken. There is no unfavorable reaction from such a stimulus. It is in keeping with nature's great remedies and her methods of healing are the best yet known, though often the least appreciated. Many who resort to medicines would derive more benefit from pure air, nutritious diet and duly regulated exercise. But how difficult it is to analyze the healthful results which follow nature's processes; they are so complex and so lap on to each other at every point.

Not only the lungs and heart do their work better, but the results of exercise are to be traced in that important organ, the skin, spread out over the whole surface of the body. It becomes more active, the pores are opened, copious moisture is eliminated together with other waste products which tend to embarrass the system. Every organ of the body is stimulated to a more healthy performance of its functions.

It is not easy to enumerate in detail what exercise can do in the way of maintaining or restoring the health. It increases the demand for nutrition, hastens digestion, aids absorption, promotes sleep and increases the energy of mind and body. It acts like a balance wheel to regulate, equalize and preserve the health. The many ailments of the sedentary which render life a kind of prolonged misery can be largely prevented, or if in more advanced stages can be cured by means of exercise intelligently prescribed and conscientiously administered in appropriate and regular doses. Many sedentary persons are subject to headache, nervousness, sleeplessness, neuralgia, disordered stomach, biliousness, constipation, piles and a long list of such allied miseries which could be alleviated, if not wholly cured by systematic exercise. It is a powerful factor not only in the preservation of the health and the prevention of disease, but also in diminishing the bodily weight when such result is desirable, in reducing deformities and overcoming the weakness of nerves, muscles, parts or organs.

The use of physical culture in all the public schools should be encouraged. While the practice is a splendid discipline it also serves to relieve the weariness of close application or prolonged study and restraint in one position. School children thoroughly enjoy such drill and student life is rendered far less tedious than under the old methods.

Feeble persons must omit out door exercise in bad weather and be contented with home gymnastics, which can readily be devised with a little ingenuity.

Of two medicines possessing equal virtue that is to be selected which is the more pleasant. On the same principle that exercise is preferable which will be relished, which possesses the element of diversion and combines the cheerful employment of the mind and body. That exercise which is not enjoyed, like bad-tasting medicine, is more likely to be omitted than taken. It is quite essential in order to obtain the best results that exercise should be agreeable and much enjoyed.

Public gymnasiums are preferable to private because the feeling of compulsion and restraint experienced causes a more regular and systematic pursuit of their benefits.

The danger of carrying exercise to excess must be guarded against. It is well known that professional athletes suffer unpleasant consequences from their occupation. Even the bones suffer injury, the joints after a time lose their mobility, the muscles are over-taxed, the heart valves are strained and often permanently injured. Exercise should be regulated in order to stimulate the body and brain in the right proportion. The energy must not be wholly consumed in muscular exertions. Exhaustive exercise may affect unfavorably not only the muscles, joints and heart, but also the brain and nervous system.

School boys and college students are especially liable to carry physical exercise to excess. The vying with each other and the powerful stimulus to excel often result disastrously. Football is an exercise of such severe nature as to be dreaded by the friends of those who participate in the game, and it is doubtful if such immoderate exertion is ever beneficial, while it often results in minor accidents and sprained ankles if nothing more serious.

Prize contests on the part of athletes should not be encouraged; for the nervous strain is injurious even though the muscles appear to endure it unharmed. Out-door games when there is no especial element of rivalry are healthful and invigorating and should be encouraged. Walking is good exercise though not vigorous enough to develop the chest and upper extremities. It may be carried to excess by beginners.

Horseback riding has much to commend it as healthful exercise. It should alternate with walking as it does not sufficiently exercise the muscles of the legs. Walking makes up the deficiency. Rowing should be added when practicable, to develop the chest and its muscles. No one kind of exercise serves for complete development. In winter skating is admirable exercise for boys and girls; it should not be too long continued. Bicycle riding is an ideal exercise in which all the members of a household can join. From the bicycle, women learn the important lesson of controlling the nerves. "It is a fine sight," says a recent writer, "to see in 1896 a woman weaving her wheel in and out among the loaded teams who in 1894 would hardly have dared to cross the same street without a policeman's arm. When the mother of a family can strap a lunch box to her handle bar and convey a brood of young cyclists for a day at the seashore or in the woods there is a decided gain in the average health of women. The girls, not a few but nearly all of them, are getting out-of-doors which is precisely what has been wanted for the last two generations to give the American race a fighting chance to survive."

After exercising, the pores of the skin become relaxed and care must be taken not to cool off too suddenly. Draughts of air should be avoided and friction of the skin with a coarse dry towel is advantageous.

The following health code by an unknown writer contains a practical summing up of the whole subject.

> "Take the open air, the more you take the better,
> Follow nature's laws to the very letter;
> Throw the drastic pills in the Bay of Biscay,
> Let alone the gin, the brandy and the whiskey.
>
> "Freely exercise, keep your spirits cheerful,
> Let no dread of sickness make you ever fearful,
> Eat the simplest food, drink the pure, cold water,
> Then you will be well, or at least you ought to."

X.—LONGEVITY.

> "Years steal fire from the mind as vigor from the limb;
> And life's enchanted cup but sparkles near the brim."
> —*Byron.*

It is the duty of all mankind to apply their knowledge so far as possible to right living. Longevity is promoted by a proper observance of health laws, but the strictest observance of these laws cannot guarantee health or long life to every one. In attempting to discover the secrets of longevity, if secrets there are, our research must be extensive enough to include certain exceptions, found in the foot notes, under all rules.

For those who inherit a debilitated constitution, a deficit in physical force, the problem of longevity appears to be a very difficult one and its working out seems to promise only uncertain results. It is well known by medical men and actuaries that there is no factor so prominent in the subject under consideration as heredity, and yet it would be useless to pause and discuss it so far as the present generation is concerned, since no one can rectify the mistakes of his progenitors. It is everywhere admitted that those who have descended from hardy stock, who are by nature strong and vigorous, have the advantage, and it would seem as though predictions could be made in their favor with great certainty, but we have all noticed that the strong are often rash and fail to conserve their health, while those naturally frail may be so cautious and temperate as to outlive them and reach a ripe old age.

There can be no system of living which everyone can adopt to insure longevity, but there are many aids which if brought into constant service offer the best prospect for reaching up to and beyond the average expectancy. There are certain general principles that experience has taught the thoughtful in every age, which it is advantageous to learn early and practice persistently. These have almost become proverbial and can be stated in a few brief sentences thus: take plenty of exercise; bathe often; keep the head cool, the feet warm and dry; avoid unwholesome food, impure water, unventilated rooms, foul air, damp dwellings, etc. Any discussion of health subjects can be but little more than the elaboration of these hackneyed expressions made interesting and impressive simply by the earnestness with which they are enforced.

We announce no new discovery, only an open secret, when we say that the body and mind are in the most favorable condition for the maintenance of health when occupied by some congenial employment. Work is not unhealthy. Many of the hardest workers the world has ever known have lived beyond their allotted threescore years and ten; and it would be a great misfortune for the masses to be relieved of the necessity of toil. The diligent live longer and enjoy more than the indolent whose time is a burden and who squander it in nursing imaginary evils and complaints. Idleness is destructive of human happiness and the welfare of both individuals and nations. It tends to effeminacy and immorality.

There is not so much danger of over work as is popularly supposed; but there is far greater danger of violating those general health principles to which reference has already been made. The great danger is not from hard work but from worry, anxiety and constant vexation, which are largely the outcome of our present methods of business in which competition is often so selfish, fierce and heartless. It is no wonder that in this desperate struggle many are crowded to the edge of the precipice and that occasionally some poor disheartened victim, prodded till his brain whirls and reason gives way, is tempted to leap off. These unnatural burdens of anxiety make the heaviest draft upon the reserve, exhaust the brain and are detrimental to health and bloom.

Self regulation is one of those fundamental principles which if learned by experience may come too late. It is necessary to avoid that stress of business which interferes with digestion and refreshing sleep. There are many who do not allow sufficient time for eating; "five minutes for refreshments," then the rush and scramble are renewed. We must not permit ourselves to get into a chronic state of hurry and fly around as if there was only another moment to live. Take time to eat, masticate your food thoroughly; for this is the only process by which it can be prepared for digestion and otherwise you will pay the penalty, which is dyspepsia.

Take time to sleep. It has been learned that eight or nine hours out of the twenty-four are essential for this purpose. Sleep is a period of recuperation during which repairs are in progress. Unless compensation is made during sleep for the wastes of the body an equilibrium of its forces cannot be maintained.

History appears to coincide with experience and proves that man needs, in addition to sleep, an occasional day of rest from his labors and there is probably no better arrangement than the one which already exists, of one day out of every seven.

It is important to cultivate a cheerful disposition and not allow despondency to obtain control of the spirits. Cheerfulness quickens the circulation, adds warmth and vitality to the blood, sends a thrill of health to every fiber of the body and stimulates all the functions of animal life. Whatever banishes cheerfulness upsets the digestion, obstructs nutrition, makes the liver sluggish, renders the blood impure and riles up all the foundations of life. Cheerfulness purchases contentment, that perpetual feast for the mind, while its violation breeds discontent and may eventually end in suicide or insanity.

There is no doubt but what great emotions overtax the nerve force, disturb the stomach, the brain, the heart, and should be avoided. There can be no emotion that does not reach the heart and brain. You cannot even run or hurry without compelling the heart to beat faster in order to provide the necessary force. There is nothing in the line of emotion or effort which does not affect the heart and consequently no organ is so liable to overwork. When the heart is overburdened and begins to fail the stomach becomes feeble, digestion is disturbed; the brain suffers from want of nutrition, the memory falters and unmistakable signs of age or exhaustion quickly follow.

It has been observed that strong emotions affect unfavorably the secretion of the mother's milk and it is a matter of record that adults have sometimes fallen dead in a fit of anger. How important it is then to regulate the emotions, to control the feelings and practice self-management.

Excesses of all kinds squander the vital forces, hence are debilitating. They destroy the natural and normal equilibrium of the body and ought to be strenuously avoided. The control of self demands that reason have sway even if it makes you a tyrant over your passions. When reason presides there will be contentment, order, sobriety and happiness; where reason is violated discontent, misery, intemperance and anxiety reign. Be on the outlook in regard to over-indulgence at the table and late suppers. In some things abstinence, in others moderation and in all things a life pure and constant, is consistent with longevity.

Temperance and sobriety are among the open secrets of a long life. The most natural drink for mankind is water and there is no more healthy beverage when all other things are considered. The prolonged use of alcoholic stimulants inflames the stomach, congests the brain, excites and overworks the heart, produces vascular excitement of all the organs and at length leads to alteration of their structure.

All powerful or narcotic drugs should be avoided except under skilled direction for the amelioration or cure of disease. Those who resort on every trifling pretext to the use of such agents, unless restrained, will shorten life and fill its brief remnant with untold bitterness.

All fatigue should be counteracted by rest or sleep and not by a resort to stimulants. When temporarily wearied a warm bath will be found refreshing; to the bath may be added with benefit a tablespoonful of aqua ammonia or a little common salt. Friction of the skin with a coarse towel should follow the bath; if this is thoroughly done it will draw away surplus blood from the overtaxed brain, equalize the circulation, invigorate the system and promote rest.

Harmless recreation, without making pleasure the aim in life, should be sought, for it is exhilarating. Change of place and rest from the drudgery of a continued and harassing occupation is refreshing. It is beneficial to body and mind to breathe the sea air, to look upon the vast ocean, for the sight is both grand and inspiring.

Travel is beneficial in many ways. It enables one to mingle with diverse classes of people, observe their habits, their hardships, their undesirable methods of living and teaches lessons of gratitude and contentment. Such experiences broaden and quicken the mind, increase its capacity for enjoyment and bring us into touch with all the world outside ourselves; they help us to avoid excessive thirst for wealth and assist us in the cultivation of charity, liberality, magnanimity. They illustrate the folly of the miser's stinginess, the unfriendliness of the selfish, the emptiness of pride and enforce more just and correct views of life.

Finally it should be borne in mind that there are more desirable attainments than old age with its infirmities, its waning strength and weakened intellect. Many have succeeded in crowding a short life full of glorious achievements.

> "We should count time by heart throbs. He most lives
> Who thinks most, feels the noblest, acts the best."

CHAPTER III.

GENERAL TOPICS OF INTEREST IN MEDICINE.

I. Home Prescribing.—II. Strange Delusions.—III. Patent Medicines.—IV. Medicines.—V. Doses.—VI. Household Remedies.

I.—HOME PRESCRIBING.

IF you can diagnose disease and determine from the symptoms what particular disease you have to treat and not confuse one disease with another, then the matter of prescribing for the members of your family will be quite a simple matter in ordinary cases. But if on the other hand you are unable to distinguish between things that differ and cannot recognize even the simpler forms of disease, you will be able safely to do but very little home prescribing. You cannot prescribe unless you will learn to read and interpret symptoms. This book will help you in this matter if you will give to its pages your earnest attention.

The trouble with home prescribing is apt to be that you consider the patient dangerously ill when the ailment is simple, almost trifling; and then your imagination helps to exaggerate the case, you allow your good judgment to be dethroned by fear, you first get nervous, then frightened and the whole household becomes demoralized. The reverse is still more unfortunate; for perhaps the disease is really serious, but being unable to interpret the symptoms you consider it slight and unimportant; time is lost and evil consequences are averted with difficulty. Every physician encounters cases where the household is misled in these different ways. The author has often been called to attend children sick with lung fever (pneumonia), some of them in great danger. It is quite usual to find some neighbor present whose reputation is extensive for experience in sickness perhaps some old lady, wise in her own estimation, who with a knowing look and positive utterance hastens to display her cunning by remarking that "nothing but worms ails that child," and she usually feels quite humiliated when the doctor fails to confirm her diagnosis. There is no disease among children which deceives the household more often than pneumonia; in another place you will find a full description of the symptoms. These can be easily learned if you will give heed, but if you cannot or will not learn these positive symptoms then you will be obliged to depend upon some one whose knowledge is not guesswork. Above all, do not trust to some wiseacre who will declare every ill of childhood due to worms.

There are many mild diseases which can be intelligently treated if you will only give heed to their symptoms and learn their simple management; there are other diseases you could not treat after a thorough medical education unless you had supplemented it with years of observation and experience.

Diseases too difficult for home treatment will be outlined and the hint properly given, so that having recognized a serious malady you will see the need of experienced counsel and direction. It is far better to employ a skillful physician and pay him cheerfully than to run a serious risk and imperil the life of yourself or others for lack of knowledge.

It is expensive to employ skillful counsel, but that is little compared with the heartache which would fill your life with a never-ending regret, if a dear friend or child were the victim of your ignorance or prejudice.

II.—STRANGE DELUSIONS.

Many persons otherwise intelligent adopt a strange course when sickness overtakes them. As drowning men catch at straws so sick people are often the victims of lying pretenders. The belief that the gift of healing is a natural one is a relic of the past. In olden times disease was a demon, to be cast out by those who were especially gifted in prayer and in other mysteries which the common people did not understand. Superstition and pretence come nowhere to the front at the present day, so much as in attempts to deceive and work the miracles of healing. Some people seem to be ever courting deception, ready for the silvery words of flattery and pretence. A good and competent man must live a long time in a community and win the confidence of the people little by little, but let some brazen-faced deceiver come to town with flowing locks and advertise himself as the most wonderful healer of modern times, and it is astonishing how credulous the people are and how cheerfully they will bring forth their hidden shekels and how enthusiastic they will become over the greasy locks and swarthy complexion of such an ignorant fraud. Men of honor and attainment stand a poor show in comparison with the boasting seventh son of a seventh son, a natural healer or perchance a natural bone-setter.

Does a person know any too much about the practice of medicine who has made it a thorough and conscientious study, and who has pursued a complete course of medical study in a college of recognized merit? Ask the opinion, if in doubt, of men of good judgment and experience who are leaders in their profession, if it is possible for a man to be a natural healer of diseases or a natural bone-setter or surgeon. You would not employ a man to build a house because his only qualification was that he professed to be a natural carpenter. You would not think of employing a man to shoe a valuable horse because he pretended to be a born blacksmith. No man would pretend to be a natural carpenter or blacksmith because his works would condemn him and prove him a humbug. But there is something so mysterious about the art of healing, nature is so prompt and efficient in her work, that a humbug or fraud can point to her incomparable art and shout, "Behold my skill, I can work miracles." People often employ these frauds who have almost no qualifications to treat them, because they boast unceasingly of some special and peculiar or inherited power over disease, without making any effort to ascertain whether they can perform a tithe of what they pretend. The following code is a good one to remember:

True wisdom is always quiet, modest and unassuming, makes no boast, is cautious about promising a cure for disease and free from pretence.

Those who know nothing fear nothing. Ignorance is loudmouthed, shouting to attract attention, full of boasting and pretence and rushes into print to make impossible statements. The pretender in medicine always heralds his coming with no little splurge, he hesitates not to boast of marvelous and impossible achievements. He can always cure consumption or Bright's disease in their last stages, anything, no matter what. The truth probably is that his medical knowledge is so scanty, that he knows almost nothing except a little smattering gleaned from the medical almanacs; his medicines are receipts that he has copied or stolen or obtained in questionable ways, yet what miracles they will perform, warranted to cure every disease flesh is heir to. What a shame it is that in some of the states the tramp, the jail-bird, the cowboy, any ignorant pretender, male or female, can enter a community and announce himself as Doctor Blank without fulfilling a single requirement as to medical study or graduation.

The pharmacist must be registered, else he cannot put up your medicines; the dentist must be licensed, else he can neither fill nor extract your teeth; the peddler who sells tin must have a license and even the man who picks rags from the gutter. But in some of the states no restriction is deemed necessary to protect citizens from self-styled doctors. A diamond in his shirt front, a dashing manner and a loud mouth are all some people demand as evidence of ability.

III.—PATENT MEDICINES.

"Canst thou not minister to a mind diseased?"

Patent medicines like advertising doctors should be avoided. If you are in health you do not need them and if you are sick you need something better. A few of these shop remedies may possess a small amount of virtue, and even when taken at random may occasionally benefit, especially if the taker has a large degree of faith in their potency. It is usually the mysterious make-up of these compounds, coupled with the wondrous stories of the advertisement which excites the curiosity of the credulous. If they could only see the formula written out in full upon the bottle and know how small the grain of truth the advertisement contains the spell would be broken and their faith shattered.

The inspiration of all this vast business is not, as pretended, to alleviate human suffering and cure the ills of mankind; for it is a money-making scheme. Vast fortunes have been made out of the selling of mixtures for one dollar which cost about ten cents. Patent medicines are usually concocted out of inexpensive drugs and many of them contain an objectionable amount of alcohol and vile whiskey. Their great item of cost is not in the making of them but in advertising them. It is easy to see why the press rarely criticises with severity this nefarious business of selling nothing for something, inasmuch as about fifty per cent. of the income of advertising doctors and their remedies is paid to the newspapers. It is a matter simply of millions to the income of the press, and hence, no public sentiment is awakened and no attempt is made to instruct the people in regard to these important health matters.

The field for this patent medicine business is an extensive one, for the American people are largely overworked and nervous. In this condition they easily fancy themselves ill, and if they can be induced to read and ponder the worthless literature of the medical advertising page, this fancy will soon take a deep root and become an actual growing reality. More than half the dosing of the people is for fancied illness. If the mixtures they buy and prescribe for themselves were only as harmless as they are worthless little would need to be said.

Even when you are really sick it is not much medicine you need, but a little, and that of the right kind. Do not pervert your stomach with base and uncertain mixtures; for it was never intended to be converted into an apothecary's shop.

There are strong reasons for believing that patent medicines do a great amount of harm in the aggregate. They are often the cause of dyspepsia, constipation and a host of other functional disorders. Many people exercise about the same grade of intelligence in regard to medicine, as a certain family who called one doctor to see their sick child, and after his departure called still another doctor. Acting on the theory that if one doctor knows a little, two know more, they alternated one's medicine with the other's. Acting also on the theory that if one spoonful of medicine is good, two are better, they doubled each dose. As a result the child died.

The following recent incident illustrates the danger of the patent medicine business: A hard-working butcher who inherited a taste for alcoholic liquors moved from the city to a small town to avoid temptation. In this village to which he had come was a certain groceryman who had decided to sell out his stock of goods, and in order to do so offered them at reduced prices. The butcher bought a list of necessary goods and at the suggestion of the grocer, added to his purchase one of the compound sarsaparillas. He took his goods home and soon commenced taking a dose of his sarsaparilla each morning, as he was obliged to go to work early and work a long time before breakfast. He soon noticed however that if he failed to take the medicine for a single morning he felt depressed and unequal to the work to which he had been accustomed. His next step was to resort to whiskey drinking for which the medicine had prepared the way. There is no question but what patent medicines under the names of bitters, tonics, etc., have often led the way to the dramshop, hence on this ground, if no other, they should be avoided.

IV.—MEDICINES.

Medicines are substances used to accomplish certain objects, as the prevention or cure of disease. They also help to produce changes in the body or in some tissue or part and bring about results more or less definite.

Medicines possess certain properties which aid in their identification as color, taste, odor and weight.

They also possess chemical properties some of which are similar and some are antagonistic or incompatible. Advantage is taken of the various properties of medicines by the prescriber. He sometimes unites remedies which aid each other and gets much better results than could be obtained by a single remedy. In order to do this successfully he must have an acquaintance with their chemical properties, otherwise medicines might be placed in combination which would render the mixture worthless or even dangerous. Acids are neutralized by alkalies, and a knowledge of this fact enables one sometimes to relieve suffering or save life. A single medicine sometimes contains several active principles or medical properties.

The action of medicine often depends upon the size of the dose. Ipecac, in large doses, excites the mucous and muscular coats of the stomach and causes vomiting; while in very small doses it may be successfully used to allay vomiting. It has other properties which render it valuable as an expectorant, an astringent and to check hemorrhage. Rhubarb has a double action, in the first place as a cathartic, in the second as an astringent. Opium is made more efficient for relieving pain by combining it with belladonna, while the action of the two remedies upon the pupil of the eye is antagonistic, the one contracting and the other dilating it. A great number of similar illustrations might be brought forward to prove that medicines are capable of accomplishing a great variety of results, if their properties are familiar, and when they are administered in the correct dose and proper combination.

The insolubility of certain remedies must not be overlooked. Many are freely soluble in water, others in glycerine, others in acids, others in alcohol, still others in ether and some are not soluble in any of the substances mentioned. In order to prepare suitable combinations it is necessary to know about the chemical properties and solubility of medicines, as this cannot be learned except by extensive study of chemistry and other branches, it has been deemed essential to include under the treatment of diseases, suitable prescriptions with complete directions for their use, in addition to the list and doses of household remedies in this chapter. Such an arrangement renders this work as complete as possible for the household purposes for which it is designed.

Some medicines enter the blood and assist in removing from it morbid material, or add to it some property of which it is deficient; thus the quality of the vital fluid is improved, purified or enriched and made efficient to work a renovation of the system. In this way disease is cast out, normal processes are invigorated and health is restored. Such medicines are known as *hæmatics*.

Another class act upon the nervous system and exert their influence upon some special nerve or nerve center, or upon all the nerve centers and the numerous nerve fibers by which they are connected. Medicines which work changes in the blood accomplish their mission in a deliberate and permanent manner, but those which influence the nervous system work quickly and the effect is often temporary and fleeting, requiring a repetition at stated intervals to continue the result. Such medicines are known as *neurotics*.

Another class act upon the muscular system and cause contraction of the muscular fibres and are often used for allaying hemorrhage, or for toning up the system weakened by debilitating discharges; and they also diminish the secretions of the glandular system. These are known as *astringents*.

Another class excite the secretions by stimulating the action of the glandular system. They aid in removing those morbid products which ought to be cast out of the body. They are known as *diminutives*.

These classes are again divided and subdivided. It is necessary to consider later on some of these subdivisions in order to learn more about the action of various remedies.

Medicines are introduced into the system in several ways, the most common of which is by the mouth and stomach. Medicines introduced into the stomach are acted upon, absorbed and enter into the circulation just in the same way as food, after it undergoes solution and digestion.

Some medicines, like some foods, are not soluble in the stomach but only in the small intestines. The quickest and most positive action of certain medicines is obtained by injection into the cellular tissue under the skin. This is the modern and well-known hypodermic method. The injected medicine must be in solution so that it can be quickly taken up by the absorbent vessels which are numerous in this vicinity. This method is scarcely suitable for household practice as only a few of the most powerful remedies are so used, and usually by physicians in cases of emergency where there is intense suffering and speedy relief is essential. Only about half the dose is required when medicine is introduced by this method. The needle of the syringe must be cleansed each time, before and after use, to avoid inserting any septic material which would result in a painful swelling or abscess. The hypodermic method has certain advantages.

When medicine is administered by the mouth it may offend a sensitive stomach and vomiting may ensue; or it may pass through the alimentary canal without being absorbed. Medicine injected under the skin exerts its full force, for it cannot be rejected nor expelled from the system without being absorbed.

In some cases such remedies as liniments, lotions and ointments are advantageously applied to the integument. When it is necessary to treat a burn, a wound, parasitic affections and certain other diseases of the skin or to cause the destruction of some superficial growth, as a wart, medicines can be applied locally with success. There is considerable virtue in the well-known and much-used mustard poultice, when applied to relieve inflammation and pain in some neighboring part. Medicines applied externally, except to denuded surfaces, can be much stronger than those taken internally.

The application of medicine to a surface, blistered for the purpose, is not of sufficient importance to receive detailed notice, and is rarely employed except in some case of emergency and would be of doubtful utility.

Medicines are applied successfully to the mucous membrane of the eye, nose, throat and various other mucous surfaces. Diseases of the air passages are often benefited by the inhalation of medicated vapors sprayed by an atomizer. This method yields excellent results in catarrh, bronchitis and other inflamed conditions.

Medicines are used advantageously in enemas or suppositories. This is an efficient method of treating diarrhœa, dysentery and various other diseases of the bowels, bladder and other pelvic organs. When the stomach is inflamed or too irritable to retain medicines or even nutrients, they are often introduced into the rectum, for a time, and the result is sometimes quite satisfactory. The indications for these special methods are noticed under the affections which indicate their use and need not be repeated here.

There are a great variety of circumstances and conditions which modify the action of medicines and these must be kept in mind. The medicine suitable for an adult is often unsuitable for a child.

Habit diminishes the susceptibility to certain remedies; for instance, the opium taker uses a quantity with impunity often sufficient to destroy the life of a person not addicted to its use.

Children are easily impressed with the action of an emetic or cathartic. Opiates should rarely be given to children and then with the utmost care or under the direction of a competent physician.

Blisters should be employed, if at all, with great care in the case of children or delicate persons. The nervous system is especially sensitive in many such patients as well as the integument.

Climate modifies the action of medicines considerably. It is found that remedies and doses used in one part of the world often produce unsatisfactory results in other parts, owing to the modifying influence of heat and cold upon the nervous system.

The condition of pregnancy is one which should receive careful consideration when medicines are required, as much injury might be done by the administration of powerful or unsuitable agents. Medicine should be given to a nursing mother with unusual care, as enough of a powerful narcotic might be absorbed and become an ingredient of the milk to injure the child. The medicine suitable for one stage of a disease is often unsuitable for another stage.

There are many individual peculiarities which must be regarded. Some persons are always harmed by certain medicines which prove for other people ordinarily beneficial. Some conditions increase while other conditions diminish the action of medicines. To appreciate all these modifying influences it will be necessary to give earnest attention to this part of the work.

EMETICS.

Emetics.—There are many medicines which excite nausea and vomiting. They are often indicated to rid the stomach of poisons, to remove some obstruction in the trachea or œsophagus, to expel secretions from the air passages, to relieve convulsions in children or headache and hysteria in adults.

When an active poison has been swallowed death may result before a physician could arrive, or so much poison may have been absorbed into the system that his efforts would be unavailing. It is well to have some efficient remedies at hand to produce vomiting. A teaspoonful of ground mustard and the same amount of common salt mixed up in a cup of lukewarm water, will usually act promptly and is harmless

Ipecac is a harmless emetic but is rather slow in action. It is a good remedy, especially for children, when vomiting is indicated in bronchial diseases, to relieve the air passages. It is useful in croup and whooping cough. It is much used in small doses in colds and coughs, in bronchitis and other diseases of the air passages, for its expectorant effect. The emetic dose for a child is one teaspoonful or more of the syrup.

The compound syrup of squill (Hive Syrup) may be used to produce vomiting. It owes its chief action to the small amount of tartar emetic which it contains, each teaspoonful containing one-eighth of a grain. The dose for a child is from eight drops to a teaspoonful. It produces considerable nausea and is consequently quite depressing. It should be administered to a feeble infant, if at all, with considerable care, in small and repeated doses.

Alum in powder is an excellent remedy in croup to promote vomiting. It has considerable reputation for dislodging the false membrane which is characteristic of this disease and in preventing it from reforming. It is prompt, thorough and without depressing effects. A teaspoonful of the powder may be administered in syrup and repeated every half hour till it causes free vomiting. The action of emetics is favored by a free use of lukewarm water.

Cathartics.—These are medicines which cause the bowels to act, usually by irritating their muscular fibers, thus stimulating the normal peristaltic action. Cathartics are often serviceable but no remedies are more abused in domestic practice. The custom of buying cheap pills composed of aloes, gamboge and such like drugs cannot be too severely condemned. They cause an evacuation of the bowels in consequence of their irritant action; but constant repetition renders their action less satisfactory and the bowels finally lose their normal vigor or tone and will not respond to the natural stimulus.

In this way the habit of constipation is often induced and becomes chronic. It is always detrimental to the comfort and health of the individual. Constipation and its attendant evils and sufferings are largely the result of the cheap and drastic pills bought in the shops; for they produce an over stimulation of the bowels and reaction is sure to follow. They are called mandrake pills and liver pills to give them popularity and increase their sale. They often bring a large fortune to the proprietor, who has little regard for the injury they cause. Simple remedies to produce daily and normal evacuation of the bowels are preferable to harsh and irritating medicines.

Regulation of the diet, the eating of fruits or the occasional injection of water or soap water or a small dose of nux vomica daily, to improve the action of the muscular coat of the bowels, are simple remedies but much more satisfactory in the long run than harsh cathartics.

Among medicines the granular effervescent citrate of magnesia is a mild though excellent cathartic. From a teaspoonful to a dessertspoonful in a half glass of water can be taken each morning or oftener, as needed.

The sulphate of magnesia (Epsom Salts) is an old and cheap remedy and in certain cases where there is a tendency to dropsical effusions it is especially valuable. It has been recently prepared in the granular effervescent form which adds not only to its cost but to its elegance. The dose of this is one or more tablespoonfuls in water.

The infusion of senna is a safe and valuable physic. It is liable to produce griping pains and hence should be combined with such carminatives as ginger, peppermint or camphor. Its taste is rather unpleasant. It is prepared like a cup of tea by pouring a little boiling water upon a generous pinch of the leaves.

Castor oil is a well-known domestic remedy, somewhat difficult to take but an excellent physic for many conditions. It is soothing in its nature, it does not produce nor aggravate inflammation and is sure to act if given in sufficient dose and allowed a proper time. It may be given on the top of a cup of milk, coffee, chocolate or soda water or with lemon juice and be scarcely tasted. There is no better physic for children in summer nor for women after confinement. The dose for children is one to two teaspoonfuls; adults can take one or two tablespoonfuls as needed.

Of the many remedies used as cathartics reference will be made here to only one other, namely, podophyllin. This is a remedy of great potency in curing constipation. It stimulates the liver to a healthy action, increases the flow of bile and in small doses is one of our most valuable remedies. Its efficiency will be improved by combining it with nux vomica. It is usually taken in too large doses. It can be obtained in little sugar-coated parvules containing one-twentieth of a grain. From one to two of these may be given to a child as needed. If the parvules cannot be obtained it may be used in the following prescription:

℞   Podophyllin   six grains
    Alcohol   one ounce

Mix. Dose, six drops in sweetened water for a child one year old and for other children in proportion each day as needed.

The following makes an excellent pill for general cathartic use:

℞   Podophyllin   one grain
    Hydrastin   ten grains
    Leptandrin   five grains
    Ex. Nux Vomica   three grains
    Ex. Hyoscyamus   five grains

Mix. Make twenty pills. Dose, one each night or one each night and morning as needed.

The dose in the above pills is small, the design is not to overstimulate the action of the bowels but to bring about a natural and healthy condition when their use is to be diminished or discontinued.

Diuretics.—Diuretics are medicines which increase the action of the kidneys and consequently augment the flow of urine. A very intimate relation exists between the skin and kidneys. In hot weather large quantities of fluid escape from the body through the pores of the skin, while in cold weather the kidneys are more active and secrete a larger quantity of urine. Diuretics are made use of not only to increase the flow of urine but also the solid constituents which it holds in solution. It is for this reason that diuretics are administered in gout; for they assist in carrying off the uric acid and the other waste products which clog up the system and produce disease. They are much used to carry away the excess of fluids in dropsical effusions. They are prescribed in rheumatism for the purpose of eliminating the lactic acid, which if retained in the blood in excess is thought by some to be a common cause of this disease. Diuretics are numerous and it will not be difficult to select a few suitable for domestic use.

Some mineral waters, as the Bethesda, are given with excellent results as diuretics.

An infusion of buchu or uva ursi leaves are serviceable diuretics and easily prepared as needed. The dose of the infusion is two or three tablespoonfuls.

The following combination is much more efficient than one remedy alone:

℞ Acetate of potash   one ounce
    Ext. Buchu fl.   one ounce
    Sweet spirits of nitre   one-half ounce
    Syr. Tolu.   two ounces
    Wintergreen water sufficient to make eight ounces.

Mix. Dose, one or two dessertspoonfuls three times a day taken in water.

The following is an efficient diuretic:

℞ Juniper berries   two drams
    Cream of Tartar   two drams
    Boiling water   one-half pint

Mix. Flavor with wintergreen and use as needed to increase the flow of urine.

The granular effervescent citrate of potash is an excellent diuretic drink. Dose, a dessertspoonful in a glass of water and drink while effervescing.

In dropsical conditions, digitalis combined with caffeine are very efficient, but such remedies are not suitable for any but physicians to administer.

Sudorifics.—These are medicines which stimulate the sweat glands and produce copious perspiration. The action of sudorific remedies is retarded by cold and favored by warmth; and when such remedies are administered they will be assisted to produce their best results by bathing the feet or body in hot water, drinking hot drinks, covering the patient with blankets and by the application of hot poultices and artificial heat. Sweating medicines are made use of in domestic practice to break up colds. They are beneficial in the early stage of fevers, measles, scarlatina, pneumonia, pleurisy and other affections of the lungs and throat; also in dropsical affections. Hot sage or catnip tea, hot drops, pepper or composition tea will often promote profuse sweating without resort to more positive remedies.

Opium is a valuable remedy to produce perspiration. The dose is one grain. Still better than opium alone is its combination with ipecac in the familiar and widely-used Dover's powder, the adult dose of which is from five to ten grains.

Aconite is much used in the early stage of fevers and is especially valuable to produce sweating in children. Ten drops of the tincture of aconite can be added to two-thirds of a tumbler of water, one teaspoonful of which can be given every half hour or hour till it thoroughly moistens the skin, when it may be continued at longer intervals as needed to allay fever.

Jaborandi is a popular remedy with physicians but is hardly a household medicine.

The tincture of lobelia may be given in doses to adults of from ten to sixty drops every hour or two and will be found efficient if not too depressing for the patient.

The following is a good prescription in the early stage of pneumonia or other acute diseases, to favor sweating:

℞	Liq. ammonia acetate	one ounce
	Tincture of aconite	fifteen drops
	Syrup of ipecac	two ounces
	Water sufficient to make four ounces	

Mix. Dose, one teaspoonful every two or four hours.

The sweet spirits of nitre in doses of from one-half to one teaspoonful is a valuable domestic remedy.

Quinine in five to ten-grain doses lowers the temperature and produces perspiration. If threatened with some acute disease, as pneumonia or pleurisy, I should have more faith in this remedy to abort it than in all the others. It would be necessary to make the dose large enough to produce a decided impression upon the system, and to take it in the first stage of the disease.

Astringents.—These are medicinal substances which cause contraction of the muscular fibers and soft tissues of the body. They have a puckering taste and coagulate albumen. They are used both internally and externally.

There are two varieties of astringents, vegetable and mineral. The vegetable astringents owe their virtue to tannic or gallic acid. The mineral astringents as alum, sulphate of zinc and the sub-sulphate of iron are more styptic in their nature and the last is so powerful in its action that it not only contracts the tissues, but instantly coagulates the blood and can be used to arrest hemorrhages from the vessels of small caliber with considerable success.

Astringent remedies are applied to the mucous membrane of the nose, throat, the eye, the bowels, the urethra, vagina and wherever there is inflammation, congestion and a relaxed or swollen condition of the mucous surfaces.

Tea and coffee are somewhat astringent owing to the tannin that they contain. Persons not accustomed to their action will find the first use, especially of strong tea, attended with marked constipation.

Ergot powerfully contracts unstriped muscular fibers and hence its ability to control hemorrhage by diminishing the caliber of the blood vessel. It will contract the uterus when it is in a relaxed condition. It has considerable power to relieve diarrhœa and hemorrhage of the bowels or lungs and also congestion of the brain.

The sulphate of zinc is much used as an astringent in conjunctivitis, gonorrhœa and vaginitis.

The subnitrate of bismuth is regarded as of great value in summer diarrhœa, especially in cholera infantum.

Blackberry root is also a vegetable astringent which enjoys considerable reputation in diarrhœa. The infusion, fluid extract, syrup or wine, are all efficient. It may be prepared domestically and enough brandy added to the infusion to keep it. The brandy improves its medical action in weakened and relaxed conditions.

Witch-hazel owes its popularity to its astringent action. It has some virtue in the treatment of piles, mild hemorrhages, varicose veins and ulcers and chronic throat affections.

Gallic acid is administered for internal hemorrhages.

Nitrate of silver in suitable solutions is an astringent of great efficiency. In some cases of persistent diarrhœa, combined with opium, it has cured cases in the author's practice that have resisted every other method of treatment. It is not a domestic remedy.

Tannin in some cases of painful hemorrhoids (piles) has been used in combination with cocaine and other remedies (in suppositories) with almost magical results.

The list of astringents has only been touched upon here. They form a very large class of remedies; but those suggested are in common use and represent the whole class sufficiently for these pages.

Astringents when taken internally should not be brought in contact with the stomach or food, just before eating or during the process of digestion, they should be taken in a pill or else well diluted.

It may be noticed that some of the remedies mentioned, as the sulphate of zinc and the sulphate of copper, act as emetics as well as astringents. Many other remedies possess properties which belong to two or more classes.

Tonics.—Tonics are medicines which impart strength and energy to the system. They quicken the appetite, aid digestion, stimulate the various functions of the bodily organs, improve the quality and quantity of the blood and thus increase the strength and build up the general health.

Tonics like other remedies have a wide range of action, some exerting their influence upon the blood, as iron, others upon the nervous system as phosphorus and strychnia and others as the simple bitters upon the stomach. Tonics can be used but little in acute diseases or inflammatory conditions; but for the most part they are appropriate in the debility which follows prolonged sickness and in chronic disorders.

Tonics must be selected with reference to the particular condition it is essential to reach and improve, but the dose must not be too large as there is danger of disarranging the digestion instead of strengthening it.

Tonics designed to improve the appetite should be taken before meals. Medicines designed to aid digestion, like pepsin, or to stimulate the flow of gastric juice should be taken at meal time or directly after. The simple vegetable bitters which have the reputation of stimulating the appetite and improving digestion are represented by gentian, colombo, nux vomica, motherwort and boneset.

There is no single tonic equal to iron in a large number of cases especially where anæmia is marked. It improves the blood, adds to its richness and renders it able to carry to the cells which are elaborating the tissues, the materials which are essential to growth or health. The slow recovery which is liable to follow fevers, pneumonia and other severe sicknesses is often hastened by iron in some suitable form or combination.

Salicin is of marked benefit in cases suffering from chronic rheumatism.

Cod liver oil is sometimes indicated in wasting diseases and in scrofula. It enriches the blood and aids in the reproduction of tissues; hence the body shows that it is better nourished during its use. It combines the virtues of a food and medicine. It contains bromine, iodine, phosphorous and iron in small quantities in addition to a large amount of nutrition. Its use has been so extensive that it has often been prescribed where it was neither indicated nor tolerated and in this way it has sometimes been brought into disrepute. Notwithstanding all this there are cases, especially of wasting diseases, where it serves an admirable purpose.

The following is an elegant emulsion :

℞	Gum Tragacanth	two drams
	Cold water	one pint
	Oil sweet almond	sixteen minims
	Cod live oil	one pint

The directions for combination must be observed. Place the tragacanth in the water and let it remain for twenty-four hours, stir occasionally, then place it on the back of the stove, warm it a little and sweeten to taste with sugar, then add one pint of pure cod liver oil and mix thoroughly, adding the oil of sweet almond. If preferred the oil of peppermint, wintergreen or lemon may be used instead to flavor.

Wild cherry bark is a good tonic. It possesses sedative properties making it popular in coughs. Quinine enjoys the distinction of being a tonic almost specific in malarial troubles, it is also indicated in enlarged spleen of malarial origin. Other tonics possess properties of a stimulating character and will be noticed under the head of stimulants.

Antispasmodics.—These are remedies which allay the excited condition of the nervous system as seen when the muscles are thrown into a state of spasm or convulsion. They are very similar in their action to nervines. They quiet and soothe the nerves which are unduly excited, relax the muscular condition and secure rest which is often the prelude to recovery.

They are necessary in treating the convulsions of children, hysteria, chorea, tetanus (lockjaw), and diseases of this class. Among the vegetable antispasmodics may be mentioned lobelia, camphor, valerian and assafœtida. Other remedies are ether, chloroform and chloral-hydrate. The latter remedy is elsewhere recommended for the convulsions of children and its method of use and administration will be found under that head.

Assafœtida is an efficient remedy for hysteria. It is a safe medicine with disagreeable odor and taste and is usually prescribed in pills containing two or four grains.

Stimulants.—Stimulants increase the heart force and are indicated in the condition known as shock. When a severe injury has produced a powerful and depressing effect upon the nervous system or where disease has been so prostrating as to cause a marked decline in the heart force and threaten failure in that vital organ, the condition is similar to that known as shock and usually requires stimulants.

Ammonia acts quickly in emergencies and in cases of fainting is often serviceable. Its inhalation is beneficial. It may be given internally and in weak conditions it has been injected hypodermically.

The carbonate of ammonia is a reliable stimulant of the lungs in pneumonia and other diseases where the lung capacity is greatly diminished.

Alcoholic liquors are much used for their stimulating effect in cases of emergency and in some diseases which depress the vitality by the action of poison upon the nerve centers.

Turpentine has considerable reputation as a diffusible stimulant, a carminative, a diuretic and anthelmintic.

Digitalis stimulates the heart's action and in suitable cases is a remedy of decided value but it is in no sense a household remedy.

Nitro-glycerine in doses of one one-hundredth of a grain exerts a powerful and almost instantaneous exhilaration of the heart's action. It can be obtained in tablets of the above dose.

Sedatives.—These are medicines which lessen the heart's action as aconite, gelsemium, veratrum, tartar emetic and prussic acid.

They are dangerous remedies except in small and suitable doses, and poisons which cannot be trifled with. In fevers and acute inflammations they afford the prescriber some of his most valuable weapons for combating disease. When the pulse is rapid, strong, full or bounding, no remedies are administered with greater satisfaction and with more certain results. In the early fever stages, in pleurisy and pneumonia, aconite and veratrum are remedies of efficiency.

Aconite has come to be so widely known and so generally recognized and employed as a domestic remedy that it is necessary to know when and how to administer it. It produces the best results in small doses. It lessens the frequency of the pulse, calms the excitement of the heart, relieves the circulation, relaxes the skin and produces moisture in febrile conditions.

Veratrum is given in the same dose as aconite and by some is considered preferable in the early stages of pneumonia and other inflammatory conditions. It should not be used if the heart is weak or if the condition shows signs of depression and exhaustion. It may be as successfully used as aconite or any other powerful remedy. Put ten drops of the fluid extract or fifteen of the tincture in half a glass of water and give one teaspoonful every hour till the pulse rate declines near the normal.

The leaves and bark of the peach tree contain a trace of prussic acid and are consequently sedative. One or two tablespoonfuls of the infusion are said to be serviceable in irritable stomach, with nausea and vomiting. Dilute prussic acid in small doses is often added to cough mixtures for its sedative effect.

Gelsemium is a valuable sedative to the nervous system. It allays congestion of the brain and is especially serviceable in meningitis and is reported to have cured cases of lockjaw. It is a valuable remedy in neuralgia of the face, the pains of menstruation, also the after pains following labor. It is serviceable in inflammation of the lungs and has been highly recommended in bilious and malarial fevers.

Expectorants.—Expectorants are remedies which act on the mucous membrane lining the throat and bronchi and modify the character and quantity of the secretions. They are sometimes useful in acute and chronic bronchitis, but they should not be too long continued. Some of the more common and efficient expectorants are the syrup of tolu, syrup of ipecac, syrup of squill, sanguinaria, chloral hydrate and muriate of ammonia.

Antipyretics.—Antipyretics are remedies which antagonize febrile conditions and lower the temperature. Acetanilide and phenacetine are members of this class. They may be safely given in five-grain doses if there are no signs of heart weakening.

Alteratives.—Alteratives are medicines which affect the bodily nutrition, stimulate the secretions, aid elimination of waste products and cause improvement in the health. They are closely allied to tonics, stimulants and laxatives. An alterative remedy often possesses the property of several other classes.

Podophyllin acts favorably upon morbid conditions of the system, removing the effete materials and stimulating the secretions; hence it is not only a cathartic but a powerful alterative.

Yellow dock, burdock and bloodroot are among the most useful and efficient vegetable alteratives.

The iodide of potash, lime and iron are often used with the most happy effect. The administration of such remedies cannot be recommended for domestic use except in some combination. The following prescription is a reliable blood purifier and an efficient alterative.

℞ Iodide of potash two drams
 Ext. sanguinaria, fl. one dram
 Ext. yellow dock, fl. one ounce
 Syr. sarsaparilla comp. one ounce
 Spirits gaultheria two drams
 Elix. cinchona q. s. to make four ounces

Mix. Dose, one teaspoonful three times a day after meals. This may be given where the condition of the system requires thorough renovation.

Antiseptics.—Antiseptics are remedies which prevent putrefaction. Some of the more commonly used are chlorine, creosote, carbolic acid, salicylic acid, boracic acid and corrosive sublimate.

Escharotics.—Escharotics are applied locally to destroy some growth or unhealthy tissue. They are the strong acids, especially nitric, nitrate of silver, caustic potash, chromic acid and carbolic acid.

Anodynes.—These are used to relieve pain. At the head of the list stands opium and some of its alkaloids as morphia and codeina. Belladonna and its alkaloid atropia, especially where associated with opium or morphine, assist in relieving pain. Henbane and its alkaloid hyoscine are also included in this list. The alkaloid is given in doses of one one-hundredth of a grain. Opium and its helpers ought not to be prescribed on every pretext of pain. Prescriptions containing them ought not to be repeated except by the advice and consent of the physician who first ordered them. Too little attention is given to the danger of the morphia habit. A resort to opium or morphine on every occasion is reprehensible; and yet at times their use is demanded and to withold such agents is unwise, but their use should be discontinued as soon as the condition of the patient will admit of it. In peritonitis there is no remedy which can take its place. It should be given in this fearful disease boldly and unsparingly till the danger is over. It has saved many lives.

Properly used opium is one of the most valuable remedies known but it is not a remedy for domestic use, except perhaps in the form of paregoric, Dover's powder and Tully's powder. It requires much experience and skill to know when and how to use an agent so potent for good or for evil.

Anodynes should be sparingly administered to children and only in minute doses as their nervous systems are powerfully impressed by this class of remedies. When a very sensitive stomach will not tolerate morphine from an eighth to a fourth of a grain inserted under the skin will produce speedy relief.

Anaesthetics belong to this class. They are taken by inhalation and produce such a condition of unconsciousness that a tooth can be extracted or a limb amputated without any feeling of pain whatever. Their discovery has accomplished much for the progress of surgery as well as for the amelioration of human suffering.

Other minor classes of medicine as *carminatives* allay pain in the stomach and bowels from flatulency; *anthelmintics* destroy worms. These require mention merely as the remedies referred to are sufficiently mentioned in connection with the treatment of the various diseases in other sections of this work.

Emmenagogues are remedies which favor the appearance of the monthly flow.

Aphrodisiacs are remedies which stimulate the sexual organs and their functions.

Infusions are generally made by pouring boiling water upon medicinal substances, whether bark, leaves, roots or seeds and allowing it to cool. Then it is strained. An infusion should be made in small quantity and fresh as wanted as it does not keep well.

Tinctures are prepared by soaking the medicinal substances in officinal or dilute alcohol. The dilute alcohol dissolves medicinal principles, which water will not, and its preservative qualities are a great advantage.

Syrups are simply medicated fluids added to a sugar solution. Many of the medicated syrups are useful in the preparation of prescriptions, some adding more to their flavor than to their virtue.

Some medicines are best given in powder form but when they are very bitter or bad tasting they are better in the form of a pill, tablet or capsule, so that they can be swallowed without tasting. The preparation of medicines has become an extensive business and requires an acquaintance with a great variety of processes. Anyone wishing to give the subject thorough study should consult the United States Dispensatory or other books on the subject of pharmacy.

Many medicinal substances like opium, contain several distinct alkaloids or active principles. The separation of these active principles from drugs as strychnia from nux vomica, atropia from belladonna, quinia from cinchona and morphia from opium provides the physician with a list of efficient medicines in concentrated form always reliable in dose and action. This is a great benefit both to the patient and physician. It does away with the administration of large draughts of nauseating mixtures as well as with the doctor's saddle-bags. In the ordinary pocketcase containing only one or two dozen little bottles, can be stored more medicinal virtue at the present day than could be placed in the oldtime attic filled with herbs, roots, plants and barks from meadow and woodland.

The following abbreviations commonly used will be found convenient :

aq.	stands for	the	Latin	aqua	and	means	water
carb.	"	"	"	"	carbonas	"	"	carbonate
co. or comp.	"	"	"	"	compositus	"	"	compound
cort.	"	"	"	"	cortex	"	"	bark

dil.	stands	for	the	Latin dilutus	and	means	dilute
dist.	"	"	"	" distillatus	"	"	distilled
emp.	"	"	"	" emplastrum	"	"	plaster
ext.	"	"	"	" extractum	"	"	extract
fort.	"	"	"	" fortior	"	"	stronger
inf.	"	"	"	" infusum	"	"	infusion
lin.	"	"	"	" linimentum	"	"	liniment
lot.	"	"	"	" lotio	"	"	wash
mist.	"	"	"	" mistura	"	"	mixture
mur.	"	"	"	" murias	"	"	muriate
nit.	"	"	"	" nitras	"	"	nitrate
ol.	"	"	"	" oleum	"	"	oil
pul.	"	"	"	" pulvis	"	"	powder
rad.	"	"	"	" radix	"	"	root
sol.	"	"	"	" solutio	"	"	solution
spts.	"	"	"	" spiritus	"	"	spirits
sulph.	"	"	"	" sulphas	"	"	sulphate
suppos.	"	"	"	" suppositorium	"	"	suppository
syr.	"	"	"	" syrapus	"	"	syrup
tr. or tinc.	"	"	"	" tinctura	"	"	tincture
ungt.	"	"	"	" unguentum	"	"	ointment
vin.	"	"	"	" vinum	"	"	wine

The following are the more common abbreviations used in prescriptions:

a a	stands	for	the	Greek ana	and	means	of each
ad	"	"	"	Latin adde	"	"	add
chart	"	"	"	" chartula	"	"	a small paper
collyr.	"	"	"	" collyrium	"	"	eye water
D.	"	"	"	Greek dosis	"	"	dose
div.	"	"	"	Latin divide	"	"	divide
fl.	"	"	"	" fluidum	"	"	fluid
ft.	"	"	"	" fiat	"	"	make
M.	"	"	"	" misce	"	"	mix
pil.	"	"	"	" pilula	"	"	pill
q. s.	"	"	"	" quantum sufficit	"	"	sufficient quantity
sig.	"	"	"	" signa	and	"	write
ss	"	"	"	" semis	"	"	one-half
t. i. d.	"	"	"	" ter in diem	"	"	three times a day
gr.	"	"	"	" granum	"	"	a grain

gtt.	stands for the Latin				gutta	and means	a drop
m.	"	"	"	"	minimum	" "	a minim
℈	"	"	"	"	scrupulum	" "	a scruple
ʒ	"	"	"	"	drachma	" "	a dram
℥	"	"	"	"	uncia	" "	an ounce
O	"	"	"	"	octarius	" "	a pint

℞ This sign is placed at the head and left hand of each prescription and means recipe or take, the remedies to be taken or used usually follow in Latin, taking the genitive termination, while the quantity if written out would take the accusative case. In practice a prescription is never fully written out; it is abbreviated and the directions are written in plain English. For the sake of ease in reading it has seemed best to discard in this work the use of Latin and symbols for the most part and use English words.

one minim is equivalent to about		two drops	
one dram	"	one teaspoonful	
two drams	"	one dessertspoonful	
four drams	"	one tablespoonful	
sixty minims		make one dram	written thus: ʒ¹
eight fluid drams		" " ounce	" " ℥¹
sixteen fluid ounces		" " pint	" " O¹
twenty grains		" " scruple	" " ℈¹
three scruples		" " dram	" " ʒ¹
eight drams		" " ounce	" " ℥¹
sixty grains		" " dram	" " ʒ¹
four hundred and eighty grains		" " ounce	" " ℥¹

A little time and study devoted to the above symbols will render them plain and well repay one interested in medical literature for the labor.

V. DOSES.

The dose of any medicine is the average quantity, ascertained by experience as necessary to produce a desired result. No more of any medicine should be administered than the necessity of the case requires, nor should its use be needlessly prolonged.

A powerful, dangerous remedy should not be chosen when a mild and harmless one will answer just as well.

Any remedy should be avoided which is liable to produce results more desperate than the condition for which it is to be administered.

Age is an important factor in regulating the dose of medicines. The chief difficulty in household prescribing is to determine the proper dose for the different ages. How much ought to be given to an infant or a child one or two years old? In administering medicines, the dose for an adult is taken as the standard, and when a dose is recommended, unless otherwise specified, an adult dose is always to be understood. The following will be helpful in ascertaining the dose for different ages:

An infant from one to three months old requires about $\frac{1}{30}$ the adult dose, six months old $\frac{1}{20}$.

Give a child one year old $\frac{1}{13}$ of the adult dose.
" " two years " $\frac{1}{7}$ " " "
" " three " " $\frac{1}{5}$ " " "
" " four " " $\frac{1}{4}$ " " "
" " six " " $\frac{1}{3}$ " " "
" " twelve " " $\frac{1}{2}$ " " "
" a person fourteen " " $\frac{2}{3}$ " " "
" " from eighteen to twenty nearly the full dose.
After fifty reduce the dose $\frac{1}{4}$
" seventy " " $\frac{1}{3}$
" ninety " " $\frac{1}{2}$

There are some exceptions to the above rules which should be borne in mind. Persons under size require a smaller dose than those over weight; those in a debilitated or feeble condition require a smaller dose than the robust and strong. Persons engaged in indoor work, or those of sedentary habits require a smaller dose than those engaged in manual labor, and who are exposed to the weather at all seasons.

Medicines should be prescribed for feeble infants and very old people with especial care. The nervous system of an infant is easily impressed, therefore opium or morphine, if given to very young children, should be in smaller doses than those indicated by the foregoing rules, and such remedies ought not to be prescribed by inexperienced persons.

Owing to the sensitive condition of the mucous membrane in young children, emetics and cathartics act with proportionably greater energy than in the case of adults, so that the administration of such remedies should be cautious and guarded; and the harsh and more irritating remedies should consequently be avoided. For domestic use choose those remedies which are simple and whose effects are well known. Many harmless medicines are the most efficient, and it is not necessary to be as particular in their administration. They can be given in much larger doses to children than indicated by the above rule. It is not necessary that a remedy should be expensive in order to be efficient. In using a remedy with which you are but little acquainted, choose the minimum dose; this rule is imperative in the case of energetic and powerful drugs.

Small doses, frequently repeated generally give better results than large doses at longer intervals, except where vomiting is the object aimed at.

A dose table for the more common remedies, and the diseases for which they are chiefly used, is here appended, while valuable medical combinations with full directions for their use, is to be found under the treatment of each disease.

In addition to the following doses those remedies advised for household practice will each receive still further notice to render their use intelligent and successful.

REMEDY.	INDICATED FOR WHAT.	DOSE.
acid, carbolic	vomiting	1 drop well diluted with water
" " solution	disinfectant wash	q. s.
" " ointment	sores, burns, itching, etc.	q. s.
" hydriodic syrup	asthma, hay fever	1 teaspoonful in water
" phosphoric dil.	exhaustion of brain	10 to 30 drops in water
" salicylic	rheumatism	5 to 10 grains
" tannic	piles in suppositories	2 to 3 grains
acetanilid	rheumatism to reduce temperature	2 to 5 grains
aconite tinct.	fevers	1 to 2 drops in water
" fl. ex.	" .	¼ to 1 drop in water
alum pulverized	croup, (emetic)	10 to 60 grains in water
ammonia—carbonate	pneumonia	5 to 10 grains
" aromatic spirits	fainting	¼ to 1 dram
ammonia valerianate elixir	hysteria	1 dram
anise water	colic	1 to 4 drams

REMEDY.	INDICATED FOR WHAT.	DOSE.
anise oil	colic	1 to 4 drops
arnica tinct.	bruises	externally
" "	concussion of brain,	5 to 20 drops internally
arsenic	cancers	$\frac{1}{60}$ to $\frac{1}{20}$ grain
" sulphide	skin affections	$\frac{1}{100}$ grain
atropia	catarrh	$\frac{1}{100}$ grain
" with morphine	severe pain	tablets internally or hypodermically, $\frac{1}{100}$ gr. atropia and $\frac{1}{4}$ gr. morphia
belladonna tinct.	scarlet fever and many other diseases	1 to 3 drops
bismuth subnitrate	diarrhœa	3 to 60 grains
" subgallate	stomach distress	5 to 10 grains
blackberry root, tinct. wine or syrup	diarrhœa	one teaspoonful
buchu fluid extract	irritable bladder or gravel	$\frac{1}{4}$ to 1 dram
burdock root—fl. ext.	chronic skin diseases	$\frac{1}{2}$ to 1 dram
caffeine	weak heart or dropsy	1 to 5 grains
calcium sulphide	abcesses, carbuncles and acnae	$\frac{1}{4}$ to 1 grain
camphor	chordee, after pains, cholera	1 to 5 grains
castor oil	laxative and cathartic	1 to 8 drams
chalk mixture	antacid, summer complaint	1 to 8 drams
charcoal of wood pulverized	flatulence	10 to 20 grains
chloral hydrate	convulsions, sleeplessness	5 to 20 grains
chloroform	convulsions	3 to 10 drops cautiously inhaled
Dover's powder	cold, to ease pain	5 to 10 grains
elaterium	dropsy	$\frac{1}{8}$ to $\frac{1}{4}$ grain in pill
Epsom salts or sulphate of magnesia	cathartic	1 to 4 drams in water

REMEDY.	INDICATED FOR WHAT.	DOSE.
ergot fl. ext.	hemorrhage	10 to 30 drops
gentian tr. comp.	dyspepsia	1 to 2 drams
ginger tr.	colic, dysentery	10 to 30 drops
gold thread	sore mouth, wash	$\frac{1}{2}$ to 20 grains
grindelia robusta fl. ext.	asthma	$\frac{1}{4}$ to 1 dram
henbane tr.	diseases of bladder	10 to 60 drops
" fl. ext.	mania	2 to 10 drops
iodine	enlarged glands	externally
ipecac, wine of	cough, bronchitis	1 dram
" syrup of	expectorant, emetic	$\frac{1}{2}$ to 4 drams
iron tr. chloride	anæmia, erysipelas	5 to 20 drops
iron reduced	blood tonic—in pill	$\frac{1}{2}$ to 2 grains
lavender spts. comp.	flatulence	$\frac{1}{2}$ to 2 drams
lactucarium syrup	cough	1 to 2 drams
laudanum or opium tincture of	pain, enemeta	10 to 30 drops
lime water	antacid	1 to 4 drams
lobelia tinct.	expectorant, antispasmodic	10 to 60 drops
magnesia cit. granular effervescent	laxative and cathartic	1 to 4 teaspoonfuls
menthol	neuralgia, burns	externally
morphia	pain	$\frac{1}{16}$ to $\frac{1}{4}$ grain
niter, sweet spirits of	diuretic, in fevers	$\frac{1}{4}$ to 1 dram
nux vomica, tinct.	anæmia, dyspepsia and constipation	3 to 10 drops
" " ext.	" "	(pills) $\frac{1}{8}$ to $\frac{1}{4}$ grain
opium	cholera, peritonitis	1 grain
pepsin pure	dyspepsia	1 to 3 grains
paregoric	cough	$\frac{1}{2}$ to 1 teaspoonful
peppermint spts.	nausea, colic	20 to 30 drops
phenacetin	pain and rheumatism	5 to 10 grains
pink root, and senna fl. ext.	worms	$\frac{1}{2}$ to 2 drams
podophyllin	biliousness, constipation	$\frac{1}{20}$ to $\frac{1}{2}$ grain
quinine	malária, fevers	1 to 20 grains
rhubarb, syr. aromatic	laxative for children	1 to 4 drams

REMEDY.	INDICATED FOR WHAT.	DOSE.
salol	rheumatism	5 grains.
santonin	worms	1 to 3 grains
soda bicarb.	antacid	5 to 60 grains
soda, bromide of	nervousness	5 to 20 grains
squill, syrup of	expectorant	½ to 1 dram
squill syrup comp.	croup	8 to 30 drops
strychnia	paralysis, alcoholism	$\frac{1}{100}$ to $\frac{1}{60}$ grain
sulphonal	sleeplessness	5 grains
Tully's powder	after pains, stomach ache or pain in bowels	5 to 10 grams
wild cherry syr.	cough	1 to 2 teaspoonfuls

VI.—HOUSEHOLD REMEDIES.

It is unnecessary to have constantly on hand all the remedies mentioned in this book, some of them are rarely required and it is better to obtain them fresh as needed. There are a few remedies, however, which should be kept in every family to meet cases of emergency, especially if beyond the easy reach of a competent physician.

This article follows the general description of medicines, and proposes to select from them a small list of those efficient remedies which are appropriate for domestic use, tell you when they are indicated, and give all necessary instruction in regard to their action, so that you can practically have the doctor with you to consult on all occasions.

Household medicines should be kept together in some secure place, away from the reach of children, distinctly labeled with the name and dose. They should be kept tightly corked and excluded from the atmosphere as much as possible. It is a good plan to have the powerful remedies and poisions like aconite in round, two dram vials, and conspicuously labeled poison or caution.

Liniments and external remedies, being used more freely, can be placed in square bottles, holding six ounces. A cough and diarrhœa mixture can be put in four ounce bottles. Some such plan, modified to meet the tastes and requirements of each family, will prove convenient and satisfactory.

This list might be easily extended, the chief difficulty being to keep it within reasonable limits. These remedies are not expensive, yet often worth a hundred times more than they cost, if at hand as needed. They can be used by an intelligent adult person who will give attention to simple details and make use of good judgment.

This list does not contain anything like all the good remedies, but what it contains are efficient to accomplish the purposes for which they are directed, in so far as it is possible with a list of domestic remedies. Experience and careful attention to the other portions of this work will enable you to add other remedies to the list, or in some cases to substitute, for those suggested, others better adapted to special cases.

Tincture of Aconite Root.—This is an excellent and powerful remedy, to be used in the early febrile disturbances of children or adults. It moderates the heart's excitement, relieves the congestion of the blood-vessels, checks the process of inflammation, and can be used with the best results by any intelligent person. Its effects should be watched, for it should be given less often when the pulse has declined to its normal condition and when free perspiration has been produced. The dose is from one to five drops of the tincture in water. One drop every hour is usually sufficient to produce the characteristic results.

For a child one year old, put five drops into one half glass of water, and of this mixture give one teaspoonful each hour or half hour, depending upon the urgency of the case, till sweating is produced and the fever symptoms abate, when it may be continued at less frequent intervals or discontinued as indicated by the symptoms.

Tincture of Belladonna.—This is a remedy much used and popular among the people who prescribe somewhat for their own family. The tincture can be used in the same dose and manner as aconite. Belladonna renders good service in the collapse of cholera infantum. It increases the capillary circulation, and relieves congestion of the internal organs. It improves the depth and character of the respiration and hence is much employed in inflammations of the lungs and air passages. It is used in asthma, whooping cough, catarrh with profuse secretions of mucous, in headache, in neuralgia, and nocturnal incontinence of the urine in children. It flushes the face in full doses, dilates the pupils, causes dryness of the mouth and throat, and excites the nervous system. Atropia is the best form of using this powerful remedy. It can be obtained in soluble tablets containing one one-hundredth of a grain, one of which is an adult dose. For a child one year old, one of these tablets can be dissolved in ten or twenty teaspoonfuls of water, of which one teaspoonful is a sufficient dose, given every one or two hours. It may also be alternated with aconite, with good results, in fevers and inflammations of the lungs and air passages, or pleurisy. It is made use of extensively in eye practice, also in connection with morphia hypodermically, to relieve sciatica and other severe neuralgias and cramps; also colic, either bilious, intestinal, uterine or renal.

Atropia is an efficient remedy for night sweats. Belladonna ointment is a valuable application to an inflamed breast. It is also used locally to check the secretion of milk.

Alum.—Pulverized alum is a serviceable and safe emetic in case of croup. It would be well to keep it on hand if there are children in the family liable to attacks of this urgent disease. The dose is one teaspoonful in water, to be followed by free drinking of warm water.

Ammonia.—It is known also as hartshorn, or smelling salts, and is a convenient stimulant for inhalation in cases of fainting. A small glass-stoppered bottle of strong aqua ammonia will answer as well. If used internally it must be well diluted. A teaspoonful in a half glass of water and given in teaspoonful doses every half hour would be appropriate in an emergency, requiring the use of a stimulant. A teaspoonful dose of the aromatic spirits, if at hand, would be preferable. Some care must be exercised in the inhalation of ammonia, otherwise it might injure the mouth and produce inflammation of the glottis.

Tincture of Arnica.—This is much employed domestically as a remedy for bruises. In case of much soreness or pain equal parts of the tincture of arnica and the tincture of opium form a valuable external application. It may be applied freely, as needed, on a piece of clean muslin.

Spirits of Camphor.—There are but few households probably where camphor is not included among the domestic remedies. It is a sort of habit to have a camphor bottle, even when no attempt is made to keep any medical supplies. A few drops will often relieve hysterical vomiting; it is also serviceable in flatulence. The dose is eight to twenty drops, well diluted with water. Camphor is serviceable in summer diarrhœa, but as it enters into the composition of Tully's powder, which is given later, it requires no further mention here.

Camphor Liniment.—(Camphorated oil.)—This is camphor gum, dissolved in sweet oil. It is an excellent emollient for many purposes. In pleurisy or inflammation of the lungs it can be used externally on flannel, or added to a flaxseed poultice just before applying it. It is somewhat warming and stimulating, it keeps the poultice warm and soft, and is a reliable and safe remedy. It is excellent to apply externally to all glandular swellings, such as appear in the neck in diphtheria and scarlet fever. It may be applied to bubo swellings in the groins and any acute glandular enlargements. It penetrates such indurations, softens them, relieves the congestion and inflammation and often prevents suppuration.

Camphor Liniment Compound.—This is composed of camphor liniment three parts and chloroform one part. This mixture has been prescribed and used for years by the author with the most happy effects. It makes a clear mixture and does not, like most liniments, separate. It is a liniment of great efficiency to apply to painful joints in gout and rheumatism, to painful swellings, sprains or wherever a soothing application is needed.

Castor Oil.—This is a valuable laxative for children, and it can be used with safety in the early stages of all diseases when there is inaction of the bowels. A small teaspoonful for a child is the proper dose. It is used in cholera infantum, combined with the tincture of opium or paregoric with happy results. (See cholera infantum.)

The following elegant and palatable prescription may be used for giving castor oil:

℞	Castor oil	two ounces
	Saccharin	two grains
	Syr. acaciæ	half an ounce
	Syr. of liquorice	half an ounce
	Wintergreen water	one ounce

Mix. Shake before using. Dose, one to four teaspoonfuls as needed.

Tincture or Essence of Jamaica Ginger.—This is a good domestic remedy for colic in the bowels, or cramps in the stomach;

also diarrhœa with griping pains. The dose is ten to thirty drops or more in hot water. A teaspoonful of paregoric may be added for an adult and increases its efficiency in all the range of its employment.

Tincture of Iodine.—This is an excellent remedy for application to corns, bunions and chronic swellings of the glands or joints. It may be painted over such enlargements once or twice a day. It favors the absorption of chronic swellings.

Ipecac. The Syrup of.—This is a convenient emetic and expectorant. It is given in colds, croup, coughs, or bronchitis in minute doses and for vomiting. The dose is from one-half to two teaspoonfuls, repeated as necessary. The larger dose is for emetic purposes. It is a perfectly safe remedy.

Menthol Liniment.—This is a very efficient remedy for headache, neuralgia, and superficial pains. The formula is as follows:

℞	Menthol	one dram
	Alcohol	two ounces
	Oil of clove	twenty minims
	Oil of cinnamon	twenty minims

Mix. This is to be applied externally as needed.

Pills. For a safe and efficient pill see formula under constipation.

Podophyllin.—This remedy in little granules or parvules, containing one-twentieth of a grain, is an excellent cathartic for children; one or more can be given at night, or night and morning, as required.

Quinine.—This is a remedy that ought to be kept on hand in malarial regions. The dose is from one to five grains in pills or powders. It is often given in much larger doses. It should be taken in connection with the podophyllin parvules, if the liver is inactive. (For formula see Malaria.)

Syrup of Squill Compound.—(Hive Syrup.)—There is no better household remedy for sudden attacks of croup. It should be used with caution, as it is somewhat depressing in its action. It may be given with excellent results in acute colds, bronchitis and croup. It may be given in small and often repeated doses, or if it is desired to hasten vomiting, increase the dose till such result is obtained. As soon as it has caused vomiting the dose, if continued, should be considerably reduced. The dose is eight to twenty drops. It should be given to feeble infants cautiously.

A few other remedies are handy in case of emergency.

The Oil of Clove.—A dram of oil of clove is a convenient remedy to have on hand in case toothache should occur suddenly at night. A piece of cotton saturated with the oil and placed in the cavity of a tooth affords temporary relief. Creosote is more efficient, but is a less safe remedy to use, and if handled carelessly burns the lining of the mouth and the skin. The two remedies may be combined. A prescription for toothache is found under that head.

Lime Water and Sweet Oil.—Have a four ounce bottle of equal parts of lime water and sweet oil on hand to apply to burns and scalds. It is an efficient remedy and affords marked relief from pain. The old name for this remedy is Carron oil.

Carbolized Ointment.—Prepare this useful ointment by adding ten drops of strong, pure carbolic acid to an ounce of vaseline; if you wish a stronger ointment twenty drops may be added to an ounce of the vaseline. This makes an inexpensive domestic ointment which may be applied to burns, chapped hands, cracked lips, cold sores, itching of the skin and to other abrasions and sores as they occur.

Ground Mustard.—This is an excellent domestic remedy. Do not allow yourself to be without it in the family. A teaspoonful, mixed with lukewarm water and taken, will produce speedy vomiting and often perhaps relieve a person choked with a chunk of meat or piece of bone or other substance. Ground mustard is excellent to add to a foot-bath in case a person has been much exposed and has had wet feet during the day. Cloths wrung out of hot mustard water are excellent to apply to the surface in case of pain, vomiting or to stimulate the skin and bring out the rash of scarlet fever. It is useful in convulsions. A mustard poultice is a well-known and much-used counter-irritant. It is used to allay vomiting, applied over the stomach.

It is serviceable in the first stages of pneumonia, pleurisy and to relieve many conditions of internal congestion and deep-seated pain. It will often relieve lumbago. The strength of a mustard poultice can be reduced by mixing it in any desired proportion with flour; and it can be prevented from blistering by mixing with the white of an egg. A mustard poultice is much improved by adding to it a teaspoonful or more of sweet oil. For small children the strength of a mustard poultice should be considerably reduced as the skin is very sensitive.

Hot Water.—This has many uses both externally and internally. It has a large range of uses in the household. Taken internally it often relieves pain in the stomach, vomiting and dyspepsia. It can be safely used in fevers if it has been previously boiled, and in the chill stage of many diseases. It is useful for injections to allay hemorrhages; it must be used as hot as it can be borne for that. It relieves congestions and inflammations. A hot foot-bath often relieves slight congestion of the brain by drawing the blood away from the upper extremities to the general circulation. It is an excellent dressing for slight wounds, sprains, bruises and the attendant pain. It should be used in the form of a hot pack, wrapped outside with flannel or oiled silk.

Notwithstanding the numerous valuable prescriptions contained in this work, the following for cough and another for diarrhœa will not be out of place to complete this list of domestic medicines.

COUGH MIXTURE.

℞ Muriate of ammonia   two drams
   Muriate of morphia or codeina   two grains
   Spts. of chloroform   two drams
   Syr. of wild cherry   two ounces
   Anise water enough to make   four ounces

Mix. Dose, one teaspoonful, and repeat in four hours as needed:

DIARRHŒA MIXTURE.

℞ Tincture deodorized opium   sixteen drops
   Subnitrate of bismuth   two drams
   Syrup of blackberry root   one ounce
   Cinnamon water   two ounces

Mix. Dose, a teaspoonful every two or four hours.

This list of remedies, recommended for household use, contains about twenty medicines and ought not with the prescriptions for cough and diarrhœa to cost more than two or three dollars.

Tully's Powder or Paregoric.—For stomach ache so common among small children it might be well to add Tully's powder. The adult dose is ten grains, for an infant under a year old one-half a grain is a sufficient dose. If preferred a few drops of paregoric can be used instead but the common and constant use of paregoric or soothing syrup to quiet cross children and keep them sleeping to avoid a racket is reprehensible. In sickness attended by pain it is admissible but in health it is injurious.

CHAPTER IV.

POISONS AND THEIR ANTIDOTES.

1. Poisons in General.—II. The Mineral Acids.—III. Oxalic Acid.—IV. Carbolic Acid and Creosote.—V. Acetic Acid.—VI. Ammonia.—VII. Prussic or Hydrocyanic Acid.—VIII. Arsenic and its Preparations.—IX. Copper, Mercury and Zinc Compounds.—X. Tartar Emetic. XI. Lead Compounds.—XII. Nitrate of Silver.—XIII. Phosphorus.—XIV. Opium and Morphine.—XV. Chloral Hydrate.—XVI. Strychnia.—XVII. Aconite and Vegetable Poisons.—XVIII. Poison Ivy.—XIX. Poison Gases.

I.—POISONS IN GENERAL.

IT is somewhat difficult to give a satisfactory definition of poisons because there are so many vegetable, mineral and animal substances which come under this head and because there are so many substances, like the chloride of sodium, (common salt,) which are poisonous in large doses and yet harmless or essential to life in small quantities.

There are some substances which are poisonous only when separated from the inert material by which they are diluted. Oxygen, which is always essential to the maintenance of life is poisonous when separated from the nitrogen which dilutes it sufficiently for breathing purposes. A person inhales enough carbonic acid during twenty-four hours to destroy life if breathed alone by itself.

Some of the properties of plants are harmless in their natural combinations but when their medicinal virtues are concentrated or their active principles separated they may act as violent poisons. The common sorrel and pie plant contain oxalic acid; and the leaf and bark of the cherry and peach trees, also the pit of the latter, contain prussic acid, a most deadly poison.

The active principle of aconite, known as the alkaloid aconitia is a fatal poison in the dose of one-twentieth of a grain, the medicinal dose being from one two-hundredth to one four-hundredth of a grain.

Some substances are poisonous simply because their strength is concentrated but when sufficiently diluted are harmless. Muriatic acid is a powerful common poison, burning and destroying the tissues, yet in diluted form it is a useful medicine and it is also a constituent of the normal gastric juice.

Phosphorus is an energetic poison but its compounds exist in many articles of our daily food and it is essential to the growth of the bodily tissues, the bones containing it in large quantities.

We shall simply regard poisons as those substances which destroy life, without attempting a comprehensive definition. There are three classes of poisons, mineral, vegetable and animal. Some of the most active as prussic acid, strychnia, aconite, hyoscine and many others are obtained from the vegetable kingdom.

Poisons usually act upon the system in one of two ways; chemically or physiologically. By the first method they unite with the fluids of the body with which they come in contact and corrode a layer of the tissue leaving it as if charred; the vitality is destroyed as deeply as the corrosive substance can penetrate and there is superficial death of the corroded layer. By the second method the poison is absorbed, enters the circulation and produces some definite condition or physiological result.

The strong mineral acids are poisonous by means of their corrosive action. They produce death of the soft tissues to which they are applied. Opium illustrates the action of the second method. It does not act chemically. It has no power to destroy the life of a tissue but it is absorbed into the system and in poisonous doses stupefies the brain and certain nerves whose action is essential to the process of respiration and the continuation of life. The processes of life become fainter and fainter, the breathing takes place at unusually long intervals until it ceases altogether and the whole machinery stops.

There are several ways by which poisons may enter the system, the most common method is by being taken into the mouth and stomach. Some poisons exist in the form of vapor and gas and enter the system by being inhaled. The vapor of prussic acid cannot be safely inhaled; even the smallest amount is not without great danger. It produces fatal results almost instantly and where a case of poisoning occurs from this powerful agent the physician rarely has an opportunity to reach the victim before death has occurred.

Some poisons are occasionally introduced into the system through an abrasion in the skin, or a wound, or it may be injected into the cellular tissue beneath the skin. The poisons of rabid animals and serpents are introduced by means of a wound or bite.

Some poisons reach the system simply by contact with the skin. Poison ivy acts in this way. Lead is absorbed into the system from hair-dyes and mercury from cosmetics.

Cases of belladonna poisoning have occurred from its extensive application externally in the form of plasters.

ANTIDOTES.

Antidotes are substances which antagonize the action of poisons and render them more or less harmless. Some of the antidotes for the mineral acids are alkalies which neutralize their action by contact. Other poisons are antagonized by physiological antidotes. These set up an action in the system which is opposed to the action of the poison and thus its effect is counteracted until nature can eliminate it.

There are some general principles to be observed in treating those who have taken poisons.

It is necessary in the first place to get rid of the poison as soon as possible. Nature often accomplishes this end by means of vomiting and thus irritating poisons are often expelled. The process of vomiting is favored by the abundant administration of lukewarm water. If the poisonous substance does not itself produce vomiting, administer an emetic. The sulphate of zinc is an excellent emetic in doses of from five to twenty grains. It is rapid in its action and it does not produce depressing effects like many other emetics. Ipecac, either the syrup or teaspoonful doses of the fluid extract, stands second on the list, or from fifteen to thirty grains of the powder may be stirred into warm water and drank freely. Ipecac can be taken in considerable quantity as it does no injury and the dose can be frequently repeated till it acts. When these cannot be obtained do not wait for their arrival but use ground mustard, a teaspoonful or more in warm water and repeat frequently. Common salt may be used in warm water. Vomiting is hastened by tickling the throat or fauces with the finger or a feather, also by the copious administration of lukewarm water. In the hands of a physician apomorphine may be used to cause vomiting. It is a certain emetic. The dose is from one-tenth to one-twentieth of a grain injected under the skin.

Poison introduced by the bite of a rabid dog requires energetic treatment (see hydrophobia); the wound should be speedily and thoroughly cauterized. It is customary to recommend sucking a poison wound immediately. This can be done without danger if there is no abrasion about the mouth to favor the absorption of the poison and if the wound is not extensive.

It is seldom that all the poison taken can be expelled by vomiting hence other measures are made use of, as the administration of an antidote. There is no universal antidote for all poisons, but the special antidote to be used in each case will be mentioned in connection with each particular poison or group of poisons.

Antidotes should be such remedies as can be freely administered without further danger. They should act quickly and be able to counteract the danger which arises from the use of the poison. It often happens that too much time has elapsed between the taking of a poison and the administration of an emetic or an antidote. The poison which has been absorbed and sent all over the system cannot be expelled by vomiting, and antidotes in these cases will not always avail.

In many instances it is necessary to combat the unfavorable symptoms which arise by stimulants, or remedies which produce upon the system the opposite effects of the poison. When poisons suspend the act of respiration artificial respiration performed for a certain time as indicated is sometimes sufficient to avert death. Life sometimes trembles in the balance and a little prompt action is often the means of changing the result from death to life.

II.—THE MINERAL ACIDS.

Sulphuric acid		Bicarbonate of soda
Muriatic acid	Antidotes	Chalk
Nitric acid		Magnesia
Nitromuriatic acid		and other alkalies

In poisoning from the mineral acids vomiting will not avail. It is necessary to neutralize the acids with alkalies; prompt action is essential. In case cooking soda is not at hand make a solution of soap by shaving it up, mixing it with warm water and administer quickly. After the copious use of the antidotes give milk, olive oil, mucilage or whites of eggs. These substances can be mixed with the antidotes and given together.

For acid in the eye use a wash of common baking soda (bicarbonate of soda) and then use oil to allay the irritation.

These acids taken into the stomach are corrosive and produce inflammatory conditions of the alimentary canal of a severe type. Great pain in the mouth and distress in the stomach are experienced. It is difficult to administer the antidotes quickly enough to prevent serious results.

III.—OXALIC ACID.

Antidotes { Chalk
Whiting
Lime
Magnesia }

Occasional poisoning from oxalic acid has occurred on account of its great resemblance to Epsom salts. Druggists have in occasional instances sold oxalic acid by mistake for Epsom salts. The tastes of the two drugs are different. Oxalic acid has a sour taste and the well-known saline purge is extremely bitter; but many times a dose of salts is mixed with water and swallowed too quickly to recognize the difference even when a mistake has been made. It is a violent poison and produces the following symptoms: Great anxiety, extreme pain, great thirst, swollen tongue, violent efforts to vomit, marked debility and prostration. The mouth and throat appear as if scalded, and the mucous lining of the stomach is more or less injured or destroyed by a fatal dose.

The antidote must be used with haste. Chalk or magnesia, mixed with milk or water, should be drank freely. Vomiting may be encouraged by drinking a teaspoonful of mustard mixed with warm water. Also tickle the throat with the finger or a feather. In case no other remedy is at hand, take lime from the walls of the house, crumble it into water and drink it. Stimulants are necessary to combat the depression of the vital forces. The much used pie plant contains oxalic acid, and children are sometimes made sick by its extensive use in the spring when it grows abundantly.

IV.—CARBOLIC ACID AND CREOSOTE.

Antidotes. { Olive oil or whites of eggs.
Saccharate of lime (lime and sugar). }

If strong carbolic acid or creosote is taken internally, it acts as an irritant and corrosive poison. A teaspoonful has been known to produce fatal results. Olive oil should be freely used. The saccharate of lime is the best antidote, but not likely to be at hand. Mustard and warm water should also be given to provoke vomiting. Obtain the saccharate of lime, if possible, and give it in solution. A dose of Epsom salts should be given, and hot applications and stimulants as demanded. The symptoms are violent vomiting and purging, burning pain in the stomach and bowels, a pinched look, weak pulse, difficult breathing and collapse.

V.—ACETIC ACID, OR STRONG VINEGAR.

Antidotes.
- Baking soda
- Lime water
- Carbonate of magnesia.
- Soap water.

After neutralizing the acid, administer olive oil, flaxseed tea or mucilaginous drinks.

VI.—AMMONIA. QUICK LIME.

Lye of wood ashes. Caustic potash or soda.

Antidotes.
- Vinegar
- Lemon juice.

When ammonia has been taken by mistake it produces irritation and caustic action upon the mucous membrane. Give diluted vinegar, olive oil, and milk.

VII.—PRUSSIC ACID, OR HYDROCYANIC ACID.

CYANIDE OF POTASH.

Antidote.—There is no chemical antidote.

Ammonia or chlorine are recommended.

This is the most potent and speedily fatal of all the poisons, acting almost instantly in many cases.

The symptoms of poisoning by prussic acid are loss of sense, difficult breathing, coldness of the extremities, weak pulse and convulsions. The poison is absorbed with great rapidity and the victim often drops dead with a gasp. If life continues for twenty or thirty minutes it is to be regarded as a favorable sign.

Peach pits, bitter almond oil, cherry laurel water and some other vegetable substances, as peach tree leaves and wild cherry, contain prussic acid. Twenty peach pits have been known to fatally poison a child, eaten upon an empty stomach. The treatment indicated is the best that can be used for this class of poisons.

Throw cold water on the face, use inhalations of ammonia, also give ammonia internally; see that it is properly diluted; use friction over the chest and abdomen; keep up the respiration by artificial means; apply warmth. Moisten chloride of lime to liberate the chlorine, and cause the gas to be inhaled. Atropia, hypodermically, would no doubt prove beneficial, as it increases the respiration. A physician rarely has the opportunity to treat a case of poisoning by this agent, so speedily fatal is its action. Other remedies could be suggested by a medical man, as the sulphate of iron, but those suggested above are the most practical, and the easiest to obtain in haste, which is a good point in the treatment.

VIII.—ARSENIC AND ITS PREPARATIONS.

Antidote.—The hydrated sesqui-oxide of iron with magnesia.

Arsenic in large doses usually excites vomiting. This action is to be favored by the administration of ground mustard mixed with warm water. Also tickle the throat with the finger. The stomach should be washed out by the stomach pump. Dialyzed iron, a fluid and somewhat feeble preparation, may be used as an antidote to arsenic in doses of from fifteen to thirty minims. The usual antidote to arsenic is the hydrated sesqui-oxide of iron, and it is prepared thus:

Take a pint of the muriate tincture of iron, add to it ammonia or magnesia to precipitate the iron; strain off the liquid through a muslin and wash out all the ammonia; this leaves a sediment like iron rust, which is harmless and can be administered freely. This antidote may be administered with magnesia, which is also an antidote.

The symptoms of arsenical poisoning are violent gastritis, with vomiting and purging, cramps, great pain in the stomach and abdomen. The bowels are denuded of the mucous membrane, which passes off in shreds. To meet these conditions, opium should be given to allay pain and vomiting, or still better, morphia, hypodermically. Milk, olive oil and the whites of eggs should be taken internally. Fluids should be freely used to enable the kidneys to eliminate the remaining poison.

Death may occur from arsenic several days or even weeks after the poison has been taken and when there appears to be promise of complete recovery.

IX.—COPPER, MERCURY AND ZINC COMPOUNDS.

The more common of these poisons and their names are: Blue vitriol, verdigris, corrosive sublimate, vermilion, the white and red precipitate, and white vitriol.

These poisons coagulate albumen and enter into combination with it. Therefore give the whites of eggs freely, then warm mustard water to excite vomiting. After free vomiting, give the whites of eggs and milk, also olive oil, and apply mustard poultice over the stomach to relieve the gastic symptoms.

Copper salts in poisonous quantity cause violent, burning pain in the stomach, and metallic taste in the mouth, the vomiting of glairy mucous, great exhaustion, and also convulsions. Corrosive sublimate in overdoses causes violent pain, vomiting of mucous and blood, metallic taste in the mouth, and an eroded condition of the mucous lining of the mouth, purging of mucous and blood, collapse and death.

X.—TARTAR EMETIC.

ALSO KNOWN AS TARTARIZED ANTIMONY.

Antidote.—Tannin in large doses.

As tea and coffee contain tannin, strong infusions of either may be used instead, unless the symptoms are severe. Warm water freely taken will render the process of vomiting more tolerable, also extreme heat should be applied, stimulants, and perhaps morphine, hypodermically.

The symptoms of antimony poisoning are violent vomiting of mucous, fluids, bile and blood, also violent purging. Later the rice water stools appear, very similar to those in Asiatic cholera. The pulse is rapid, feeble and flickering. The respirations are faint, fluttering and shallow. The temperature falls if death approaches, and cramps in the legs attack the patient on account of the removal of liquids from the tissues.

XI.—LEAD COMPOUNDS.
SUGAR OF LEAD, WHITE LEAD, LITHARGE.

Antidote.—Epsom salts (sulphate of magnesia.)

Give an ounce of Epsom salts dissolved in water. But first promote vomiting by giving ten to fifteen grains of sulphate of zinc dissolved in water, or mustard water. Hot applications should be applied to the feet and hands, and the pain and irritation relieved by doses of opium. Milk and eggs are serviceable and soothing. The symptoms of lead poisoning are obstinate constipation, pain in the stomach, vomiting, rapid pulse, anxious face, thirst, cramps and muscular twitching.

XII.—NITRATE OF SILVER.

Antidote.—Common Salt (Chloride of Sodium).

Common salt solution neutralizes the action of this poison. The whites of eggs and mucilaginous drinks or olive oil should be given, after vomiting has been provoked by warm mustard water. The symptoms are pain in the abdomen with vomiting and purging. The face is anxious and covered with perspiration. The lips are stained brown or black and convulsions may occur.

XIII.—PHOSPHORUS.

There is no certain antidote for this poison. It should first of all be removed from the stomach by vomiting and other available means. Emetics of mustard and warm water or ipecac should be administered. Vomiting should be followed by giving calcined or carbonate of magnesia or cooking soda. Mix a teaspoonful of either with water or gruel and give as soon as vomiting has taken place. Nothing containing oil or fat is admissible in phosphorous poisoning. It is to be remembered that oils are serviceable in every other kind of poisoning, especially when the tissues are corroded, but as oil favors the absorption of phosphorus it should never be given after accidental poisoning by this agent. Turpentine formerly regarded as an antidote is no longer used.

The symptoms of poisoning by phorphorus are so violent that it is never taken intentionally for suicidal purposes but only by accident. The symptoms are violent pain in the stomach, vomiting, diarrhœa, great distress in the stomach and bowels, and convulsions with the approach of death.

Care should be taken in every family to keep matches out of the way of children. A phosphorous paste is used for the destruction of rats. Such active agents should be used if at all with especial caution.

XIV.—OPIUM AND MORPHINE.

The first indication is the removal of the poison from the stomach. Give twenty grains of the sulphate of zinc or strong mustard water to provoke free vomiting. Prevent the patient from going to sleep. Give ammonia by inhalation and keep the patient aroused by dashing cold water on the face or making the patient walk to and fro. Flagellations are sometimes employed. Administer tannin or strong coffee and in extreme cases resort to artificial respiration. One one-hundredth of a grain of atropia should be given hypodermically. Stimulants may be necessary. Efforts should not be relaxed until the patient is out of danger or so long as life continues.

The symptoms are drowsiness, deep sleep, slow pulse and contracted pupil. In the worst cases the face becomes pale, the respirations decrease sometimes to four or five a minute, the breathing becomes very shallow and in fatal cases the patient becomes so deeply narcotized that no effort can arouse him from this condition. Death results from the failure of respiration.

The tincture of opium (laudanum) is often used with suicidal intent. Soothing syrups have sometimes destroyed the lives of children by means of the large amount of opium or morphine which they contain. Carelessness in constantly repeating prescriptions containing opium is to be observed by watching the drug business and is censurable.

XV.—CHLORAL HYDRATE.

Promote vomiting by the administration of warm mustard water or fifteen to twenty grains of the sulphate of zinc dissolved in water. Give strong tea and coffee. Artificial respiration must be employed if necessary. Stimulants with the exception of ammonia are indicated.

Strychnine should be given to stimulate the respiration; one-fortieth to one-twentieth of a grain will be needed in these cases, or atropia may be used for the same purpose in doses of one-ninetieth of a grain.

The symptoms of poisoning which develop from a fatal dose are sleep followed by coma, the respiration becoming slow and labored and gradually getting shallow and feeble. The pulse becomes thready, flickering and at length ceases at the wrist. The face is pale, the body is covered with a cold sweat and the pupils are widely dilated. The whole muscular system is in a state of marked relaxation and sometimes no effort succeeds in arousing the patient.

XVI.—STRYCHNIA.

(The alkaloid of nux vomica.)

In treating strychnia poisoning nitrite of amyl is an excellent remedy to control convulsions. Three or four drops as needed may be placed upon a handkerchief and inhaled. Excite vomiting by means of strong mustard water and tickling the throat. Give tannin in water. This is a chemical antidote. After the stomach has been emptied by vomiting give bromide of potash, thirty grains and chloral hydrate, fifteen grains, in water sweetened to taste. Chloroform may be inhaled to relax muscular spasms. If relaxation does not occur the injection of nitrite of amyl hypodermically should be tried. The symptoms of strychnia poisoning are convulsions. The contractions of the muscles are attended by pain and the patient dies from spasm of the chest muscles which prevents respiration.

XVII.—ACONITE AND VEGETABLE POISONS.

There is still a large list of vegetable poisons, but as they are rarely used with suicidal intent, and not as likely to be used accidentally as those already mentioned, it will be unnecessary to describe each one by itself. Aconite well represents this class. When any vegetable poison has been taken, excite vomiting as quickly as possible, then give milk, or strong coffee, also stimulants, if necessary.

XVIII.—POISON IVY.

Poisoning by this agent needs to be noticed because of its prevalence. Ivy is a climbing plant, very common in hay fields, and about old walls and fences. Some are more severely affected by coming in contact with it than others. It produces a fiery inflammation of the skin, characterized by itching, redness and the formation of vesicles. It should be treated with soothing lotions, as equal parts of lime water and sweet oil, or a solution of bicarbonate of soda, or either of the following:

℞   Hyposulphite of soda   one ounce
    Carbolic acid   one and a half drams
    Glycerine   two ounces
    Water enough to make   eight ounces

Mix. Apply upon cloths and repeat frequently.

℞   Benzoinal   four ounces
    Carbolic acid   one dram
    Cocaine   thirty grains

Mix. Apply as needed.

There are a number of occupations which, if long continued, result in a chronic condition of poisoning; the most common among which are those occupations which require the use of phosphorus, lead and mercury.

Those who work in match factories, thermometer manufactories, paint shops and similar places, should exercise all the more generally known precautions, and abandon the occupation for one more healthful if symptoms of poisoning appear.

Poisoning of chronic form has occurred from the use of cosmetics, hair dyes and fabrics colored by the arsenical pigments.

Lead, mercury and arsenic are the three poisons which are most used in a great variety of ways, and concerning which it is necessary to be on guard. Most of the hair dyes contain lead and are dangerous to apply to the scalp; and much ill health and some cases of lead palsy have resulted from their use.

The best way to escape the dangers that lie concealed in preparations for the hair and complexion is to avoid them. In the long run, cosmetics injure and destroy the complexion more than they beautify it. There is really no sufficient excuse for the use of such preparations as involve the risk of poisoning.

XIX.—POISON GASES.

Gases with few exceptions have a poisonous action when breathed into the lungs or inhaled.

The severity of the condition manifested usually depends upon the concentration of the gas and the length of time it has been inhaled.

If sufficiently mixed with atmospheric air no evil consequences except headache, vertigo, pallor and nausea may be experienced.

Danger attends the burning of coal and charcoal when used for fuel in rooms unventilated and having no chimney exit; for death has frequently resulted from the gas escaping from these substances under these circumstances.

Sewer gas has caused death when its inhalation has been prolonged as in the case of workmen engaged in the construction of the Thames tunnel.

Illuminating gas being made from coal is quickly poisonous when inhaled in concentrated form. If well mixed with atmospheric air its action is less speedy and fatal.

The gas fixtures in houses should be so constructed as to preclude any possible danger from escaping gas.

Gas has a peculiar and offensive odor, easily recognized when a person first enters a room, going from the outside air; but the gradual escape of gas into a room may be unperceived by the occupant, and more especially if sleeping.

Persons, unaccustomed to the use of gas, visiting a large city for the first time have sometimes lost their lives by blowing out the flame instead of turning it off.

When gas escapes into the atmosphere of a room it forms with the air an explosive mixture; hence when a strong smell of gas is perceived in any room no lighted flame should be introduced until the main supply has been turned off and the room ventilated.

TREATMENT.

When a person has been overcome by gases, whether illuminating, coal, or charcoal gas, he should be removed from the poisoned atmosphere to the fresh air and placed in a reclining position. Cold water, if the patient is warm, should be sprinkled or poured over the head and spine, or if the external surface is cold, warm water should be preferred.

Artificial respiration (see drowning) should be performed until respiration is established or the patient's condition is known to be hopeless.

Other measures such as stimulants or the subcutaneous injection of atropia and strychnia will be instituted by the medical attendant upon his arrival. Each case must receive the treatment favoring recovery which the patient's condition requires.

Poison gases the product of the laboratory in limited quantities need no attention here, as they are demanded only by scientific workers who know how to handle them. They are often so irritating that their inhalation is avoided and if a single breath is inhaled the victim rushes to the fresh air which is in most cases the only needed antidote

CHAPTER V.

THE USE OF ALCOHOL AND OTHER DANGEROUS OR NARCOTIC DRUGS.

I. Alcohol, Its Use and Abuse.—II. Chronic Alcoholism. III. The Morphine, Cocaine and Chloral Habits.—IV. The Effects of Tobacco.

I.—ALCOHOL, ITS USE AND ABUSE.

IT is to be regretted that a large portion of the civilized world makes a common use of alcoholic drink. The daily use of such beverages is superfluous and harmful. The healthy individual does not need them and they cause in the aggregate a large amount of mental and physical disease which frequently terminates in death.

Alcohol is a necessary medicinal agent and is often beneficially though perhaps too frequently prescribed by the physician, but when habitually used by the individual it is the most unsuitable and harmful of all remedies.

It will be necessary to consider the action of this agent in health and in disease in order to understand its proper and improper use.

The first action of alcohol upon a healthy person is as a stimulant. It powerfully forces the heart and when taken in considerable quantity increases its action several beats each minute. It is difficult to compute the excess of work which it is obliged to perform urged on by this agent. The face is flushed and all the blood vessels are in a condition of temporary congestion. The brain, spinal cord, liver, lungs, spleen and kidneys are also in a state of temporary congestion, a condition which becomes chronic after long continued use.

It is well known that the harder a machine is driven and the higher the rate of speed the greater the wear and tear, owing to the increased amount of friction developed.

Alcohol increases the speed of that human machine, the heart, causing strain and overwork of that organ, also congestion of the blood vessels of the various organs of the body and hence is detrimental and dangerous to the healthy man.

Alcohol itself like many other things used medicinally, may be regarded as an active poison, for fatal cases sometimes occur among children who accidentally find and drink it. It may produce such severe inflammation of the stomach or such violent congestion of the brain or such abnormal disturbances of natural processes as to cause death on the part of those unaccustomed to its use.

The proper use of alcohol as a stimulant is seen in depressing sickness and in emergencies. In these cases it can be used to antagonize the tendency to heart failure and maintain life till nature is able to assert itself.

The action of poison upon the system may seem to paralyze the life forces. The heart stroke becomes feeble and threatens to fail altogether. Then this agent is the most reliable antidote known.

There are a few diseases or stages in certain diseases when it is sometimes strongly indicated and its use becomes a necessity, but it is ever to be remembered that its administration must be carefully guarded and cease as soon as it can be safely omitted.

In the late stages of typhoid fever and pneumonia, after the excitement of the inflammatory stage has subsided, it may be needed to prevent heart failure and its wise administration may sometimes save life. In the acute stages of most diseases it is uncalled for and is capable of producing harm; for it quickens the pulse too much, increases congestion of the internal organs, augments inflammatory action and aggravates many of the early symptoms. Its use must be reserved for strengthening the waning life forces as manifested by the flagging of the heart.

In some conditions, however, when used medicinally, it exerts another important and almost contrary action to what it does in health. In these cases, when its use is demanded, it prevents the rapid waste of muscular tissue, thus conserving the strength. It may so strengthen and steady the pulse which has become excited, rapid and thready from exhaustion and weakness, that it declines in frequency and manifests greater energy. The flickering, weak action of the heart is changed to a nearly normal condition.

Alcohol used medicinally in appropriate cases may be said to have an effect directly opposite from what it has when used in health or injudiciously and inappropriately. It has its true place in medicine as well as arsenic, strychnia, aconite and other powerful remedies.

It is no wonder that some persons have acquired such a prejudice from its destructive and demoralizing action upon the human family, through its misuse, that they deny that it has a legitimate place even when judiciously prescribed. The successful practitioner cannot fail to recognize this fact, and he must only make use of this powerful agent in such a way as commends itself to his conscience, reason and experience.

Ordinarily, alcohol as a stimulant or nutrient is rarely required in the diseases of children. It is more often appropriate and serviceable in the diseases of the aged, the infirm, and those greatly debilitated, where the circulation is sluggish, and all the processes of life are verging towards the minimum.

From the standpoint of the moralist alcohol is appropriately regarded as a great evil. Its wrecks lie thickly about us on all sides, like the driftwood along the river banks after a freshet. From the standpoint of the conscientious physician, alcohol is a medicine, injurious in health, destructive to honesty, reliability, morality and character; the defamer of home, the blighter of prospects, the sorrow of wifehood and motherhood, the parent of filth, disorder, rags, poverty and dishonor, but on the other hand, a remedy whose judicious employment by skillful hands may save the inestimable life of a father, mother, brother, sister, husband, wife or sweet infant. It is a remedy, like strychnia, to be relegated to its appropriate sphere, and confined and limited to its legitimate place; a remedy which, if persistently used, will easily make you a slave, and slowly and surely work your destruction.

Owing to the dreadful danger which lurks in the stimulating cup, which first fascinates and then intoxicates, the author earnestly advises that alcohol in all forms be shunned except in dire emergencies, or when recommended and employed by the cautious and conscientious physician.

II.—CHRONIC ALCOHOLISM.

When alcohol is indulged in habitually, it works a great variety of changes, some of which occur in the corpuscles of the blood, and others in the tissues of the body. The rapidity of these changes cannot be foretold. They depend upon individual traits, constitution, temperament, occupation, habits, and the inherent tendency to weakness on the part of certain organs. The extent and degree of these changes depend upon the amount consumed and the duration of its use.

The early effects produced are functional changes, such as derangement of the digestive system. The mucous surfaces are irritated and congested, a condition which is liable to be followed by catarrhal inflammations. These functional changes at length interfere with the normal action of the various organs. The tissues are perverted, their thickening, shrinking and inaction follow.

When structural degeneration takes place, the functions of the bodily organs are more seriously interfered with. Years may intervene before well marked organic changes follow these functional disturbances.

The system for a time becomes somewhat accustomed to its use, and in spite of it is able to maintain health, sometimes for a long period, but injurious changes are sure to come, for they are slowly and steadily advancing. They are none the less real or injurious because insidious in their approach.

Among the earlier symptoms which awaken attention are dyspeptic troubles. All forms and every degree of gastritis accompany alcoholic excesses. The small vessels of the mucous coat of the stomach are dilated, congested and at length inflamed. The glands of the stomach are enlarged. The appetite is variable and irregular, there is a distaste for food in the morning. Flatulence, sour stomach and heart burn are common. Gastric ulcers are not infrequent, and permanent changes in the mucous membrane take place.

Next to the stomach the liver is disturbed by the excessive use of alcohol. The injury to this organ is usually serious and severe. Alcohol is taken up by the absorbent vessels and carried by the portal circulation directly into the circulation of this organ, where it induces prominent symptoms and serious changes, depending upon the amount and quality of the stimulant which is consumed. Diseases of the liver are far more numerous among hard drinkers, especially those who consume the strong beverages as whiskey, brandy and gin than among any other class. The first action which alcohol produces in the liver is congestion, next inflammation, then at length follow those characteristic changes which are so well known to medical men as Bright's disease, yellow atrophy of the liver, fatty degeneration and perhaps diabetes.

Some of the symptoms of these diseases which alcohol drinkers manifest are vomiting, headache, constipation or diarrhœa, muscular tremor, vertigo and mental depression. Still more suggestive symptoms are jaundice, dropsy, hardening of the liver (cirrhosis), producing emaciation and interfering with the function of every bodily organ. These severe symptoms commonly progress slowly and almost always lead to a fatal termination.

Alcohol drinkers are especially liable to that dreaded disease, pneumonia. Owing to the fact that alcohol produces congestion of the capillary blood vessels it predisposes to attacks of pneumonia, which are especially fatal in such subjects as is well known. Fatal attacks of bronchitis are also common among hard drinkers.

The blood vessels suffer from the effects of the drink habit. There is degeneration of their tissues especially in the arteries, their elasticity is lost, the walls become thin and allow extreme dilatation and under severe pressure the vessels give way and death ensues. This is the case when apoplexy terminates their career.

The heart usually suffers to a greater or less extent. There may be hypertrophy of this organ or fatty degeneration. The heart power is enfeebled and there is degeneration of the heart muscle. The stimulant at length fails to stimulate and when such is the case the vital powers must soon fail. Such persons after a brief illness are prone to die with symptoms of heart failure. As the stomach, liver and heart undergo structural changes so the kidneys suffer degeneration, the vessels lose their elasticity, the membranes become weakened and permit the albumen of the blood to drain away through them. Fatty degeneration of the kidneys as of other organs is liable to take place. From the organic changes which take place in the liver and kidneys diabetes may result, as an enormous quantity of grape sugar is manufactured by the liver and eliminated by the kidneys.

The derangements of the nervous system are numerous and prominent. In the early stages of this trouble the heart is unduly stimulated and drives too much blood to the brain. The blood vessels of the brain are in a condition of chronic congestion. The effect of this unnatural blood supply to the brain produces a sense of dullness or confusion, headache, varied mental disturbances, disorders of motion and sensation. Unnatural noises are sometimes heard, spots and imaginary objects appear before the eyes, buzzing noises are heard in the head and cramps and pain in the feet and legs are not unusual. Sleep is disturbed and troubled with dreams and hence fails to bring suitable refreshing. Insomnia is sometimes very troublesome. The mind is depressed and melancholy and undue irritableness are experienced. The nerves are in a state of partial paralysis and the face and ears are red and congested, owing to the relaxation of the nerves which control the blood supply.

Perspiration is abundant owing to the loss of nerve control over the opening of the sweat glands. The eyes are sometimes red, the muscles are trembling, the pulse at length become feeble, skin clammy, tongue coated, voice husky, breathing irregular, heart weak, overworked and more or less used up. The mind loses its vigor, the moral sense deteriorates, the conception of duty, honor and justice are lost, and crimes are often committed the thought of which would not have been entertained for a moment previous to the formation of this debasing habit.

Family obligations are overlooked. Moral energy is lost, physical energy is reduced so that the usual occupation is abandoned. Self-respect is at last lost if the body has not succumbed to previous organic derangements. The memory fails and life is warped in all its relations. There is degeneration of the brain and perhaps insanity. Asylums contain many alcoholic wrecks. The best way to avoid the evils of drink is to wholly abstain from its use. There is no other safeguard. Do not trust yourself to use it moderately. Any indulgence is unsafe and prevention is better than cure.

III.—THE MORPHINE, COCAINE AND CHLORAL HABITS.

The morphia habit is frequently formed as the result of being obliged to take this agent continuously to relieve pain in cases of severe injuries, painful growths and affections. Those persons for whom morphia has been thus prescribed, often persist in having the prescription refilled until they acquire this fascinating habit. It is often continued in this way for years after the necessity for its administration has ceased. In order to maintain the exhilarating effects of this drug, the victim is obliged to increase constantly the amount taken, and ere he is aware of it he has become a slave to a habit, which becomes persistent and exacting in its demands.

The prominent effects of using this drug are impaired appetite and digestion. The functions of the liver are diminished; the secretion of bile is lessened, and constipation ensues. The lips and tongue are dry, because the glandular activity is reduced, the body is more or less fevered, the eye is dull, and there are signs of premature old age.

The most noticeable and pitiable result, however, is the loss of will power. This becomes so enfeebled, that it is usual for a person addicted to this unfortunate habit to resort to every method of intrigue and deception in order to gratify the terrible cravings of the system for the accustomed stimulating dose. The victim of this habit occasionally resolves to break away from its use, but is so desperately wretched and unhappy that the attempt is soon abandoned, and the practice of using the drug becomes so fixed, that it is more desired than food, clothing, honor, or anything else. Sometimes the unfortunate victim of this habit has learned to use it hypodermically, and practices self-injections with great regularity at short intervals and with increasing doses.

TREATMENT.

This consists in abandoning the use of the drug, which can be accomplished in two ways, either by taking away the drug abruptly or gradually. According to the first method the suffering will be intense for a short time. The struggle will be terribly severe. The patient must have every moral aid, and especial care must be taken that the patient is placed where it is impossible to obtain the longed-for stimulant. When the habit is of long standing, there are only a very few persons who have sufficient will power left to continue such a struggle to a successful termination. It is usually necessary to place a person addicted to this habit under the full supervision of a competent physician, who will supply those efficient sedatives which will render the struggle less terrible. A competent attendant or nurse is also essential, who will keep close watch of the patient and give all necessary aid, by strengthening the patient's determination, diverting the diseased appetite, cheering up the despairing and despondent victim, who will profess to desire either death or a dose of morphine.

The second method is by diminishing the dose gradually for a period of three or four weeks until it can be omitted altogether, without shock to the patient's system, or detriment to his health. The latter method is preferable where the habit is of long standing, the dose taken large and the patient's health not robust. The same supervision is necessary in either case until the victory is won. Only those who have treated these cases can comprehend the strength of the appetite and the intense craving for its gratification. Imagine a person otherwise healthy, so disconsolate and so distressed for the accustomed opiate as to approach you, with a trembling voice, a haggard countenance, feigned weakness and nausea, and pitifully begging you for one more good dose, saying: "I would give my life for one dose of morphine."

There is nothing but the thirst of the drunkard for just one drink which can approach this desire for a little more morphine. Where the gradual method is pursued the suffering is less severe, but the struggle is perhaps of somewhat longer duration. The result in each case is the same, however. By combining with the gradual method the temporary use of caffeine, Indian hemp, strong coffee, or avena sativa, and such other remedies as the patient's condition requires, this terrible habit can be broken up with the minimum amount of inconvenience, and the patient will bless the day which emancipated him from his slavery.

With respect to cocaine and chloral little need be said. Where these drugs have been used until an insatiable craving for them has been established their speedy abandonment must be considered. Other agents must be used to strengthen and give tone to the shattered nervous system. Sleep must be induced by natural means. Baths, tonics, agreeable occupation of the mind, exercise in the open air, healthy food, massage, and a great variety of healthful agents can be suggested. The same principle applies in each case, but the abandonment of the injurious drug is preeminent.

IV.—THE EFFECTS OF TOBACCO.

That the action of tobacco upon the system is hurtful might be inferred from its effect upon those unaccustomed to its use. It excites in such pallor, nausea, vomiting and the condition of marked debility and prostration. This is due to the action of nicotine, a powerful narcotic poison which it contains.

If tobacco is the friend of man it certainly does not manifest its friendship upon the first introduction. Use however establishes a condition of tolerance and familiarity and leads to a more amicable condition of affairs.

Let us inquire concerning some of the more common effects of tobacco on the part of those who continue its use habitually.

It impresses the brain and nervous system and appears to soothe this important organ in conditions of weariness and exhaustion. We should naturally infer that its long-continued use would impair the activity of the brain, which is true. All stimulants produce in health but a temporary feeling of relief, which is followed by reaction, and unless administered in increasing quantity the last state is less tolerable than the first; hence the tendency in all habits which involve the use of stimulants or narcotics to increase more and more the amount and frequency of the dose.

The habitual use of tobacco affects the taste and relish of food and also the appetite. It interferes with digestion and consequently is a frequent promoter of dyspepsia. It excites the secretion of the salivary and other glands of the mouth and throat, reaction follows and a dry and irritable condition of the throat is produced, characterized by redness and dryness, a condition which is known as smoker's sore throat. The most unpleasant action of tobacco is upon the nervous system. It is through the nerves that it produces the well-marked disturbances of the heart in inveterate smokers. These disturbances are palpitation, irregularity of action and in some instances tremor, faintness, fits and paralysis.

The poison is rapidly eliminated from the body and does no permanent harm unless the indulgence is excessive. Tobacco does not produce organic trouble of the heart, merely functional disturbance; but in some instances this is very well marked and often so severe as to require the abandonment of the habit. Some other minor symptoms to which the use of tobacco occasionally gives rise are vertigo, impaired hearing and smell. It is agreed that the use of tobacco is especially injurious to the young, causing impaired growth, premature development and physical degeneracy.

The effect of tobacco upon the race as a whole is unfavorable. It augments the tendency to nervous troubles and its influence is given to the production of a debilitated and inferior progeny. The young ought not to acquire the habit of using tobacco and those who have acquired a habit of such pronounced detriment should be induced to abandon it at once. The odor of tobacco in the clothing and breath renders the user especially disagreeable to persons of refinement. While it is not so destructive as alcohol, its effects upon the heart and nervous system are so unfavorable that its use should be voluntarily restricted or abandoned.

CHAPTER VI.

ACCIDENTS.

I.—Drowning. II.—Fainting. III.—Burns and Scalds. IV.—Lightning Stroke. V.—Sprains and Bruises. VI.—Frost Bite. VII.—Bites of Serpents. VIII.—Stings of Insects. IX.—Poisoned Wounds. X.—Hemorrhage from Wounds, and the Treatment of Wounds in General. XI.—Incised Wounds. XII.—Scalp Wounds.

I.—DROWNING.

A DROWNING person should be removed from the water as speedily as possible, and efforts immediately instituted for reviving the patient. Simple rules are more easily remembered and applied than others.

The first thing to do is to drain off the fluid from the lungs and stomach. This is accomplished by placing the patient face downwards, the abdomen resting upon a big, hard roll of clothing, for in this position the mouth is the lowest point. Pressure is then made upon the spine and back to drive out the water from the lungs and stomach. Having thoroughly accomplished this, the patient should be turned over and artificial respiration performed. Have the same roll of cloth or clothing now placed under the back, below the shoulders. Begin by placing the hands on each side of the patient's chest, then press in the chest walls, increasing the pressure gradually as much as the age will permit. Then suddenly relax the pressure, wait two or three seconds, and perform the same movement again, repeating it ten or twelve times each minute.

If necessary, draw out the tongue from the mouth, and do not abandon the case for some time. A slight gasp should be regarded as hopeful, and should be persistently encouraged till breathing has been fully established.

Persons have been revived after remaining in the water several minutes, perhaps fifteen or twenty, but in most cases from two to five is the extent. It is not easy to determine how long a person can remain in the water, and yet be revived, as the time depends upon the amount of air in the lungs at the time of entering the water; the more air the chest contains, the longer life will be maintained.

A person falling into the water from a bridge or other elevation and being stunned or knocked senseless by the fall, can be revived after a longer interval than one who is making an effort to breathe.

When the rescued patient has been restored, or when breathing has been established, put the patient in bed and surround with abundant warmth, using blankets and hot water bottles freely. Give hot drinks, as beef tea, coffee, a teaspoonful of aromatic spirits of ammonia, or an ounce or half ounce of brandy and hot water.

II.—FAINTING.

This is due to some sudden impression upon the nervous system which depresses the heart and for the time being it is so overwhelmed that it nearly or quite ceases to contract. At once the brain fails to get its accustomed supply of blood and there is a cessation of consciousness. The breathing is slow or may be suspended.

Such a condition can last only a short time. If it is long continued death results.

CAUSES.

The cause of fainting is anything which temporarily arrests the action of the heart. It may occur from loss of blood in profuse hemorrhage, excessive emotion, starvation, fear, harrowing sights, blows upon the stomach and poisons which depress the heart.

SYMPTOMS.

The face becomes deathly pale, the pupils are enlarged, the pulse is feeble, the breathing is labored and gasping or apparently ceases. Consciousness is lost and the muscles of the body are relaxed. These symptoms are more or less intensified as the condition of fainting is more or less complete.

TREATMENT.

It is imperative to place the patient upon the back with the head low. The dress or clothing about the neck or waist should be loosened. Ammonia of suitable strength may be applied to the nose or a few drops of nitrite of amyl may be inhaled from a handkerchief. Cold water may be sprinkled upon the face to incite reaction and fresh air should be admitted. Brandy or other stimulants may be administered by the mouth or hypodermically.

These means usually avail to restore a person who has fainted, but when the swoon is profound and threatens to destroy life the electric battery may be applied or artificial respiration may be resorted to, and brandy with warm milk may be thrown into the bowels by the aid of a syringe. The patient must be kept in a reclining posture till recovery has taken place.

When the fainting is due to hemorrhage lift the bleeding limb higher than the head and proceed to stop the flow of blood as by direction given for such an emergency. The head should be placed lower than the heart so that what blood remains in the body may be used by the brain. If the hemorrhage is uterine lift the foot of the bed six or eight inches.

III.—BURNS AND SCALDS.

"What wound did ever heal, but by degrees."

Burns are caused by dry and scalds by moist or liquid heat. The amount of injury produced depends upon *two* factors; the first is the degree or intensity of the heat and the second is the extent of surface involved.

A slight superficial burn or scald involving only a small area of surface is a very common injury and one that is comparatively void of danger. There is usually only slight redness of the surface of the skin with a somewhat persistent, smarting sensation. The application of a soothing lotion gives relief and the injury is soon forgotten.

Then again the injury may be so deep and extensive as to produce death in a short time, and between these two extremes there may be every grade of injury.

In instances of mild injury, only a superficial layer of the skin is destroyed, beneath which blisters which fill with serum form, or the whole thickness of the true skin may be burned owing to the intensity of the heat applied.

In addition to the external injury there may be internal injuries from the inhalation of steam, hot smoke or flames. A superficial burn which involves a large surface is often far more serious than a deep burn of only small area. Even a superficial burn or scald disables the functions of the skin which are essential to the continuance of animal life.

It is a common rule that when from one-third to one-half of the surface of the body is burned or involved in the injury the case is fatal, even though the degree of injury may not be severe.

The skin is very liberally supplied with nerves and for this reason a burn or scald of wide area produces that condition of the system well-known and recognized by medical men as *shock*. This is a depressed condition of the system in which a person may die without rallying.

Severe burns are sometimes followed by ulceration and other serious disturbances of the bowels and other internal organs.

Burns and scalds result from a great variety of causes among which are the accidental contact with molten metals, explosions of steam, gas and gunpowder, the accidental ignition of cotton garments about a stove or range, the falling of children or workmen into tubs, tanks or vats of boiling water, hot fat and other liquids too numerous to mention.

TREATMENT.

When the clothes are on fire a person instead of fanning the flames by running into the street should lie down and smother the flames with a rug, blanket or whatever is within reach. If a second party is present he should dash water upon the flaming victim or extinguish the flames by means of a shawl or blanket. Success depends upon instantaneous action governed by good judgment and courageous methods.

In removing partially burned clothing from a person exercise much care not to remove the injured skin. Blisters should be carefully pricked at the lowest point and their contents allowed to escape without the removal of the superficial layer of the skin which forms the best covering for the injured surface.

If the person is suffering from shock a little stimulant may be appropriately administered; if from severe pain and anguish morphia should be administered hypodermically, for this will relieve the pain and also stimulate the action of the heart. If the injury is extensive it may be dressed in sections, one part at a time. The dressing should be put on in a warm room or near the fire and the parts not necessary to expose covered by warm blankets. The dressing should seek to exclude the air from the injured surface, hence oleaginous dressings have been extensively employed.

A very soothing application for a burn is the following old but efficient remedy. It is composed of equal parts of lime water and linseed or sweet oil. This may be applied upon lint and covered over with a layer of absorbent cotton, carbolized cotton or iodoform gauze. For superficial burns this dressing will answer every purpose.

Another good remedy is carbolized vaseline or oil. One-half a dram of carbolic acid to an ounce of vaseline or oil is the proper proportion to use, but where a very large extent of surface is involved other remedies are more suitable, or a less proportion of carbolic acid should be used. Iodoform and vaseline make a good dressing. If a large extent of surface is involved use less iodoform, as there would be danger of too free absorption of this remedy.

Other valuable formulæ for burns are as follows:

℞ Muriate of cocaine   five grains
   Oxide of zinc ointment   one ounce

Mix and apply as needed to a burned surface.

℞ Carbolic acid   fifteen grains
   Fl. ext. calendula   half an ounce
   Olive oil   one half pint

Mix and apply as needed.

℞ Menthol   twenty grains
   Muriate of cocaine   five grains
   Vaseline   one ounce

Mix and apply as needed.

All of the above prescriptions are of a high order.

Deep burns about the neck and joints require much care in the healing process to prevent contraction of the skin.

The modern method of skin grafting is a very flattering method of preventing unsightly contractions. This delicate operation requires the experience of the surgeon, to render its performance successful, and hence it is unnecessary to attempt a description of the process.

By this simple operation large surfaces can be healed in a brief time, and unsightly contractions prevented. No discovery of modern times yields more uniform and successful results.

Burns produced by contact with strong acids or other chemicals should be treated on the same general principles mentioned. It is well to bear in mind that the skin of infants and young persons is more easily impressed by the action of heat than that of adults, and hence extensive burns or scalds are more liable to prove fatal to such patients. In very serious injury from burns the nerves are paralyzed, and ordinarily the degree of pain experienced is less than would otherwise be supposed.

IV.—LIGHTNING STROKE.

A person receiving an accidental electric shock may be rendered unconscious temporarily, or if the current is a strong one, instantaneous death may ensue. The shock may be largely the result of fright. When this is the case recovery usually soon takes place. Insensibility may last for some time, and then be followed by recovery. There is often some paralysis of the motor nerves, usually those of the lower extremities. There may be loss of some of the special senses, as sight, hearing, taste or smell. If a person is not killed on the spot, there is a chance of recovery.

Sometimes the body is wounded or burned, and such injuries are to be treated the same as similar ones from other causes. When death results instantly, it is caused by the shock which paralyzes the brain. In some cases the blood is found to be coagulated by the electrical current.

The treatment for those not killed outright is rest and stimulants, as ammonia, brandy and other efficient heart tonics.

V.—SPRAINS AND BRUISES.

Sprains are often associated with bruises, and hence we shall consider both subjects under one head. A sprain is the over-stretching of the muscular and ligamentous tissues. It may be a slight or severe injury, or any grade of injury between the two.

In some cases the ligaments which bind the bones in place may be partially or completely ruptured and the neighboring parts more or less injured and torn.

Sometimes, in stepping down from a carriage or step, the whole weight is accidentally thrown on to one side of the foot, and the foot is turned under. This occasionally occurs in walking over rough walks, or from stepping into a hole or upon a stone. The injury caused from such a misstep may be so severe as to require several weeks for recovery. In this injury the out or inside ligaments of the ankle joint are overstrained, and in the worst cases more or less ruptured.

Many sprains are more serious and require a longer time for recovery than a fractured bone; hence a bad sprain should not be treated as a trivial affair for no one would so regard a broken bone. Sometimes the sprain or injury of a joint which at first appears to be slight will develop later serious consequences. Cases of hip joint disease in children have resulted from an injury which at first was regarded as trivial. Sometimes a fracture has been regarded only as a bad sprain and then again a sprain has been treated with splints as a fracture. It sometimes requires a large amount of experience to determine which condition exists.

The treatment is so important that a correct diagnosis should be made. In a sprain, while there is considerable swelling, the parts are not misplaced, and motion of the bone can occur without crepitus. Crepitus is the name given to the sound, when one piece of bone grates upon another, and is a certain indication of fracture. More or less weight can be borne upon a sprained joint, although movement is painful while upon a fractured limb, as a rule, no weight can be borne upon the injured part, neither can its own weight be supported without assistance.

TREATMENT.

This is all important. Rest must be enjoined for a reasonable time, depending upon the degree of injury. Cold applications such as alcohol, witch-hazel or ice are preferred by some to check the inflammation. Hot fomentations are, however, the best agents for reducing the swelling and relieving the pain. These should be applied at once and changed and re-applied for the first day with persistency to avert the inflammation. Holding the injured joint in a hot bath is beneficial. A little aqua ammonia or bicarbonate of soda added will increase the efficiency of this agent.

Hot applications are recommended because they are preferable to cold and afford a greater sense of relief. They aid the capillary circulation in the tissues and favor the rapid absorption of the extravasated blood and lymph and consequently reduce the swelling. If the lameness and swelling continue for several days the following stimulating liniment will assist the process of recovery:

℞ Camphor liniment three ounces
Chloroform one ounce

Mix and apply three or four times a day.

If the parts are much swollen a snug bandage carefully wound about the limb will give a comfortable feeling of support, and will favor the tedious process of absorption. If the swelling continues and becomes chronic in spite of such well directed efforts as have been recommended, absorption and recovery will be further aided by painting over the injury with the tincture of iodine. It is good economy to commit the care of a severe sprain to a competent medical man, as there may be earnest indications for treatment which it is impossible to anticipate, and which, if unobserved and neglected, might lead to serious mischief.

Bruises are the result of an injury, as a blow with some blunt agent, as a stick of wood, an axe, or from a fall. At the same time other injuries often accompany bruises, as lacerations of the flesh, dislocations and fractures. This is often the case in carriage and railroad accidents. The effusion of blood which follows a bruise or contusion is due to the injury either of the capillary blood vessels or, less often, to the rupture of a vein or artery. In the latter case a large amount of blood will penetrate the surrounding tissues.

In some parts of the body, as about the eye, where the cellular tissue is abundant, a bruise is succeeded by a large amount of extravasated blood. The technical term for a black eye or other extravasation of blood is ecchymosis.

TREATMENT.

The treatment of bruises is quite simple, nature being able in most instances to accomplish the cure with but little aid. Whatever the treatment, nature must absorb the extravasated blood, which always requires time; the discoloration changing in the process from black or dark purple to green, and finally yellow, gradually fading till it reaches the normal color. The process requires about two weeks. Simple water dressings, to which alcohol has been added, are serviceable, so also are hot fomentations. When soreness and symptoms of inflammation follow a bruise, equal parts of tincture of arnica and tincture of opium will usually afford relief. Slight bruises require no treatment, but sometimes the effused blood, when the injury is extensive, instead of being absorbed is changed into pus, and suppurations follow the injury. In such cases it is necessary to lance the abscess and allow the pus to drain away, and then wash out the cavity with carbolic acid water. One dram of the former to a pint of the latter, or a solution of corrosive sublimate of suitable strength.

For ecchymosis about the eye, there is no better application than the following:

℞   Muriate of ammonia   one dram
     Water   one pint

Mix and apply to a bruised surface on a cloth.

VI.—FROST BITE.

This is an injury where the cold has taken a deeper hold than in chilblains and is sufficient to arrest the circulation. Frost bite is preceded by tingling and numbness. If frost bite of an extremity as a toe is prolonged and severe, the death of the part will result. Any part which has been frosted or somewhat frozen should not be exposed to the heat suddenly as there will be an excessive reaction. The nerves in their paralyzed condition are unable to control the blood supply, the parts will suffer congestion and gangrene or death of the frozen portion will ensue.

Persons who are exposed to severe cold should not give way to a desire to sleep or fall into a state of stupor for death will certainly follow.

TREATMENT.

This must be careful and cautious. Frosted members must be restored to the normal condition very gradually, neither warm air nor warm water nor the heat of a fire should be allowed but the frosted parts should be rubbed with a piece of flannel to aid in establishing the circulation, previous to which, rubbing with snow or ice water is more suitable if the freezing is severe.

It may be necessary to administer stimulants. Especial care must be exercised to see that the return of the temperature is gradual. Remember never to apply heat to a frosted limb. After the circulation has been established warmth may be gradually added and the frosted parts should be wrapped in flannel. Portions which slough should be treated in the same way as ulcers, burns and other open sores.

Sometimes the feet are so frozen as to require amputation. In these cases a line forms between the living and the dead tissue and shows the surgeon where to draw the knife. In severe climates persons are sometimes frozen to death. Persons under the influence of liquor are often so bereft of judgment as to lie down in the snow or upon the frozen earth and if not rescued are found frozen.

VII.—BITES OF SERPENTS.

The red viper or copperhead, cobra and rattlesnake are venomous and their bites cause convulsions and death. The poison is introduced into the system in the act of biting. The bite of the rattlesnake is succeeded by pain of a pricking, burning character, which becomes more and more intensified. The tissues surrounding the bite or injury show the usual symptoms of inflammation, viz: redness, heat, pain and swelling, and there is hemorrhage into the surrounding tissues which causes their discoloration.

After the system has been inoculated by these poisons, glandular enlargements, suppuration and gangrene take place in succession. If the amount of poison introduced by the fang of the serpent is large great prostration follows, the circulation is checked or stopped in the wounded extremity in consequence of the changes which take place in the blood and death results with great rapidity.

Snake bites produce blood poisoning and the action of this poison on the nerve centers produces irritation, prostration and convulsions.

TREATMENT.

The treatment needs to be as energetic as possible in order to have a chance of success. A few seconds are sufficient for the absorption of the poison into the blood and general system. A ligature is advised to prevent the poison from reaching the circulation and nerve centers. This ligature must be placed about the injured extremity between the injury and the heart. It must be tight enough to stop both the arterial and venous circulation; the venous blood must be prevented from returning to the heart from the injured member. Then the tissues about the wound must be cut away and the whole wound thoroughly cauterized by means of strong carbolic acid or a stick of nitrate of silver. Then the blood in the wounded extremity is withdrawn by puncturing and cupping and in this way the poison with the blood is removed before the circulation is again established. In some cases it has been necessary to amputate the limb in which the poison is deposited.

As the poison is harmless when introduced into the stomach it is recommended to immediately suck the bite. Stimulants are given internally to counteract the depression and the effects of the poison, those most used being ammonia, digitalis, whiskey and strychnia. The nitrate of strychnia is reported to be an almost infallible remedy, failing in only one case out of a hundred. It is used hypodermically and repeated every few minutes as the condition of the patient requires. The hypodermic tablets are made in doses of one-fortieth, one-sixtieth and one-eightieth of a grain which are suitable doses. One of these is to be dissolved in a teaspoonful or syringe full of warm water and injected beneath the skin, watching the effect and repeating the dose as often as the patient's condition demands a renewal of the stimulant. Cases of such importance demand all the skill of a competent physician as soon as his services can be procured.

VIII.—STINGS OF INSECTS.

In temperate regions the stings of insects, unless in large numbers, are rarely severe. They sometimes cause in children fever and other constitutional disturbances of a mild character. Sometimes a wasp or bee stings the tongue, in consequence of being accidentally taken into the mouth with fruit. Should this happen there may result a rapid and extensive swelling of this organ. It has sometimes been necessary to open into the windpipe (tracheotomy) after such an accident to prevent suffocation.

The stings of insects are relieved by the application of an alkali as aqua ammonia.

The sting or bite of some of the tropical insects is more serious and is sometimes followed by pain, vomiting, nervous depression and other nervous symptoms.

The bite of the mosquito in South America is more poisonous than in North America and is sometimes followed by local inflammation and ulceration. In Africa and Asia the bite of the scorpion is so venomous as sometimes to cause death.

Large spiders are the means of many harrowing stories. They are said to have poisoned infants and small children. It is to be observed that such occurrences are usually so far away as to render verification impossible. The sad story of the death of a child from the bite of a poison spider can generally be seen in the columns of a sensational newspaper about once a year or once in six months, and if other news items are scarce, as often as every three months. The bite of a spider is to some extent poisonous but it is hardly to be believed that a spider is venomous enough to destroy even the life of an infant.

TREATMENT.

The treatment is the same for a spider bite as for that of the scorpion. Aqua ammonia is the best external application. It may be combined with olive oil as the latter is also a useful application. Menthol liniment is cooling and would be appropriate.

The principal remedies relied upon for internal treatment are ammonia and brandy if there be symptoms of prostration sufficiently well marked to require stimulants.

IX.—POISONED WOUNDS.

Many of the bites of insects, reptiles, dogs, cats, weasels, squirrels, rats, and other animals are poisonous to a greater or less degree. For the most part these wounds heal readily and occasion no special inconvenience; there are numerous exceptions, however, to this statement.

Medical students are exposed to the risk of introducing into the system poison material from dead bodies. There is especial danger of introducing dangerous poison into the body from handling or dissecting those persons who have died from puerperal and scarlet fevers, diphtheria, glanders, malignant pustule and such like diseases of a poisonous character. Even inhaling the odors from dead bodies may introduce more or less poison into the system, but this is rarely followed by anything more serious than nausea, slight malaise, and perhaps boils subsequently. Care must be exercised to prevent the inoculation of the system with the fluids of horses, cattle and other animals that have died from certain malignant diseases. It requires but a very slight abrasion for the introduction of poison into the system, and it may be so slight as to be imperceptible.

Those who have been bitten by a dog or other animal are liable to become the victims of fear, and to experience in their imagination all the horrors depicted in sensational literature. Dog bites, unless severe or by rabid dogs, usually heal kindly and are without especial danger.

TREATMENT.

Wounds made upon the hands in the dissection of dead animals should be first cleansed in the following manner: Suck the blood from the wound immediately, and then cleanse it by means of an antiseptic fluid, as the peroxide of hydrogen or a carbolic acid solution.

If the introduction of dangerous poison is suspected, cauterize the wound with the nitrate of silver pencil, or with chloride of zinc. Should inflammation follow, apply poultices, and should pus form open the abscess early to prevent its absorption into the system. After the pus has been thoroughly removed by poultices, apply carbolic salve, iodoform ointment or aristol in powder. Indurated glands may be painted over with the tincture of iodine; meantime keep the bowels free and the system in a vigorous condition.

The wounds caused by a dog's bite are to receive the same treatment as wounds from other causes, unless the animal is suffering from rabies. (See hemorrhage from wounds in the article upon hydrophobia.)

A wound caused by the bite of a healthy dog should be carefully cleansed. For this purpose use a pint of warm water to which has been added a teaspoonful of carbolic acid. The carbolized water should be prepared in a clean earthern dish. The wound may then be cauterized with nitrate of silver if any suspicion exists as to the condition of the animal inflicting the wound, but this process will somewhat retard the healing process. The wound may then be dusted with aristol powder. Gaping wounds should be brought together with plasters or stitches, as the nature and extent of the wound may require.

X.—HEMORRHAGE FROM WOUNDS,

AND THE TREATMENT OF WOUNDS IN GENERAL.

Blood flows from a wound however slight, and the amount of blood does not depend upon the size of the wound but upon the size of the vessels injured. The slightest wounds injure some of the capillary vessels, but bleeding from the capillaries is not usually attended with danger. The blood from a vein is not of a bright scarlet color as is blood from an artery. When a large vein has been cut blood flows from it in a steady stream. Pressure usually controls hemorrhage from capillary vessels and veins. If it does not dust upon it some of Monsel's salt (ferri subsulphate) which is a powerful styptic.

When an artery is cut or wounded bloods flows from it with every beat of the heart in a spurt or jet. The danger from arterial hemorrhage depends upon the size of the vessel wounded. From the

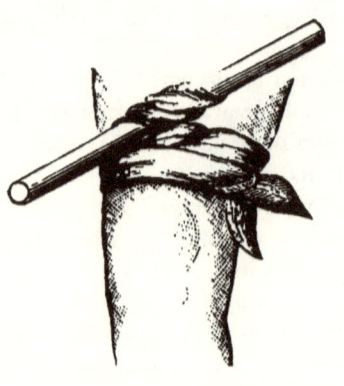

This figure shows the arrangement of the handkerchief-tourniquet to arrest bleeding from a wound below the knee. A large pad made by folding a towel, or napkin, or rolling up a woolen stocking, must first be put into the hollow behind the knee and the handkerchief applied over it.

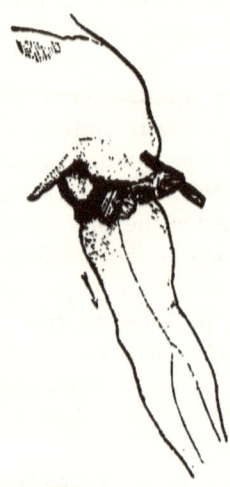

This figure shows the manner of employing the knotted handkerchief to arrest bleeding from a wound of an artery in the left upper extremity.

large artery of the leg, the femoral, one would lose blood enough to produce death in a very short time. A strip of stout cloth or a bandage can be fastened tightly enough around a limb to control the hemorrhage. This must be placed just above the wound between it and the heart. It may be necessary to place a stick under the bandage and take a twist or turn in it to tighten it enough to stop the hemorrhage especially if the blood is flowing from a large wound.

A rubber bandage, known to medical men as an Esmarch, is the best agent for controlling hemorrhage in a limb, but it is not usually at hand and so other measures must be used, as prompt action is necessary to save life. The only safe way to control a large vessel permanently is to pick it up with artery forceps, draw it out of the wound sufficiently and tie a ligature tightly about it. A white silk thread, doubled and twisted, makes a suitable ligature in an emergency. It ought to be disinfected by dipping it into a carbolic or other antiseptic solution. It must be drawn tightly enough about the exposed vessel to cut through the inner coats which are less tough than the outer. This favors the healing process. It is hardly to be supposed that anyone will attempt to ligate permanently a large vessel unless beyond the reach of medical aid, but it is necessary to be able to stop a hemorrhage for the time being till professional assistance arrives.

A torn vessel bleeds less freely than a cut one. The author has seen persons who have been run over by an engine or car wheel and the leg cut or crushed off and almost no hemorrhage follow the accident. The tissues are so crushed as to close the ends of the vessel and to favor the formation of clots in them.

Clean cut wounds bleed freely and heal more readily than mangled wounds. Such cuts often heal directly by first intention without inflammation or pus. When a cut is made through the flesh, contraction especially of the skin takes place and the wound gaps. The opposite lips of a cut must be brought close together and kept in apposition for a few days; healing is often rapid and leaves but a trifling scar which tends to disappear more and more with the lapse of time.

It is good practice to first examine and cleanse a wound and remove any dirt, foreign substance or shred of clothing. The cleansing is by a wash containing a teaspoonful of carbolic acid to each pint of hot water or a tablet of corrosive sublimate.

If pure carbolic acid is warmed and has added to it a small amount of glycerine or alcohol, it will keep in a liquid state in all temperatures and is ready for use at any moment. Antiseptic tablets of corrosive sublimate may be used, and are efficient; they may be obtained readily, for they are kept by the druggist, and directions accompany them. After cleansing a wound thoroughly bring the opposing parts close together and hold them there with strips of adhesive plaster. Plasters do not hold the parts as well as stitches, for they usually allow the wound to gap somewhat, so that as good results are not secured as by stitches. Any handy person could learn to close a wound by seeing a surgeon do it once.

Stitches should be removed after four or five days, and the parts strengthened, so as not to separate, by strips of adhesive plaster put on at short intervals. After a wound is brought together by stitches or otherwise, a piece of absorbent cotton, upon which some aristol or iodoform has been dusted, should be placed over it to seal it from the air and render it antiseptic. Iodoform is objectionable on account of its disagreeable and persistent odor.

Over all, tie a piece of muslin or bandage, or put on adhesive strips, depending upon the location of the injury. If the above directions are closely and carefully followed the results will be satisfactory.

Warm applications are excellent to improve the circulation and hasten the process of recovery. Some wounds require the attendance of experienced and professional aid, as the symptoms of inflammation, fever and suppuration are too obscure to be observed and properly headed off by the unskilled.

XI.—INCISED WOUNDS.

In general the first thing to think of in wounds of this kind is to stop the hemorrhage. This can often be accomplished by the applica-

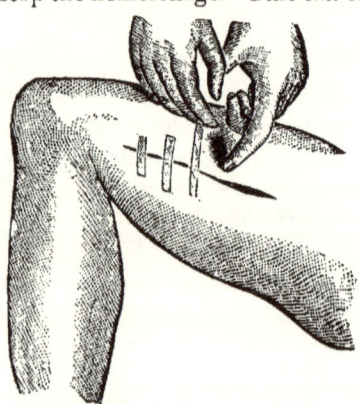

Method of applying strips of adhesive plaster to a cut or incised wound.

tion of cold or hot water, if only small vessels have been divided. It does some good to elevate the wounded part above the rest of the body. Arterial hemorrhage, when the blood spurts freely, requires that the vessel should be twisted or tied tightly with a piece of silk thread, or surgeon's silk. The wound should be cleansed thoroughly, either with a carbolized wash, containing a dram of the acid to a pint of water, or else a corrosive sublimate solution containing one tablet to a pint or quart of hot water. Plasters answer for small superficial wounds upon the surface of the body, but for wounds about the scalp, eyes, nose or mouth, stitches hold much better than plasters and should be preferred. Stitches about the face should be taken near together, and the needle and silk should both be suitably fine.

The utmost cleanliness is required in handling all wounds.

XII.—SCALP WOUNDS.

The head is much exposed to injuries from blows and falls. Owing to the hardness of the bone beneath, blunt instruments often divide the scalp and produce wounds which resemble incised wounds. The scalp is very vascular, being abundantly supplied with blood vessels, hence hemorrhage from these wounds is often profuse. It can be stopped usually by pressure and the application of cold water. Make a compress, dip it in cold water and hold it firmly over the bleeding wound with the hand.

In treating a wound of the scalp the first thing is to cleanse the wound, remove the hair or dirt and wash away the blood clots, for no foreign substance must be allowed to remain.

After cleansing the wound bring the parts into apposition and hold them there. Nothing serves this purpose so well as stitches from one fourth to one half an inch apart made with good coarse silk.

Water dressings, tint. of arnica and opium, or powdered aristol can be applied. Remove the stitches in four or five days.

CHAPTER VII.

GENERAL SUBJECTS PRELIMINARY TO THE STUDY OF DISEASE.

I.—HEALTH AND DISEASE. II.—THE TWO GREAT TYPES OF DISEASE. III.—TEMPERATURE IN DISEASE. IV.—KISSING IN ITS RELATION TO DISEASE. V.—BATHING IN ITS RELATION TO DISEASE. VI.—SYMPTOMS OF DISEASE. HOW TO READ AND INTERPRET THEM.

I.—HEALTH AND DISEASE.

THESE are relative terms since they refer to no definite condition. It is not easy to determine where health ends and disease begins because there is no well-defined border line. Health and disease are conditions which overlap each other.

In order to understand disease it is necessary first to know what is involved in the conditions which we designate health. Health may be regarded as that condition in which the various tissues of the body are maintained and all the various bodily functions are performed in a normal manner. Disease is some departure from these normal conditions; it may be only slight and temporary or severe, progressive and chronic.

So long as all the tissues of the body are maintained unimpaired and the numerous functions of all the organs and parts are performed in a regular manner, health is preserved. This leads to an inquiry concerning the process by which the tissues and functions of the body are maintained. We immediately perceive that the material for maintaining every organ and every function must be derived from the blood supply; hence this must be sufficient in quantity and quality in order to maintain health. If the blood supply should be deficient in quantity nutrition must fail to a greater or less degree and either the whole body suffers a diminished nutrition, or if only parts then these parts suffer in a more intense manner. This would mean either a departure from health, with respect to the whole body or the parts which feel the force of the reduced blood supply and deficient nutrition.

The quantity of the blood may be sufficient and still be imperfect or below the natural standard in its composition. The blood must be maintained both in quantity and quality, and constantly reinforced from the food by means of the process of digestion and absorption. It is easy to see how food, unsuitable in quantity and quality, can disorder the digestive apparatus, effect the blood unfavorably and produce disease. There may be some imperfection also in the process of elaborating the blood, some disorder of the blood making functions, even though the food supply is adequate.

Thus we perceive how easy it is for this delicate bodily machinery to fail in some fine adjustment, so that the composition of the blood may be changed sufficiently to allow departure from health and become the starting point of disease. To preserve health, an abundant supply of nutritious food is absolutely required. There must be, in addition, the inherent ability to convert the food, taken into the alimentary canal, into rich, healthy, normal blood.

The complex process of absorbing out of the food material all the fluids and salts required for the maintenance and growth of the various parts of the body must be carried on with precision and success. There must not only be digestion, but assimilation, in order to constantly manufacture within the body a perfect blood supply. Consider for a moment that over all these complex processes the nervous system must preside. Now when you remember that occupations, climate, emotions, and a thousand little things may disturb the nervous forces, is it any wonder that sickness or departure from health is common? It is by the power, not of the will, but of nerve force, largely independent of the will, that the food we eat becomes bone and muscle, nerve and brain.

So complex is the machinery of the human body, which we so little consider, and so often misuse and abuse, that the striking wonder is, not that it so often fails in its delicate and mysterious work, but that it succeeds so well and with so little of failure.

There is still another important and interesting thought in connection with the function of the blood, which thus far has escaped our notice. Not only must the blood current carry to the reach of every part the nourishment sufficient for its growth and maintenance, but it must also carry away the waste products, no longer needed. The blood supply must come to every part richly laded with nutrition, all elaborated and ready to be appropriated, and in its place must receive debris, which must be transported to some other organ for change or excretion.

If these waste products were not carried by the blood to the lungs and other organs to be changed, or to the kidneys and other organs for elimination, the whole body would soon be overloaded and overwhelmed by poisons, and the blood itself would speedily become poisoned and unfit to support life.

In certain diseases this failure of change or elimination becomes a serious complication and threatens death. The carbonic acid, the uric acid, and many other poisons, the results of the wear and tear of the human machine, must be cast out. If they remain, even in small amount, they soon disorder the functions of the body and enkindle disease.

How close then are the relations between many things which seem at first separate and distinct. Healthy blood and an abundant supply, depends upon healthy food and a proper supply, also upon exercise, which stimulates muscular action and assists the process of circulation; also upon an abundant supply of oxygen to change the impure venous into pure arterial blood. This last change takes place in the lungs, every heart-stroke sending the impure venous blood to the lungs and every breath bringing the oxygen to carry on the wonderful change.

Can we fail when we trace out these complex methods to recognize the intimate relation which always exists between health, pure food, pure air, pure water and exercise; and to observe that a correspondingly intimate relation must exist between disease, impure food, impure air or water and a lack of exercise.

It took the medical profession ages to learn what now is so simple and apparent, that disease is most successfully treated and most effectually cured by preventing it altogether. The best medical practice is the one coming everywhere to the front in the light of hygienic revelation. The physician's greatest work is not in administering pills but in disseminating such knowledge in regard to food, water, air, exercise, stimulants and various hygienic topics as will keep not only the individual, but the whole human race, in a constant and vigorous state of health.

The food which we eat may introduce poison and death, or at least sickness and functional disturbance; the water which we drink may contain germs that will work untold mischief in the human economy; the air which we breathe may be contaminated with poisonous gases or convey dangerous disease germs into the system. He is our friend who helps to eliminate the dangers to health which lurk in our pathway, and who assists in providing for the absolute needs of the race, healthy foods at a reasonable price, healthy water uncontaminated by foul pollutions, and all the requisites of health, contentment and happiness.

II.—THE TWO GREAT TYPES OF DISEASE.

There are two kinds of disease—*functional* and *organic*. Disease is always some departure from the condition of health. It is generally caused by some change in the working of nature's great laboratory, or by the alteration of the structure of some organ or organs.

We will endeavor to explain these two great general classes of disease, known as functional and organic.

When there is simply a temporary disturbance of an organ, causing a departure from health, and no alteration has taken place in its structural make up, the disease is simply functional. When permanent change has taken place in the structure of an organ, so that it has become contracted, or enlarged, and its tissues are pressed upon, causing pain and disease, this is recognized as organic.

The distinction is a very clear one, if we will only master the phraseology which describes it. A headache is often due to inaction of the liver; there is some functional trouble, the liver is not doing its customary work. This may be due to the fact that certain elements, which are ordinarily eliminated from the system, when its functions are normal, failing to be removed, are absorbed into the general circulation, and irritate the brain and nerve centers. The waste products of the system, which cannot be transformed and reused, must be cast out, or eliminated. When this process is interfered with, and these irritating substances are too long retained, they act as poisons, and give rise to a great variety of symptoms, which are known under the somewhat indefinite term biliousness. These symptoms, sallow complexion, dizziness or vertigo, headache, want of ambition, sleepiness, etc., are departures from the condition of health, but they are due to no change in the structure of the liver, and hence the disease is termed functional.

Again, a headache may be due to an entirely different cause, some growth or tumor, may press upon a nerve; the disturbance in this latter case is not functional, but due to some change of structure, and hence *organic*. Tubercles of the lungs, cirrhosis of the liver, fatty degeneration of the heart, Bright's disease of the kidneys, these are due to organic change in the structure of various organs, and are illustrations of what is known as organic disease.

Functional disease, it will be perceived, is much more satisfactory to treat than organic. The former usually responds quickly to remedies, while the latter often advances to an unfavorable issue, in spite of all remedies. A disturbance of the working or functions of the liver can be easily remedied, often without medicine, if the patient will abstain from unsuitable foods, and provide rest and favorable conditions for recovery, nature herself being able in a little time to regulate the disordered functions. Cancer of the liver is a severe departure from the health condition; organic changes have taken place in the liver which neither nature nor medicine can cure. The latter can only alleviate suffering, prolong life, and render existence tolerable.

People often get a wrong idea about disease conditions. They think the medical practitioner should be able to cope with every kind of disease. They do not see the distinctions which are apparent to the practiced eye. If they are not at once benefited by medicine, they are prone to think the doctor at fault; and they fail to realize that the trouble is not from without, but from within, and hence they fly from one to another, catching at this and that straw, hoping for health and finding none.

People seem to think that death is to be avoided at all hazards, in some way or other, that it is foreign to human conditions, and always accidental rather than natural. There is another and more rational view of this subject. Death is a natural process, a part of the great plan. To be born means to die, and the only question is *when*. Every beginning, or birth, points to an end, or death. This is true in the whole realm of the animal kingdom. It is as much a process of nature to die as to live; to cease to exist as to begin to exist.

Scarcely has the new born babe entered upon its life career before it must run the gauntlet of one disease after another; so that in a very few years half of the whole number are missing. One by one the weak and puny fall out by the way, and sometimes the most vigorous, too, are cut off by disease. The great problem before us is to strengthen the weak, to increase their power of resistance, and then to diminish the diseases that invade our pathway, to prevent disease and thus add to longevity.

Hence, whatever tends to improve the health condition of the parent contributes to the living prospects of the child, and whatever weakens and reduces the vitality of the parent reduces the health prospects of the progeny. Do we not then see how intricate and far-reaching are the subjects which we discuss with regard to health and disease? Do we not see how even our most tenable theories must be modified to account for a thousand exceptions which may occur in a field of work where all is uncertain, owing to a thousand important factors which may not only be obscure, but entirely hidden? To-day a child is born, even from healthy parents, so far as can be discovered. It may seem to have every advantage, and its prospects of a long life be excellent; to-morrow it may begin to decline, by reason of some undiscovered organic defect. The heart, perhaps, is faulty in its structure and proves unable to maintain the circulation and the infant dies.

We must not possess the confidence, that in all cases, death can be avoided, but on the other hand, the ratio of deaths can be materially diminished. How many little ones are sacrificed every summer to artificial feeding? Instead of the healthy and abundant supply nature intended, there is the improperly cleansed bottle and the unhealthy milk full of poisonous disease germs by the time it reaches the child's stomach. Thousands of children die of cholera diseases every summer that, under better conditions, might live and perhaps run the average course of human existence. This disturbance or disease is only functional, and not organic. Its cause is improper food and poisoned air during the heated term, and a lack of knowledge as to the proper care of these little patients. Its ravages are to a great extent preventable.

III.—TEMPERATURE IN DISEASE.

The temperature of the body in health and sickness did not receive very close attention and study until about thirty years ago.

The recent observations concerning the temperature of the body are due to the invention of a little instrument called the fever thermometer. This is a very convenient, but rather frail, little instrument, which consists of a graduated glass tube, in which the mercury ascends when the bottom part or bulb is exposed to heat. It is very useful in the diagnosis of disease, and discloses a large amount of information concerning fevers, the breaking down of tubercular nodules, and the formation of pus in the body, which can be obtained in no other way.

The temperature of the natural body is called the normal temperature. It is very nearly the same in all healthy persons, at all seasons of the year. The best way to obtain the temperature is by placing the bulb containing the mercury under the tongue, where it should remain four or five minutes, if accuracy is desired. It is sometimes placed in the armpit, or elsewhere, when the patient is unable, from any cause, to hold it in the mouth.

In some high fever stages, it reaches one hundred and five or six degrees; but such a temperature indicates severe sickness, and imminent danger. In acute rheumatism, a temperature of one hundred and four is quite alarming, because it indicates some complication, especially of the heart valves. In consumption, a temperature of one hundred and four degrees indicates rapid waste of tissue and a galloping progress of the disease. In typhoid fever the temperature rises slowly, and it takes a week or more for it to reach one hundred and three or four degrees, or the highest point. When the evening temperature in typhoid does not reach above one hundred and three degrees it is a mild case, if it reaches a hundred and five degrees it is a severe case, and danger threatens; a hundred and five degrees is very high temperature, it rarely goes above this except in fatal cases.

There is considerable difference between the morning and evening temperature. The case is not as favorable when the temperature is high in the morning. In fevers which pursue the ordinary course the temperature goes higher in the evening and falls toward midnight, a process which goes on until morning. When the morning temperature is as high or higher than it was in the evening it is a sign of some complication, and indicates a severe case.

In malaria and malarial fevers the temperature reaches its highest point in a few hours. A person who was well yesterday and who has a temperature of one hundred and four to-day has malarial or ephemeral fever. It is not typhoid.

In pneumonia the temperature rises rapidly from one hundred and two on the first day, to one hundred and four or five on the second and third days. In pneumonia a temperature below one hundred and two indicates a very mild case, with but little exudation into the air cells, while one hundred and four or five indicates a severe attack and a large amount of exudation, and in such a case delirium is quite likely to be present.

The temperature rises rather higher in children when sick than in adults, owing to the more active processes of the body. Each mother ought to be acquainted with the significance of temperature in disease. If a child complains of feeling ill and the temperature is under one hundred degrees the sickness is slight, while if above a hundred the case is important, and becomes more grave as the temperature ascends. The higher then the temperature goes the sicker the child, except in fever which follows malarial chills, when the temperature may ascend very rapidly and reach, for a brief time, a very high point without much significance. A rise of one degree in temperature corresponds to about ten beats of the pulse.

The temperature is high in scarlet, yellow, typhus and typhoid fevers. When the temperature rises above one hundred and five degrees the patient is usually in danger, especially if it continues elevated to that degree for any considerable period of time. When the temperature remains high after the appearance of the rash in measles some complication is indicated.

After an attack of pleurisy a high temperature generally indicates the formation of pus in the pleural cavity. After many acute diseases, if the temperature continues at one hundred and three or four degrees, it either shows that the disease is still active or that some complication exists.

In the condition of collapse, prior to death, the temperature falls below the normal. When the temperature falls below ninety degrees recovery seldom takes place. A person is sick so long as the temperature fluctuates or continues above the normal.

When, after sickness, the temperature falls to the natural point and continues there during the entire twenty-four hours it indicates that the disease has abated, and complete recovery to health may be anticipated. When, during a course of sickness, the temperature rises higher in the morning than at night the patient is getting worse, but if the decline is in the morning, it should be regarded as significant of improvement.

IV.—KISSING IN ITS RELATION TO DISEASE.

There is no especial objection hygienically to kissing on the part of equals, or friends and relatives, nor as the expression of affection and love; but for strangers to force kisses upon infants and small children, simply because the babies are sweet and the little ones cute and attractive, should be condemned as needless, and liable to convey to the child, whose ability to resist disease is especially limited, certain contagia which may prove fatal. It is also dangerous to kiss persons who are sick with certain ailments, and the practice should be restricted as much as possible.

Many persons are led by a sincere affection to kiss loved ones after death; it should be universally known that no little danger attends this practice. A dead body cannot be regarded as a wholesome object, for already the process of decomposition has commenced. We need not regard the dead with horror, nor with heathenish superstition, for the body is simply the tenement, vacated by its occupant, and it is useless to consume our emotions upon a dead and decaying body, which is not only destitute of life, but which may be capable of conveying to ourselves and others contagious diseases. Many cases of sickness and death have been traced to this revolting custom. Outbreaks of diphtheria have resulted from such a cause, and where death has resulted from diphtheria it has been found, in one instance at least, necessary to issue orders prohibiting the practice of kissing the dead.

V.—BATHING IN ITS RELATION TO DISEASE.

The frequent bathing of the body is essential to health, but in order to get the most decided benefits from the bath good sense is essential. In addition, a few common rules may not come amiss to the inexperienced. A person should not bathe too soon after a hearty meal, but an interval of two hours should occur between it and the dinner. A bath may be very injurious to a person who is very much fatigued or exhausted. Wait till a reaction has taken place. Be careful about taking a bath when the pores of the body are open and the vitality has been lowered by free perspiration. In such a condition the bath should be quite warm. Do not stay in the water after you experience a sense of chilliness. This applies more especially to open air bathing. Only the vigorous and strong should bathe in the morning before breakfast. Two or three hours after a meal is the preferable time.

A towel bath followed by brisk rubbing of the skin is very refreshing before retiring in hot weather. Bathing in the salt sea water is apt to be too prolonged and exhausting, if in the company of a large number of persons. Bathing in salt water is invigorating and enjoyable if judiciously performed at the proper season, at suitable hours, and is not indulged in too extensively. Persons who are indisposed may be injured rather than benefited by this vigorous tumble in the waves. Young people who bathe in the surf are inclined to remain too long in the water. Fifteen or twenty minutes is long enough for the most robust, except the water is delightfully warm, when a prolonged stay may be unattended by harm.

Rubbing the body after the bath is essential, and completes the act with the best results, quickening the circulation of the external surfaces. Systematic bathing, or the daily sponging over of the body, followed by friction with a coarse towel is healthful and exhilarating. The best time to do this is in the morning before dressing.

VI.—SYMPTOMS OF DISEASE.

HOW TO READ AND INTERPRET THEM.

In cases of sickness, one difficulty which confronts the ordinary individual is the inability to read and interpret the symptoms of disease correctly. No positive diagnosis can be reached except in trivial cases without giving considerable attention to this important subject. Disease symptoms must be considered collectively, as well as singly. Scarlet fever is often ushered in by vomiting, but from this symptom alone you cannot infer that you have a case, for it is very common in many other affections. It only indicates the beginning of scarlet fever, where a group of other symptoms point in the same direction, otherwise it may suggest an over-loaded stomach, the condition of pregnancy or many other varied conditions.

By going over some of the common and important symptoms of disease carefully you will be better able henceforth to determine what is the matter with the sick members of your family.

The Countenance.—The first thing we naturally notice about a person is the countenance, and by a sort of intuition we recognize the difference between that of health and sickness. The pupils of the eyes are dilated in most diseases, but contracted in opium poisoning and in certain affections of the brain. The countenance is pallid in anæmia or from loss of blood, from fright or after a fall, or other severe injury, especially if there exists the condition known as shock. The face is pale in cholera morbus, and both pale and anxious in the collapse which soon comes on, when timely relief is not obtained. There is an anxious look in diseases of the abdomen, and also in certain diseases of the heart. The face is pallid and careworn during the progress of many chronic diseases. Mania and imbecility make their impression upon the countenance. Emaciation appears in addition to pallor if the sickness is severe and of long duration. In cholera infantum emaciation comes on early.

In some diseases of the lungs or air passages, when oxygen is not obtained in sufficient amount to aerate the blood the face is pallid, with a bluish hue (cyanosis), the lips are blue, and there is a pinched look about the nose and face. The countenance bears a purple aspect in some of the low forms of fever, as typhus.

In some affections of the liver the face is sallow. This is the case in malaria which always involves the liver, and also in dyspepsia. In some of the severer affections of the liver the skin is yellow; this yellow hue, known as jaundice, is especially noticeable in the whites of the eyes.

In cancer there is a peculiar waxy, sallow countenance, which is characteristic of this malignant disorder. The face is flushed in congestions, in the early stage of pneumonia and fevers, in apoplexy, in poisoning from belladonna, and in the hectic fever which accompanies the progress of consumption.

The symptoms which appear in the countenance may mislead one who is unaccustomed to the peculiarities of an individual. Some persons in health have a flushed countenance, while others are pallid or sallow, so that these things must have due consideration. A single glance often suffices for grasping the symptoms which appear in the countenance. With these a close observer has little or no trouble.

The Tongue.—The next thing is a look at the tongue, which presents a great variety of appearances and reveals much about the condition of the individual. The natural appearance of the tongue is familiar. It is red, moist and slightly coated in the back part of the mouth, even in the condition of health. This natural appearance does not continue long after some departure from health.

In slight ailments the tongue is usually more or less furred over with a whitish or yellowish coat. This condition often indicates biliousness, indigestion or some temporary disorder of the stomach and alimentary canal. In typhoid conditions the tongue is brown and sometimes so fissured as to bleed. In scarlet fever the tongue presents a peculiar appearance, known as the strawberry tongue, because the little papillæ are swollen and look like the seeds on the outside of a strawberry.

In anæmia and malaria the tongue has a peculiar indistinct appearance and looks as though it was partially bloodless; this pale appearance of the tongue is rarely wanting in malaria. After typhoid fever the coating peels off and leaves the tongue somewhat raw and very red. This condition is known as the beefsteak tongue.

In the collapse of cholera the tongue is cold and in conditions of great weakness or extreme debility the protrusion of the tongue is accompanied by trembling. In apoplexy the tongue when protruded is inclined to either the right or left side of the face, the side opposite that half of the brain where the pressure exists which causes the paralysis.

The tongue is coated in all acute diseases as pleurisy, pneumonia and the various kinds of fever. The degree and extent of this coating, its color and the want of moisture make up a variety of suggestions which practice teaches one to interpret without mistake.

The Teeth and Gums.—While glancing at the tongue the physician also notices the condition of the teeth and gums. These parts often require special attention. Decayed teeth are unhealthy and they should be cleaned and filled or else removed except in the case of the shedding teeth, which should be allowed to remain as long as possible to prevent contraction of the jaw. Rapid decay of the teeth is often indicative of some constitutional impairment.

Certain medicines as iron injure the teeth, and when administered should be given in such a way as to prevent this unfortunate occurrence. In typhoid fever the teeth and gums are covered with a black collection of matter called sordes. This should be washed off and vaseline applied to the lips to prevent their cracking and scaling.

A blue line along the gums indicates lead poisoning. An excessive flow of saliva sometimes indicates mercurial poisoning though there are other conditions which also produce this symptom.

The Saliva and Mouth.—Some medicines, like jaborandi, increase the flow of saliva, and others, like belladonna, check the secretion, rendering the mouth and throat uncomfortably dry. An excessive flow of saliva is sometimes troublesome during the period of teething, also in pregnancy and other conditions.

The saliva is thick and *viscid* in catarrhal inflammations and in fevers. It is sometimes mixed with purulent matter in protracted bronchitis, and rust colored sputa in pneumonia.

An eroded condition of the mouth sometimes reveals the fact that poison has been taken, and the peculiar appearance of the eroded membrane indicates to the experienced eye, just what particular poison has wrought the mischief.

Appetite and Taste.—A bitter taste in the mouth usually indicates dyspepsia or biliousness, and a sour taste indicates an acid condition of the stomach, very common in indigestion. A saltish taste is noticed in hemorrhage, and a very disagreeable putrid taste from the discharge of a quinsy sore throat, when the abscess ruptures, or from gangrene of the lungs.

In most acute diseases the appetite is lost, and it is perverted in hysteria, chlorosis, and frequently in pregnancy. It is often excessive in diabetes, in certain nervous affections, and when worms infest the stomach.

Thirst is a noticeable symptom in fevers, cholera morbus and cholera infantum, and in diabetes.

Dysphagia.—In certain diseases difficulty in swallowing appears as a marked symptom. This is the case in inflammation of the tonsils, pharynx or larynx. It is usual in diphtheria, mumps, scarlet fever, abscess of the throat or neck, and many other affections which attack or infringe upon the tissues in the vicinity of the throat.

The Odor of the Breath—The odor of the breath will be noticed in many cases. It is usually offensive in fevers, quinsy and diphtheria, sour in indigestion and it has a peculiar sweetish and sickish odor in uremia. This is so marked as to be readily observed by one who has ever encountered a previous case. The odor of small pox, typhus, gout and some other affections is characteristic. In gangrene of the lungs it is so offensive as to be almost unbearable, but fortunately this putrid condition is quite uncommon.

The Pulse.—You have noticed that when a physician has been called to look you over and see what special departure from health is giving you trouble about the first thing he appears to do is to place his finger upon your wrist, over the radial artery, thus feeling the pulse. This is not the result of habit, but because the pulse reveals the action of the heart, and at the same time much concerning the condition of the patient. There are some facts about the heart beat and pulse which it is well to know. It is more rapid standing than sitting, still more rapid walking than standing, and still more rapid running than walking.

All exercise increases the action and force of the heart. The pulse is more rapid after a meal than before, owing to the energy which the digestion of food requires. Every thought or emotion of the mind correspondingly quickens the action of the heart. All excitement disturbs more or less the nervous system, and whatever disturbs the nerves disturbs the heart's action in a corresponding degree.

Exercise and thought are healthy and invigorating within certain limits, but if too prolonged and carried to excess may lead to departure from health. The relation of the mind to the bodily organs is intimate almost beyond our comprehension.

Age reveals great variation in the frequency of the pulse. In infancy the pulse is more rapid than in adult life, and this tendency is still more marked in old age. There are many individual exceptions to any general rule which could be formulated with reference to this subject. It is, however, sufficient for practical purposes to know that the pulse rate per minute in infancy is about 120, in childhood from 90 to 100, and in adult age from 70 to 80, the average being about 72. In old age the pulse declines from 70 to 60, and in some cases to 50, and even 40.

It is owing to the vigor of their circulation that children enjoy the rigors of winter, and the sports of coasting and skating, while old people cling to the warm rooms, and complain of the cold, because circulation is feeble in proportion as the heart force has declined.

The average pulse rate in females is greater than in males. This increase does not appear to indicate less vigor, but it is nature's method of compensation, for as the stroke is less vigorous a greater number are probably required to accomplish the same work. The more rapid the pulse, usually the less force in each heart beat.

In the early stages of fevers the pulse is full and bounding, the face often flushed and the eyes congested. The pulse is rapid in the acute diseases of childhood, in scarlet fever, pleurisy, pneumonia and in typhoid fever. There are, however, exceptions to this rule. In diphtheria the poison acting upon the nerve force somewhat paralyzes and retards its activity, and similar conditions exist in malaria, bilious fever and other conditions of disease poisoning.

The pulse is slow in apoplexy or in allied conditions where compression of the brain exists. The pulse is slow in cases of opium or lead poisoning. Some persons in health have a slow pulse rate without other evidence of debility or prostration, hence a slow pulse does not of necessity indicate sickness. Irregular pulse is often due to the excessive use of tobacco by smokers. Irregularity of the pulse appears to be natural to some persons and may exist without any other indication that health is impaired. In these cases some beats are more rapid or more energetic than others, a few rapid beats may occur followed by a few which are slower or more full, or a beat may be occasionally omitted. A person of ordinary skill is unable to judge whether irregular heart action is natural or the result of disease, of the brain or the heart itself. Such symptoms are of but little practical importance to the individual and to be unconscious of their existence prevents anxiety of the mind and is often favorable to the continuance of health.

In nervous diseases the pulse is usually quick or jerky showing an excited and disturbed condition of the system. In the last stages of fevers and other diseases which are approaching a fatal termination the pulse is small and thready and before death it becomes irregular and flickering. We see then how important are the suggestions which may be gained by placing the fingers upon the wrist. Practice and experience render this procedure almost prophetic.

Respiration.—The character of the breathing and the number of respirations each minute are symptoms of great importance. Normal respiration admits of quite a wide range. The new-born infant breathes about forty times a minute, a child five years old breathes about twenty-five times a minute while an adult ordinarily breathes from fifteen to twenty times each minute; the average is about eighteen for a healthy adult there being about four pulsations of the heart during each act of respiration.

In fevers the breathing is more rapid than normal except in certain typhoid conditions when it may be slower, and in profound opium poisoning it also becomes very slow or ceases altogether. The breathing is rapid and shallow in hysteria, it is short and attended with severe pain in pleurisy, it is shallow, rapid and painful in pneumonia, running up to forty and sometimes sixty a minute. It is obstructed and difficult in croup, labored in asthma, stertorous (snoring) in profound anaesthesia, in apoplexy and in the deep sleep of inebrity. In certain diseases of the heart the respiration is labored and difficult.

Cough.—The act of coughing is common to many diseases of the lungs and air passages. It is sometimes of little at other times of serious import. The character of the cough often indicates its importance as a symptom of disease. A dry, hollow or hacking cough may be sympathetic or only of nervous origin and without any very special significance. In the early stage of bronchitis the cough is tight and dry and affords no relief. This is due to the inflammation and dry condition of the bronchi; later however it becomes soft, deep, loose and brings up accumulations of thick mucous.

In the incipient stage of consumption the cough may be merely of a hacking, bronchial type, but with the advanced stages of the disease it becomes deep and often distressing.

In spasmodic croup the cough is hoarse and barking, or in advanced croup it may have a whistling sound; favorable symptoms are the softening of the cough and the secretions of mucous. In pneumonia the cough is shallow and owing to the pain a strenuous effort is made to suppress it. In whooping cough the paroxysms are characteristic and so familiar as to need no description.

The peculiar symptom known as hiccough is caused by a spasmodic action of the muscular wall which separates the abdomen from the thorax known as the diaphragm. It may be the result of exhaustion or due to indigestion or some nervous disorder. It is very common with infants but of little significance. It sometimes indicates the approach of death in serious cases and seems to be due to that final exhaustion which is relieved only by the calm and stillness which ensues.

Nausea and Vomiting.—These are symptoms of considerable importance when weighed in connection with others. They may result from many diverse causes as will be seen from the following statements. They often occur from indigestible food in the stomach especially in children who devour unripe fruits in the summer. They occur in inflammation of the muscular lining of the stomach (gastritis) whether caused by alcoholic drinks or otherwise.

They are familiar as occurring from sea-sickness, bilious disorders, pregnancy, cholera, cholera morbus and cholera infantum. They also occur in ulcers and cancers of the stomach, in diseases of the brain, in yellow fever, in Bright's disease, in strangulated hernia and from medicinal substances and various poisons. The character of the vomited matter is often of some value in diagnosis. In bilious attack the vomited matter is composed of mucous and bile, in cholera the characteristic rice-water vomit occurs, in yellow fever the black vomit appears, in ulcers of the stomach mucous, lymph and blood are vomited, in cancer of the stomach the microscope reveals cancer cells in the vomited matter, in strangulated hernia and obstruction of the bowels the vomited matter is characteristic and consists of the contents of the bowels. Vertigo is rarely due to brain disease but often to disordered stomach and liver affections of a temporary character.

Pain.—This symptom is often urgent. It must then be interpreted promptly and correctly, and in infants from their only language which is a cry. In general, pain which is relieved by pressure is not attended by inflammation. Colic causes pain of this kind and affords infants previous to three months of age most of their distress.

One of the difficulties in interpreting this common symptom is disclosed in the fact that pain is not always experienced at the seat of the trouble from whence it proceeds. In hip joint disease the pain is felt at the knee, in affections of the liver the pain is felt under the shoulder blade, in dyspepsia at the place usually described as the pit of the stomach, just under or below the sternum. In affections of the bladder and ovaries the pain is felt in the limbs and other members and parts, while uterine diseases produce headaches and pain in the top of the head.

Where pain is the product of inflammation there is usually much tenderness on pressure.

Pain may be constant or intermittent; it may be fixed at one point or wander about from place to place. The character of the pain aids in the act of diagnosis. In pleurisy the pain is located in the side of the chest, and is acute, sharp and cutting. In pneumonia it is dull, heavy and aching. In dysentery it is twisting and griping in character, while in cholera morbus it is attended by cramping. In rheumatism the pain is tearing or gnawing, while in neuralgia it is shooting and darting in character, now here and now there.

In an abscess the pain is pulsating, in erysipelas it is smarting and burning, in urticaria (nettle rash) it is stinging, in labor it is rhythmical and tends to bearing down. The pain which attends the passage of gall stones extends from the right side under the short ribs to the center of the abdomen. It is a very severe, cutting pain; a similar pain, but in a different locality, attends the passage of a calculus from the kidneys through the ureter into the bladder. It is an agonizing, tearing, cutting pain, which requires energetic measures to secure relief.

The position assumed by the patient often throws some light upon the diagnosis. Patients suffering from peritonitis lie upon the back with the limbs drawn up. This is the position which permits of the largest amount of relief from the tenderness and severe pain in the abdomen.

In asthma and in some forms of heart disease the patient is unable to lie down, and finds existence more tolerable by sleeping in a sitting posture. In the early stages of pleurisy the patient lies on the unaffected side, but later, after the effusion of water into the chest cavity takes place, changes and lies on the affected side with a greater degree of comfort. In some cases of heart enlargement and other affections of this important organ, the patient can lie only upon the right side. In the pain of colic the patient often finds a measure of relief by lying upon the abdomen.

Hemorrhage.—This is a symptom which requires deliberate judgment, unless from an injury, where its source is easily recognized, and demands prompt action. Hemorrhage from injuries is treated elsewhere. In early life hemorrhage from the nose is frequent and usually insignificant. For the treatment of serious cases, which require plugging, see Chap. XV., Art. V.

The amount of hemorrhage and the place from which it proceeds are alike important. Hemorrhage from the lungs may result from congestion caused by defect in the heart's action, or otherwise, or from tubercular disease. Hemorrhage from the lungs is frothy and bright red, and is brought up into the mouth by the act of coughing; if the quantity is large it is followed by corresponding prostration. Hemorrhage from the lips or gums is usually unimportant. It may come from the throat as the result of an abscess or ulceration.

That which comes from an ulcer in the stomach is usually dark colored and brought up by vomiting. It is never frothy nor bright colored. Blood from the nose often escapes into the stomach during the sleep of a young person, and is raised on the following morning. Hemorrhage from the ear may occur as the result of a fractured skull. Hemorrhage from the bowels may indicate dysentery or piles, or it may result from ulceration of the bowels in typhoid fever. In these cases it is not necessarily fatal unless the amount is large or the patient very weak.

Such hemorrhage is sometimes concealed and revealed only by a post mortem examination.

Hemorrhage may result from abortion or after natural labor. This may be so sudden or so copious as to endanger life. The progress of a cancer in the stomach, rectum, womb or bladder may produce alarming hemorrhage owing to the erosion of an artery. Blood sometimes appears mixed with the urine and may come from the kidneys, the bladder or the adjacent tissues. Blood may appear in the urine from congestion or inflammation of the kidneys or from a stone or cyst in the bladder. It has been known to appear in the urine in malaria and other diseases. It is sometimes of quite serious import in this connection.

Blood in the urine as a symptom would be likely to mislead persons who have not had the advantage of professional training and experience. It should be borne in mind that some persons manifest a peculiar disposition to excessive hemorrhage from the slightest causes.

Delirium.—This symptom is often observed in diseases of children associated with high temperature and does not necessarily imply an unfavorable condition. It is common in typhoid fever, malarial fever, meningitis and some other acute affections.

Coma.—This is a symptom of serious import in the later stages of acute diseases. The coma produced by alcohol is recognized by smelling the breath and is not generally fatal; that of opium poisoning is recognized by the contracted condition of the pupils of the eye and if profound requires vigorous efforts to prevent a fatal culmination. It is of serious import in typhoid and typhus fevers and other diseases which are attended by extreme prostration or disintegration of the blood corpuscles. The coma of apoplexy or from any injury or compression of the brain is generally the certain forerunner of death.

Paralysis.—This may result from a local injury or inflammation of a nerve or nerves, or from disease of or pressure upon the spinal cord or the brain itself. Paralysis of either the right or left side is known as hemiplegia, while paralysis of both lower extremities is called paraplegia.

The Skin.—The skin is usually hot and dry in fevers. In debility, prostration and consumption there is a tendency to excessive sweating. It is caused by the debilitated condition which it continually increases. In many diseases a moist condition of the skin is to be regarded as a favorable symptom. The various eruptions of the skin and their significance will be found in the chapter on the skin and its diseases.

Constipation.—This usually indicates a torpid condition of the muscular coat of the bowels. It is often associated with indigestion and sedentary habits. It indicates a deficiency in the secretions of the liver and intestinal glands.

The Eye Symptoms.—The eye symptoms which should be noticed in relation to disease are quite numerous. The pupils are dilated in many of the common diseases of childhood, also in hydrocephalus, apoplexy and from the use of belladonna and other drugs. The pupils are contracted in inflammation of the retina or brain, in profound narcotism by opium and other drugs of its class. In consumption the eyes are remarkably bright and lustrous, while in old age and in many diseases the eyes are dim and lose their lustre. The arcus senilis is a mark of physical degeneracy and of the ravages of age. It indicates that the vessels and tissues of the body are losing their elasticity and toughness.

Rolling the eyes from side to side suggests irritation of the brain. Inequality of the pupils also indicates disease of the brain.

In conjunctivitis the membrane about the eye is congested, in iritis the light is dreaded, in cataract the lens becomes opaque and the center of the eye looks milky. Many other symptoms, such as flashes of light, moving spots, double vision, etc., are of special interest to the expert, but could not be easily explained to those who have not made a special study of the eye and its diseases.

Ear Symptoms.—Ear symptoms are not so numerous. Ringing in the ears may occur from large doses of quinine, from congestion of the brain, from nervous debility, from twitching of the muscles, or from disease of the ear.

Deafness may result from cold in the head, wax in the ear, from typhus or typhoid fevers, also from disease of the ear, throat or brain.

(Abnormal Products.)—The Urine as a Symptom.—As the waste products of the system are extensively eliminated in the urine, this secretion becomes prominent in establishing the existence of many otherwise obscure and serious disorders. The normal urine is acid, and when it is found to be alkaline, dyspepsia or some disorder of the digestive apparatus may be inferred. The color of ordinary urine is amber or straw, marked departure from which suggests malaria, jaundice or other disease according as it is colored more or less highly with urates, phosphates, bile pigments or blood. The specific gravity of the normal urine ranges between 1018 and 1025; marked departure from this suggests that it contains either sugar, which may appear in large quantities in diabetes, or albumen and tube casts, which, if persistent, indicate Bright's disease.

There are many reliable tests for the various abnormal products which are occasionally found in the urine. These are contained in special works upon the subject. Inability to pass the urine is called strangury, and may be caused by a fly blister, a calculus or stone in the bladder, or by paralysis or loss of nervous control. This condition is easily relieved by the introduction of a catheter.

Suppression or failure of the kidneys to secrete urine is a serious condition, and if continued for only a few hours leads to uremic poisoning, coma, convulsions and death. Unless the uric acid is constantly eliminated from the system the blood soon becomes poisoned by it, the brain is stupefied and life continues but a brief season.

There are many other symptoms of disease which are discovered by the means employed by the skillful physician or expert who calls to his aid appliances such as the opthalmoscope, the laryngoscope, various specula and the sphygmograph. Such means, however, are not of sufficient general interest to warrant their extensive introduction in a domestic work.

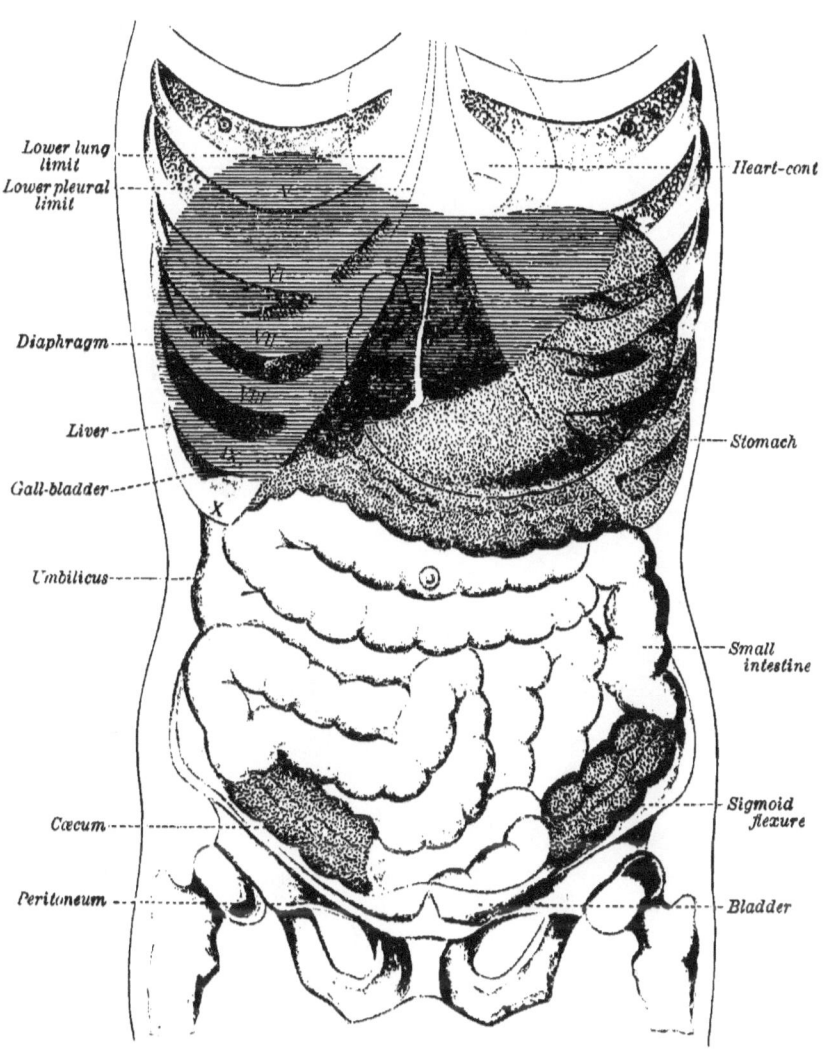

Relations of the abdominal viscera. Anterior view.

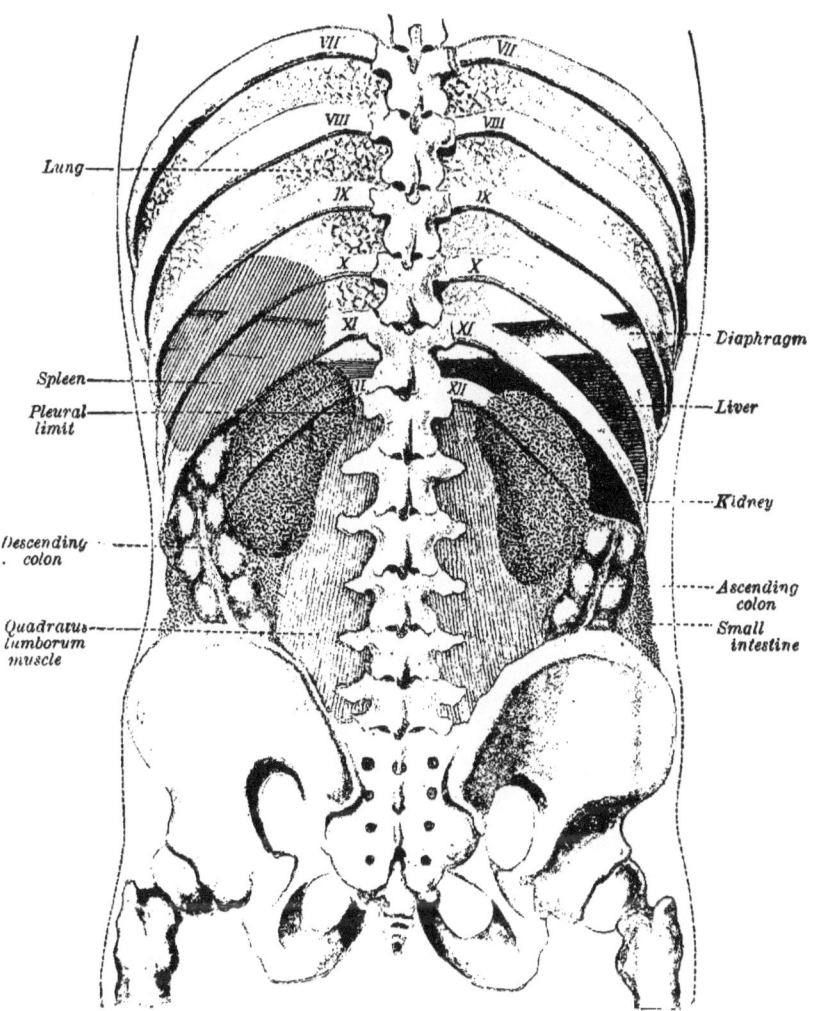

Relations of abdominal viscera. Posterior view.

CHAPTER VIII.

ANATOMY AND PHYSIOLOGY,

INCLUDING THE

BONES, JOINTS AND MUSCLES.

I.—ANATOMY AND PHYSIOLOGY. II.—THE RELATION OF PHYSIOLOGY TO ANATOMY. III.—THE ANATOMY OF THE BONES. IV.—THE BONES OF THE SKULL. V.—THE BONES OF THE FACE. VI.—THE SPINAL COLUMN. VII.—INJURIES OF THE SPINE. VIII.—THE BONES OF THE UPPER EXTREMITIES, CHEST AND PELVIS. IX.—THE BONES OF THE LOWER EXTREMITIES. X.—THE JOINTS. XI.—THE MUSCLES. XII.—NATURE'S EFFORT TO PREVENT INJURY. XIII.—FRACTURE OF BONES. XIV.—DISLOCATIONS.

I.—ANATOMY AND PHYSIOLOGY.

AN effort has been made to present the subject of anatomy so briefly and interestingly, and so associated with practical lessons, that it will be appreciated by every one. The skeleton, or framework of this wonderful human machine, known as the body, consists of a large variety of connected bones, which support it and give it form.

The human skeleton itself, when brought from the closet, awakens unpleasant associations, and is usually regarded as frightful and hideous, yet when covered and draped with the various tissues, as the muscles, and rounded out with the adipose deposits, embellished with the supple and yielding skin, and filled with animal life, easily ranks as the most beautiful work of art, or as the most intricate piece of mechanism.

The bones are developed in cartilaginous tissue, beginning at points called the centers of ossification. Bone is one of the hardest tissues in the human body, and is composed principally of lime phosphates, various salts and fat. The microscope shows that bone

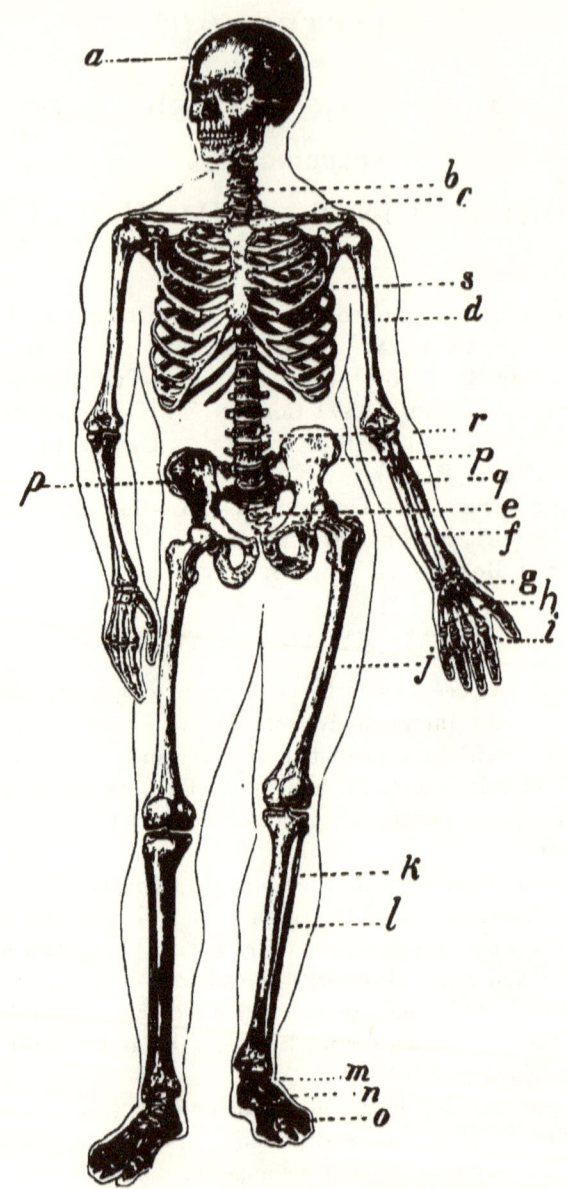

THE HUMAN SKELETON—FRONT VIEW.

a, cranial bones; *b*, cervical vertebræ; *c*, clavicle; *d*, humerus; *e*, sacrum; *f*, ulna; *g*, carpus; *h*, metacarpus; *i*, phalanges; *j*, femur; *k*, tibia; *l*, fibula; *m*, tarsus; *n*, metatarsus; *o*, phalanges; *p*, pelvis containing illum, ischium and pubes; *q*, radius; *r*, lumbar vertebræ; *s*, sternum.

tissue is not so compact as it appears, for it is traversed by numerous canals (the Haversian) which give lodgement to blood vessels and numerous nerves. There are over two hundred bones in the human body. Some are long, like the bones of the leg; some short, like the bones of the hand; and some are flat, like the bones of the skull; while others are of irregular shape, as the vertebræ which unite to form the spinal column.

The bones are connected together at the joints by strong ligaments so as to favor all necessary and graceful movements. It is customary to begin the study of medicine with the bones, because they are the foundation of the body, and without a knowledge of them it would be impossible to obtain a correct idea of the relation of other parts. It is necessary to learn the name, size, structure and position of the bones and their muscular attachments in order to be successful in repairing the injuries to which they are frequently subjected in falls and various accidents. Hence the medical student must know a great many things about the bones, muscles and nerves, which would be considered dry and uninteresting to others, and which will have to be passed over unnoticed for want of space.

It is believed that the general reader will not care to spend much time in the examination of the joists, rafters, supports and other framework of the house we live in and that far more interest will be manifested in the externals of this house beautiful, such as the clothes we wear, the food we eat, the water we drink, the cause, the symptoms and cure of the diseases to which we are subject, how to avoid sickness and live long and well.

To these practical matters it is reasonably expected that the reader will give more willing attention than to anatomical subjects. Since anatomy is fundamental it will be necessary to introduce just enough of it to render the practical portions of this work intelligible and direct those who are seeking for further light to the many special and scientific works or encyclopedias better calculated to satisfy every inquirer.

II.—THE RELATION OF PHYSIOLOGY TO ANATOMY.

The relation of physiology to anatomy is worthy of brief notice. While anatomy brings to our attention the various parts of the body their situation and relation to each other, the structure of each part by itself and of the whole combined, it lacks the charm of vitality. It presents the body very much like a machine or watch, to be taken into pieces in order to note carefully each wheel, the relation that one bears to another and to the whole.

Physiology presents the human machine not as a passive mechanism but as an acting collection of forces. It brings you the watch, not taken into pieces but in motion, every wheel moving in its proper place. It is thus that physiology studies the human body not as a dry skeleton, not a liver preserved in alcohol, but a skeleton clothed with beauty and every part animate and performing its own special functions. The lungs are breathing, the heart beating, the blood circulating, while you take note of the changes that occur during the process of its circuit in the kidneys, the liver, the lungs and back through the veins to the heart. You do not analyze the blood to see what it contains but you study it as it hurries on its way from part to part, continually acting and being acted upon. In the same manner you study the process of digestion; the food acted upon first by the saliva of the mouth, the pepsin secreted by the glands of the stomach, the pancreatic fluid, the bile and the intestinal secretions, carefully observing every change until it is taken up by the absorbent vessels and conveyed into the circulation.

The work performed by an organ is called its function, or if more than one its functions, but such work could scarcely be inferred from the mere examination of an organ. It is important to study as far as possible the organ at work and thereby learn what its functions are. Because the arteries were empty after death the ancient doctors supposed them to be hollow tubes through which air was conveyed. If they had studied the arteries in a living animal, full of blood moving always on in wave currents as propelled by each beat of the heart they would not have made such a mistake.

No one now considers that physiology is a subject devoid of interest. How interesting it is to learn that every muscular fiber is composed of a bundle of smaller fibers and that each one is accompanied by a nerve to control its action and another to preside over its blood supply and nutrition; that it may have abundant material for repairing the wastes which are constantly taking place in the fierce life struggle which causes such a constant wear and tear of this wonderful machine.

In this work anatomy and physiology will be combined, the one adding interest to and complementing the other. Some knowledge of these subjects is essential to a proper understanding of disease and its intelligent treatment and only so much will be introduced as is deemed essential for such purposes.

III.—THE ANATOMY OF THE BONES.

In life the skeleton supports the weight of the body and gives attachment to numerous muscles, which, by contracting and expanding, admit of a great variety of movements. The bones of the skull protect the brain which they surround, and the many nerves which radiate from this great center of force.

The external surface of the bones is covered by a tough, dense membrane, which aids in its nourishment, called the periosteum, and the great central cavities are lined by another similar membrane. The central cavities within the shaft of the long bones contain marrow, or material stored away for their nourishment. The ends of the bones are less compact in structure and the central opening is obliterated.

The skeleton contains about two hundred distinct bones, as follows:

In the skull, or cranium,	8
In the face,	14
In the spinal column, including the sacrum and coccyx,	26
The ribs, including the hyoid bone and sternum,	26
The upper extremities,	64
The lower extremities,	62
Total,	200

This enumeration does not include the three small bones of each ear, nor the teeth.

IV.—THE BONES OF THE SKULL.

The eight bones of the skull are the frontal, the two parietal, two temporal, the occipital, the sphenoid and ethmoid.

The frontal bone underlies and gives shape to the forehead. It has a vertical and a horizontal portion. The former extends upward from the ridges above the eyes to its union with the parietal bones on the dome of the skull, while the latter forms the roof of the orbits, and its inner surface lodges the anterior lobes of the brain.

The parietal bones extend from the frontal to the occipital, covering the center and sides of the dome. They are united in the center by the sagittal suture. They are concave on the inside surface and grooved by the arteries which lie just within, and they contain various depressions which correspond to the convolutions of the brain.

The temporal bones are more irregular in form. They are situated at the sides and base of the skull and contain the openings for the external ear.

The occipital bone forms the back part of the skull and extends forward under the base of the brain, where a great opening, the foramen magnum, exists, out through which the spinal cord and vertebral arteries pass. Its inner surface is concave and contains well marked depressions which receive the lower lobes of the brain. On the outside surface there are two smooth spots about the size and shape of a lima bean, called condyles which articulate with the first spinal vertebra or atlas. They are situated one on each side of the great opening. The occipital bone gives insertion to a large number of muscles, which are used in the various movements of the head.

The sphenoid bone is noted for its irregular shape. It touches at some point every other bone of the cranium and completes the formation of the base of the skull. Its shape resembles a bat with outspread wings. It joins all the bones which enter into the formation of the vault of the skull and binds them firmly together.

The ethmoid bone is situated between the orbits at the root of the nose. It is irregular in form and very light and spongy in its structure. It enters into the formation of the base of the skull and the central division of the nose, called the septum.

At birth these bones are incomplete in development and so separated from each other that they allow the edges of one to shut over the other, thus diminishing the size of the fœtal head in labor. At certain points where the bones unite last there is a temporary absence of bone. The most prominent of these openings, called fontanelles, is at the junction of the frontal and parietal bones. It is sometimes called the "soft spot" or anterior fontanelle and remains open for one or two years. The arteries of the brain give a pulsating movement to the scalp at this point and in some cases of severe sickness there is also noticed a marked depression.

As the osseous development extends these bones of the skull become joined in irregular lines, containing tooth-like projections called sutures, and they are so firmly dovetailed together or interlocked that the bones would break rather than separate on the original lines of union. These eight bones described above form in adult life a strong unyielding cavity which contains the brain. They are composed of two layers or plates of bone united by a bridgework of spongy structure called the "diploe." The external plate is thicker and firmer than the internal. The diploe is traversed by numerous blood vessels which carry nourishment to the structures.

On the outside of the skull there are numerous elevations known as prominences or landmarks. At these points there is great thickness of bone for the purpose of affording protection to the more exposed parts. On the inside there are various depressions which conform to the lobes of the brain and grooves for the blood vessels which bring the ever-needed supply of nourishment.

There are various small openings through the skull more especially in the region of the base for the transmission of numerous vessels and nerves.

The top, sides and back part of the head are covered by the scalp and its growth of hair, which is often luxuriant and ornamental. A broad and high forehead may indicate intelligence and a low, sloping forehead the opposite condition, but such indications are not always correct. Owing to the firm plates of bone beneath the scalp injuries usually extend down to the bone. They bleed freely but if properly dressed heal rapidly.

V.—THE BONES OF THE FACE.

The bones of the face are fourteen in number, and together with the eight of the cranium, already described, make up the complete bony framework of the head. There are two nasal, two superior maxilla, two lachrymal, two malar, two palate, two inferior turbinated, the inferior maxillary and the vomer.

The nasal bones are two small ones forming the sides of the upper part of the external nose and uniting in the center to form the bridge.

The two superior maxillary form, by meeting and uniting in the center, the bone of the upper jaw. They are of great interest to the surgeon, because of numerous diseases which develop in this region. They enter into the formation of the roof of the mouth, the sides of the nose, and the floor of the orbits. They contain a central cavity called the antrum of Highmore, and also give firm lodgment to the upper teeth.

The lachrymal bones are two very small ones about the size of a finger nail, situated near the inner angle of the eye. They assist in the formation of the lachrymal groove, which lodges the lachrymal sack and also in the formation of the lachrymal canal which lodges the nasal duct, hence their name.

The malar, or cheek bones, are two irregular prominent bones which are situated one on each side of the face beneath the eye. They enter into the formation of the orbits, they join the upper jaw bones in front, and contain an area of bone which extends to join the temporal bone just in front of the ear.

The palate bones are of irregular form and situated at the base of the cavity of the nose, filling up the vacant space and wedging together the other bones so as to complete the framework back of the upper jaw. They assist in the formation of the orbits, the nasal cavities and the roof of the mouth.

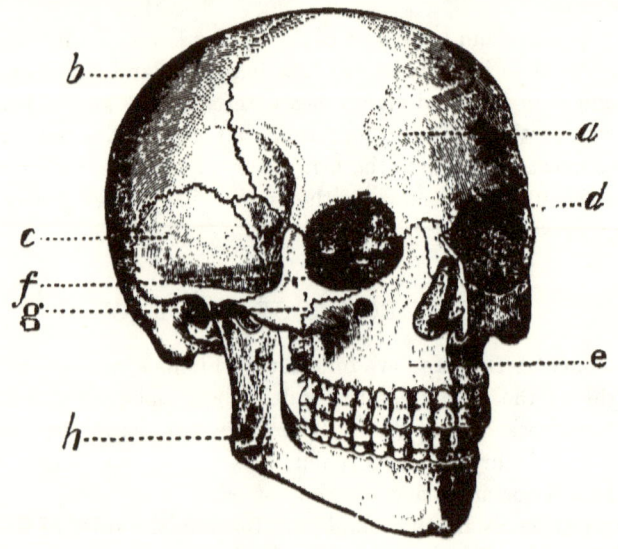

BONES OF THE SKULL AND FACE.

a, frontal ; *b*, parietal ; *c*, temporal ; the occipital is behind and out of sight, the sphenoid and ethmoid enter into the formation of the base of the skull and are not visible ; *d*, nasal ; *e*, upper maxillary ; *f*, lachrymal ; *g*, malar ; *h*, inferior maxillary or lower jaw.

The turbinated bones consist of a thin layer of bone rolled upon itself like a scroll and hence the name. They are situated on each side of the nasal cavities and assist in their formation.

The vomer forms a part of the partition in the center of the nose, and is placed vertically. It receives its name from its resemblance to a ploughshare.

The inferior maxilla is the only movable bone of the face. The main or horizontal portion of the bone is semicircular in form, and shaped like a horseshoe. It gives lodgment to the lower teeth. On each side is an upright portion which extends upward to form a joint in front of the ear; in front of the joint is a projection of bone which gives attachment to the temporal muscle. Other powerful muscles, the masseter and buccinator, are attached to this bone for the purpose of moving the jaw in biting and in the mastication of food.

At the base of the tongue is found a small bone, the hyoid or lingual, which gives support to this organ, and to which also are attached many delicate little muscles so numerous in this region. It is shaped like a horseshoe. It is not joined to any other bone, and exists simply to increase muscular attachments.

The head in man is the most prominent part of the body. It is made up of a large number of tissues, the most abundant of which is the brain within the skull. This, together with the cranial nerves, is reserved for separate consideration. We have seen that the framework of the head is made up of twenty-two bones. External to this bony framework are numerous muscles, vessels, nerves and associate tissues. The muscles of the face are numerous, and cause varied expressions which indicate fear and boldness, despair and hope, pleasure and pain, joy and grief, innocence and guilt, disgust, contempt and trouble.

Hence the face is that portion of the body which gleams with intelligence and is properly admired for its beauty. It becomes impressed with the habits of thought and the occupations of life and reveals in a tell-tale way otherwise hidden secrets. Phrenology is of trifling importance in indicating the character of a person by the external contour of the skull, but the demeanor, the general expressions of the face, the tones of the voice, these together form an array of data from which many true deductions can be made. Persons of large business capacity or those who have the reputation for great firmness or those who have been the recipients of many honors are apt to disclose without effort or intention these individual traits. Those accustomed to authority for a long time carry the head more erect until the spine becomes unyielding, the face assumes firmness and the voice becomes commanding. These are the pointers which unconsciously disclose what phrenologists profess to find in the elevations and depressions which exist on the outer plate of the skull.

VI.—THE SPINAL COLUMN.

The spinal column is made up of twenty-six bones, twenty-four vertebræ, with the sacrum and coccyx. There are seven cervical vertebræ, twelve dorsal and five lumbar. The sacrum is formed from what were originally five vertebræ, and the coccyx from four.

The vertebræ are piled into a column like empty spools upon a string, one resting upon another. This column supports the head. Behind the body of each vertebræ there is an opening which, with the others, similarly situated, forms a canal through which the spinal cord and its membrane pass from the brain, giving off branches on the way which reach every portion of the body.

Between the bodies of the vertebræ there is an elastic cushion so as to lessen jars in walking or running and prevent weariness from standing or other bodily exercise. The vertebræ are bound together strongly by ligaments, and the strong processes of bone so interlock that it requires a severe fall or injury to separate or displace them.

The upper, or cervical, is called the atlas. It supports the head, and joins the occipital bone of the skull. It is of peculiar shape, the body being absent. The occipital bone is so articulated with the atlas as to allow of nodding motion, and of throwing the head backwards. The second cervical vertebræ is called the axis, because it has a large tooth-like process which fits into the atlas. When the head turns or rotates this tooth-like process acts as a pivot and rotary motion thus takes place between the atlas and the axis.

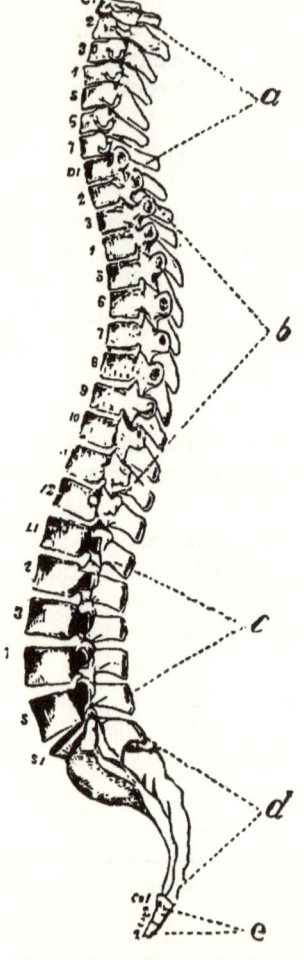

The bones of the spinal column as seen from the left side. The numbers refer to the vertebræ of the different regions.

a, cervical vertebræ ; *b*, dorsal vertebræ ; *c*, lumbar vertebræ ; *d*, sacrum ; *e*, coccyx.

The vertebræ are heavier in the dorsal than in the cervical region, and still heavier as we go downward. When the lumbar region is reached the vertebræ are very strong, thick and heavy. This is necessary to support the increasing weight of the body. The vertebræ give attachment to many muscles which control the movements in the spinal region.

VII.—INJURIES OF THE SPINE.

When a person falls a considerable distance from a tree or building the spinal column is sometimes dislocated or fractured and the cord in either case may be seriously injured. In these accidents there is paralysis of the body below the point of injury.

When such injury is in the upper region of the neck the upper limbs are paralyzed and the sufferer usually lives only a short time. The result of spinal injury varies and depends upon the amount of damage done to the spinal cord or marrow. When this is severe the cord being crushed, if the patient survives his condition is pitiable. Many of these cases terminate fatally as the result of inflammation and softening of the cord.

The spine may be sprained and the ligaments which bind the adjacent vertebræ together lacerated and yet the cord escape serious injury. When portions of the vertebræ are crushed a severe injury is indicated. The adjacent vertebræ may be dislocated. This produces pressure upon the cord and at least temporary paralysis of all the body below. The injury is recognized by a break in the continuity of the spinous processes which may be felt by running the fingers of the hand down the back. The treatment must be prompt.

Place the injured man upon his abdomen. Powerful extension must be made by four men, two at the upper and two at the lower extremities while the surgeon pushes the displaced vertebræ back into place. If this is well done and the cord is not severely injured good recovery may be expected.

The gravity of the case depends upon the amount of damage experienced by the cord. Spinal injury may result in temporary or permanent paralysis, hemorrhage or the effusion of fluid into the canal about the cord, inflammation of the cord and its membranes, and lastly softening of the cord which would be followed by hopeless paralysis. These uncertain and serious results are liable to follow an injury of the spine.

It must not be forgotten that any considerable injury to the spine renders it impossible to empty the bladder and the water must be drawn frequently by a suitable catheter. Spinal injuries ought to receive prompt surgical attendance.

VIII.—THE BONES OF THE UPPER EXTREMITIES CHEST AND PELVIS.

The scapula, or shoulder blade, is a large, flat, triangular shaped bone situated back of the shoulder. It is held in position by large muscles. At the upper, outer end it has a cup-shaped depression in which the upper end of the humerus rotates, forming a ball and socket joint. The scapula is quite thin; a large spine or brace of bone crosses the upper third and teminates in a projection, the acromion process, which helps in the formation of the cavity of the shoulder joint. There is still another projection of bone, the coracoid process, which also enters into the formation of the joint. Large and powerful muscles are attached to the sides and edges of this bone, some of which extend to the humerus and assist in the movements of the arm.

The clavicle, or collar bone, is a long bone curved like the italic letter *S*. It is situated at the top and front part of the chest above the ribs. It extends from the upper outside corner of the sternum to the acromion process of the scapula. It is a brace to hold the shoulder back in place, and its curved direction renders it more elastic, and less liable to fracture when one falls upon the shoulder. Notwithstanding this fact it is often broken, especially in childhood. Several muscles are attached to this bone, some of which aid in the movements of the head.

The humerus is a long and powerful bone situated in the upper arm and extending from the shoulder to the elbow. The upper end is a rounded head which fits into the socket of the scapula. This cup or socket is rendered deep and complete by surrounding tissues so that the head of the humerus rotates in every direction. The humerus has numerous powerful muscular attachments, large muscles coming from the front and back of the chest and top of the shoulder so as to secure a great variety of motion.

The bones of the forearm are the radius and ulna. When the hand is placed on its back these two bones are parailel, the radius occupying the outside portion. When the hand is turned over onto the palm the radius crosses the ulna obliquely. The upper head of the radius rolls upon the ulna. The ulna is large at the elbow and forms the principal part of the joint. The point of the elbow called the crazy bone is a projection from the ulna. Its true name is the olecranon process to which the triceps is attached, a strong muscle which straightens the arm.

At the wrist the radius is large and enters into the formation of the wrist joint. When one falls upon the hand the radius is often fractured near the wrist. This fracture is called a Colles fracture and is one of the most common injuries which the surgeon is called to treat. Many powerful muscles are attached to these bones which become tendons or cords as they approach the hand.

The wrist consists of eight bones arranged in two layer or rows and strongly bound together but capable of some slight movement, and hence of increasing the elasticity of the hand. The names of these are the scaphoid, semilunar, cuneiform, pisiform, trapezium, trapezoid, os-magnum and unciform. The bones of the thick portion of the hand are the metacarpal; they are five in number and they may be felt beneath the skin on the back of the hand. Four of them are parallel but the one belonging to the thumb stands out considerably from the rest.

The bones of the fingers are called the phalanges. There are fourteen in each hand three in each finger and two in each thumb. The fingers are manipulated chiefly by tendons which are the continuation of muscles of the arm.

The sternum is a flat bone in the front part of the chest. It is made up of three bones which become united into one in adult life. On each side it is joined by the clavicles and by the cartilages of the ribs.

The ribs are twenty-four in number, twelve on each side. They are long curved bones extending from the spine around to the sternum, forming the chest cavity which contains the heart and lungs.

The union with the sternum is cartilaginous. The first rib is short and crooked. The two lower ribs are not joined to anything in front and hence are called floating ribs.

The thorax, or chest, is the cavity bounded by the spine, ribs and sternum, and on the under side it is separated from the abdominal cavity by a muscular partition called the diaphragm. The ribs are so constructed that they rise and fall during every act of respiration, and thus increase and diminish the capacity of the chest alternately.

The abdominal cavity lies below the diaphragm and extends to the pelvic basin. It lies in front of the large lumbar vertebræ. There are no bones in front, but strong muscular walls. Within the abdominal cavity are the liver, stomach, pancreas, bowels and kidneys.

The pelvic cavity or basin is surrounded by strong bones, the sacrum is behind and on the sides and front are two large, broad,

BONES OF THE THORAX AND UPPER EXTREMITIES.

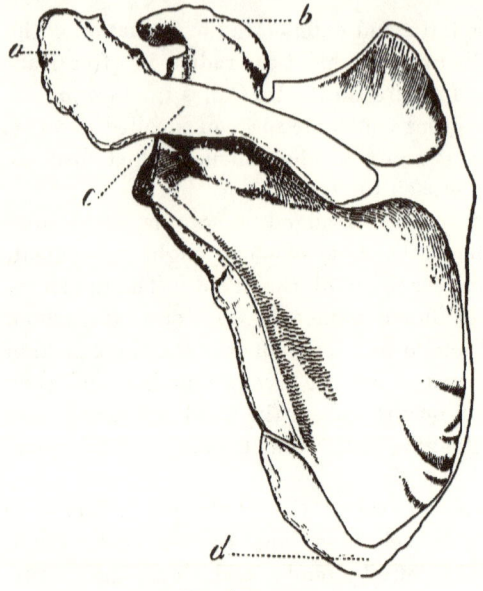

THE SCAPULA.
a, acromion process; *b*, coracoid process; *c*, spine of scapula; *d*, lower angle.

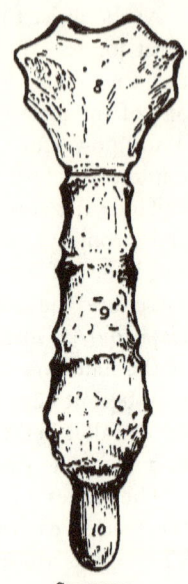

STERNUM.
The ribs are illustrated on a previous page.

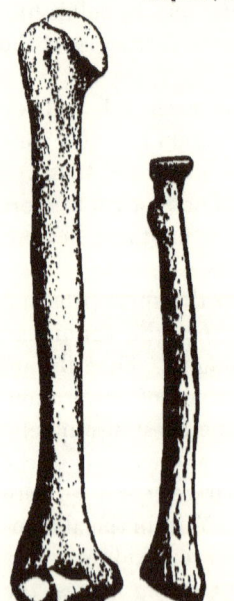

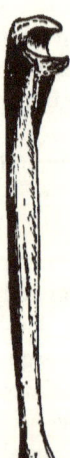

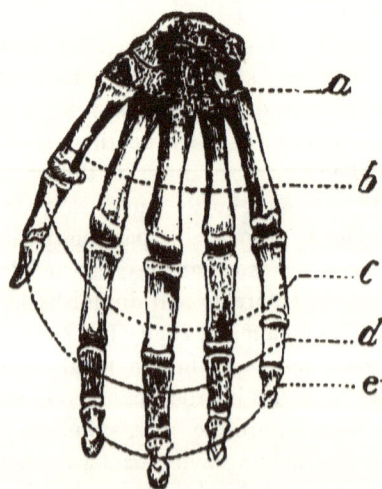

HUMERUS.   RADIUS.   ULNA.

a, 8 bones of wrist; *b*, metacarpus; *c*, *d*, *e*, phalanges.

flaring bones, and from their lack of resemblance to anything they are called the nameless bones (innominata), and they are sometimes called the haunch bones. The os innominatum in early life is composed of three bones, the ilium, ischium and pubic; these unite in adult life and form one bone.

The sacrum fits in between the innominata like a wedge. The ilium is the upper and flaring portion of the os innominatum, usually called the hip bone; the ischium is the lower portion, upon which the body rests when we sit. The rim of bone running round in front to meet its opposite is the pubic bone, and the line of union is called the symphysis. On each side there is a deep cup-shaped depression to receive the head of the thigh bone, or femur. This deep cup is called the acetabulum, and the thigh bone is held in it by a strong

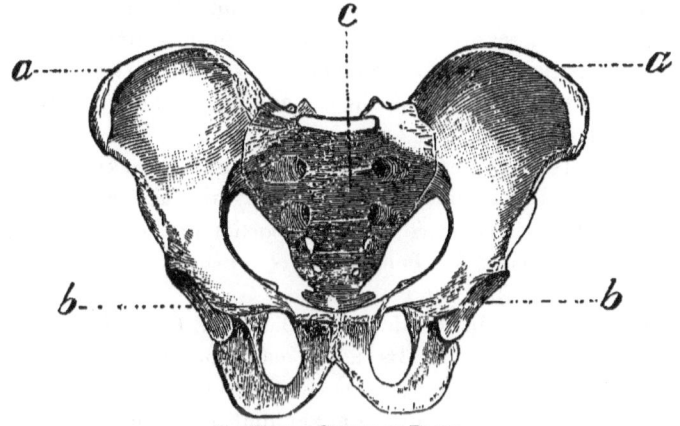

THE PELVIC CAVITY OR BASIN.
a, nameless bones (innominata); *b*, acetabulum; *c*, sacrum.

ligament, the ligamentum teres. The sacrum and innominata form the pelvis. Within the pelvis are important organs, as the bladder, the uterus and the rectum.

The pelvis is of especial interest to the physician, who must understand thoroughly its mechanism in order to be successful in conducting difficult labor or childbirth.

IX.—THE BONES OF THE LOWER EXTREMITIES.

The femur or thigh bone is the largest, longest and strongest bone of the human body. Its upper end terminates in a rounded head which rolls in a deep ball socket joint and permits of motion in several directions.

The head joins the main shaft almost at right angles. Powerful muscles from the pelvis are attached to this bone to carry out the movements necessary in walking and other varieties of exercise. The bone enlarges at its lower end to form the knee joint and the two projections are called condyles, one outer and the other the inner. The inner condyle is the larger of the two, and between the two condyles is a notch which is filled with a corresponding elevation at the summit of the head of the tibia.

The patella or knee cap covering the outer portion of the knee joint is a flat triangular one. It lies directly over the knee joint in front and is held in place by the quadriceps extensor muscle to which it gives attachment. When the leg is held in a straight position this powerful muscle is relaxed and then the bone can be moved about quite freely with the hand. It protects the knee joint which is much exposed to injuries and increases the leverage of the muscles attached to it.

The tibia is the large and prominent bone of the leg situated on the inner side of the leg. It ranks in size and length next to the femur and is the next largest bone in the skeleton. It is often called the shin bone. Its front portion lies just underneath the skin and superficial tissues and its outline may be seen by the eye or felt by the hand. Its ends are enlarged to form a portion of the ankle and knee joints. On the inside the bone projects down over the ankle and this projection is called the malleolus.

Parallel with the tibia is a long, slender, small bone of equal length called the fibula or splint. Its upper end does not enter into the formation of the joint but rests against the tibia. The lower end of this bone projects down over the ankle joint on the outside and is the outer malleolus. Fracture of this bone is often unrecognized from the fact that it is so enveloped in strong muscles that it can only be felt for a few inches above the ankle. Its chief importance is to afford attachment for the muscles of the leg and assist in forming the ankle joints.

The ankle bones are seven in number, the calcis, astragalus, cuboid, scaphoid, internal, middle and external cuneiform. These bones of the ankle together are called the tarsus, and are one less in number than the bones of the wrist, or carpus. Their arrangement is somewhat different. The os calcis forms the heel and is the largest of these bones. To it is attached a powerful tendon, the Achilles a continuation of the muscles of the calf, which raises the body upon the front of the foot in walking.

The astragalus forms with the lower end of the tibia and fibula the ankle joint. It rests upon the forward end of the os calcis. In front of the astragalus on the inner side of the foot is situated the scaphoid, while on the outside of the foot is situated the cuboid bone.

BONES OF THE LOWER EXTREMITIES.

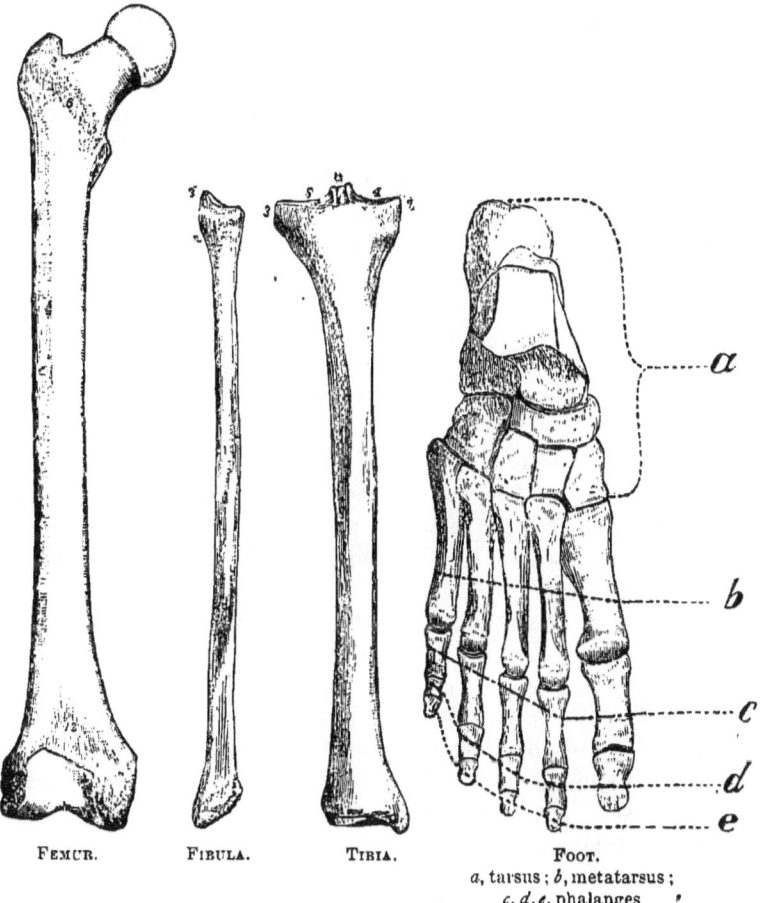

FEMUR.   FIBULA.   TIBIA.   FOOT.
a, tarsus; *b*, metatarsus; *c, d, e,* phalanges

The cuneiform are arranged in a row of three bones wedged in between the scaphoid, cuboid and metatarsal bones (see plate). The metatarsal bones are five in number and extend forward from the bones of the tarsus toward each toe.

The phalanges like those of the hand are three in number, except for the great toe, which, like the thumb, has only two. This brief description completes the bony framework of the human body; this framework gives to it form, and also gives attachment to a great variety of muscles which are essential to motion.

X.—THE JOINTS.

Nearly every bone is connected with one or more others to form a joint or articulation, which admits of varying degrees of motion to correspond to the requirements of the particular region. Indeed, some of the articulations are immovable, the bones being united so firmly in adult life as to admit of no motion. The articulation of the cranial bones are immovable, and are called sutures.

In some, only slight motion is required, and such articulations are bound together by tough, elastic fibers and cartilage, as for instance the vertebræ of the spine. In others the ends of the bones are enlarged and free motion in one direction takes place, as in the elbow and knee, which are hinge joints.

In still others there is greater freedom of motion, and the rounded head of the bone rotates in a deep depression or cup, as the shoulder and hip joints. These are known as ball and socket joints and admit of the freest motion of all the joints.

The ends of bones forming movable joints are covered over with a smooth layer of shining cartilage and bound together by ligaments, which are composed of strong, tough, elastic fibers. Around the movable joints is a thin, delicate membrane, the synovial, which secretes a thick, viscid fluid, resembling the white of an egg; this keeps the joint lubricated. Without this jointed arrangement of the bones the body would be stiff, unyielding and lacking in graceful movement. It would be impossible to sit down, to lie down, or turn either the head or body. A joint capable of motion in all directions is a ball and socket, while a joint limited to two motions, forward and backward, is a hinge joint; the elbow, knee and ankle are specimens of the latter.

XI.—THE MUSCLES.

The bones themselves have no power of motion except as they are acted upon by the muscles. Muscles possess the power of contracting when acted upon by nervous stimulus. In some muscular tissue the nerve force generated by the will causes contraction; in other tissue the stimulus is developed independently of the will power as it is necessary to keep up organic action in the digestion of food and during sleep.

There are found to be two kinds of muscular fiber; voluntary, or those controlled by the will, also known as striped muscular fibers or the muscles of animal life; and involuntary or those acting independently of the will, also known as unstriped muscular fiber or the muscles of organic life.

The muscles are composed of bundles of fibers held together and enclosed by a delicate tissue. Each bundle is composed of groups of smaller bundles and each little bundle can be separated into primitive fibers smaller in diameter than an ordinary hair.

The voluntary muscles composed of masses of fibers surround the bones and make up a large portion of the external weight of the body. Many of them are attached to the bones and by contracting cause the various movements of the body, as in walking and all kinds of manual labor. The blood supply to the muscles is abundant by means of the arterial and capillary circulation; and the nerve supply results from a profuse distribution of nerve fibers to the voluntary muscles.

There are several hundred muscles in the human body. They are attached to the bones, cartilages, ligaments and also to the skin. They vary greatly in size and form and in the manner in which their fibers are arranged. In books of anatomy the origin of a muscle refers to its more fixed attachment and the insertion to the more movable end or point; this distinction however is often arbitrary as most muscles act from either extremity. A knowledge of the action of the muscles is important to the surgeon and explains the cause of displacements in fractures and other deformities and simplifies the methods of treatment.

Some of the muscles are a guide to the course of important blood vessels and stand out as prominent landmarks of the body. The muscles have been named without reference to any particular system, some from their situation as the pectoral, temporal and gluteal; others from their direction as the rectus capitis, rectus femoris, etc.; others from their use as the masseter and the extensors and flexors; others from their shape as the trapezius, rhomboid and deltoid; others from some peculiarity of formation as the biceps and triceps, and still others from their origin and insertion as the sterno-cleido-mastoid and the sterno-thyroid.

It is necessary that one set of muscles should act in an opposite direction to another set; for instance those which bend the forearm are called flexors and those which straighten it again extensors. Such groups of muscles are termed antagonists. The muscles which close the jaw in eating must be antagonized by another set to open it.

The action of nearly every muscle in the body is antagonized by the action of some other muscle in order to produce motion in an opposite direction and establish an equilibrium. The muscles which move the eye ball form an interesting group, consisting of four recti muscles and the superior and inferior oblique.

The muscles of the arm form an important and interesting group. The deltoid rounds out the upper part of the arm, and when contracted lifts it away from the side of the body. The biceps, aided by the brachialis, flexes the forearm and hand, bending the elbow, as when a dumb-bell or weight is raised by the hand.

The triceps antagonizes the biceps and extends the forearm. The latissimus dorsi is a strong muscle of the back inserted into the humerus, or upper part of the arm. Its action carries the extended arm backwards. This muscle is antagonized by the pectoralis, a large muscle covering the upper part of the chest and inserted into the humerus, which brings the extended arm forward toward the chest. From the inside of the lower portion of the humerus, called the inner condyle, arise a group of muscles which bend the wrist and fingers, and to the outside, the external condyle, are attached the extensors, which straighten the fingers and hand, thus antagonizing the flexors.

Many other things could be said concerning the muscles, which would be of interest to those possessing professional or technical knowledge, but for general purposes the subject is too complicated for more extended consideration.

XII.—NATURE'S EFFORT TO PREVENT INJURY.

In connection with a study of the bones, it is well to notice nature's efforts to prevent injury. Nature possesses a great variety of means both for warding off injury and preventing disease. We have seen how strong and thick the bones of the skull are in order to thoroughly protect the soft tissues enclosed within. Notice the prominent ridges of strong projecting bone which surround the eyeballs to protect them from injury.

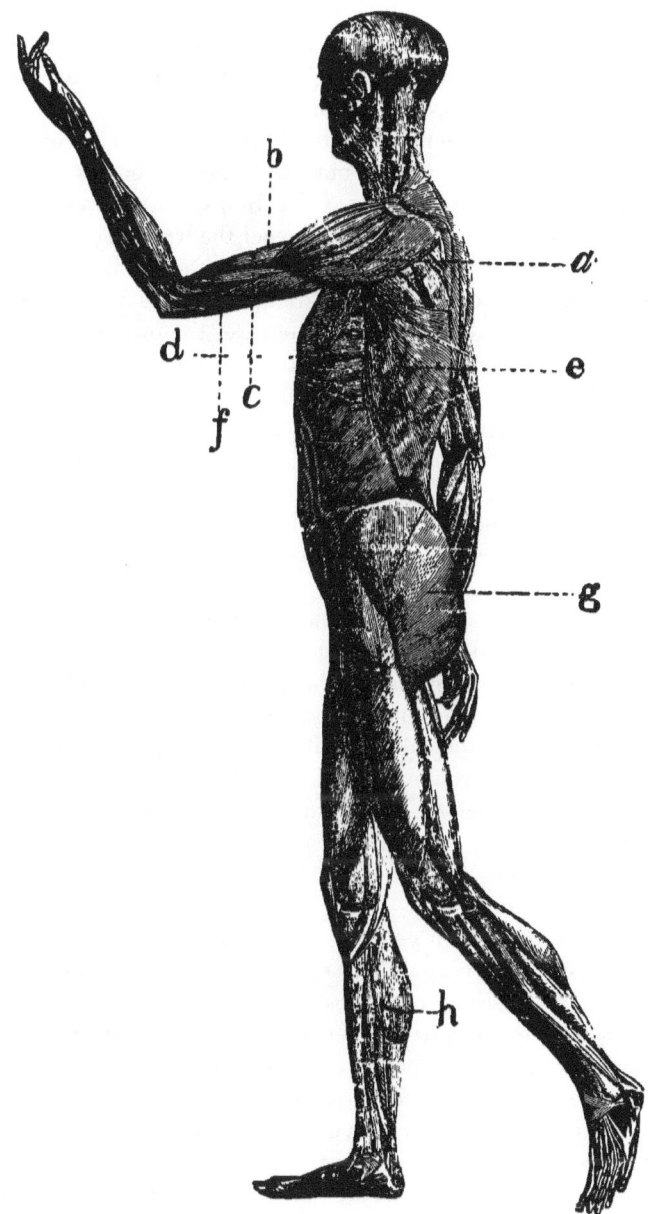

THE MUSCLES.

a, deltoid ; *b*, brachialis ; *c*, biceps ; *d*, pectoralis ; *e*, latissimus dorsi ; *f*, triceps ; *g*, gluteus ; *h*, gastrocnemius.

See the sensitive eyelids guarded by a row of long hairs along the margins to announce danger and close up the eyes so that dust and other injurious substances cannot enter.

Notice the act of vomiting, nature's process to expel disturbing substances and poisons. When mucous or foreign bodies occupy the nasal passages and the bronchi of the lungs, nature causes you to cough or sneeze violently in order to expel the irritating and harmful substance. When heat or exhaustion causes the bodily temperature to rise above the normal nature gradually opens more than two millions of little pores, by which she increases the process of evaporation, equalizes the temperature and prevents the heat from working injury, and at the same time that this evaporation is going on she takes occasion to send out noxious elements from the blood, which would have to be eliminated in other ways, or else remain to poison the system.

Did you ever think what a complex machine the human body is, and what a variety of processes are going on all the time within it?

Have you ever thought how when you climb a mountain and the air becomes more and more rarefied and nature requires an increased amount of oxygen to keep the machinery running smoothly, that the response to her call comes in more rapid breathing?

Suppose you are obliged to suffer hunger being allowed only short rations. Have you ever considered the resources of this wonderful something which we call nature, how she slowly and cautiously consumes the surplus fat laid up in the tissues, drawing upon her reserve very much as you draw upon your surplus in the bank under the force of necessity?

Suppose for any reason you are obliged to encounter exposure and severe cold, can nature again come to your rescue? Her resources are legion; she closes up the pores of your skin to prevent evaporation and the escape of heat and sends word to the kidneys that they must carry off the waste products which are eliminated ordinarily with the perspiration. In addition to this she consumes more of the reserve fat and takes in more oxygen into the lungs.

What happens when we overtax nature and she is unable to meet all the demands we make upon her? It is at this point that we begin to be made the victims of disease. Nature has great force to resist but she is not all powerful. She cannot always resist disease. She can cast off some contagious germs and resist a certain amount of poison but when each breath is loaded with poisonous germs they may get the mastery and effect an entrance into the blood where they multiply like yeast in the moistened flour and so fermentation ensues accompanied by fever and prostration. If nature becomes weakened in any way so that she is unable to eliminate the poison products of the system the avenues of the body soon become clogged and disorder follows. Biliousness, uræmia and other troubles manifest themselves.

Should nature become unable to secure sufficient nutrition to make healthy blood anæmia, atrophy, fatty degeneration and many other diseases might result.

When nature is unable to obtain sufficient oxygen to purify the blood impurities accumulate and there follows disturbed bodily functions and disease. In these cases it is not so much medicine that is required as improved sanitary conditions which will contribute to the restoration of health.

It is necessary to learn something about the complex working of nature in order to help rather than hinder her in her difficult work. Medicines cannot do the work of nature for they can at their best only assist her as oil does the machine to run more smoothly.

It may be seen from the article which follows that nature in addition to warding off injury has marvelous power to repair injuries when they have occurred and can readily accomplish a task so apparently difficult as the union of fractured bones.

XIII.—THE FRACTURE OF BONES.

Fractures are broken bones, often the result of a fall or other accident. They are known as simple, compound and comminuted.

A simple fracture is not complicated by any external wound. A compound fracture is where the skin and soft tissues are broken through by the ends of the severed bone. When the bone is broken into several separate pieces or small fragments the injury is known as a comminuted fracture. Other distinctions are also recognized by surgeons. A fracture is complete when the bone is broken clear across or severed in twain; it is incomplete when cracked or partially broken. Incomplete fractures are common in children, because the bones are more elastic, and, like a green stick, they bend rather than break. The term green stick fracture is sometimes applied to the incomplete fractures of children. A fracture is transverse when the bone is broken at right angles or straight across. When the fracture is slanting it is known as an oblique fracture. Fractures occur at all ages. In infancy the bones are flexible, and usually bend rather than break. The bones of adults are more brittle, and a complete fracture is more likely to result. The bones of old people are often quite brittle, and break from slight falls and injuries. Sometimes muscular action is sufficient to produce a fracture. In certain diseased conditions, as rickets, in some forms of atrophy, and when the bones are very much weakened by tumors or syphilis, fractures result from slight causes. A fracture may be complicated by injury of the joint, and then always awakens unusual concern on account of the liability to a stiff or anchylosed joint.

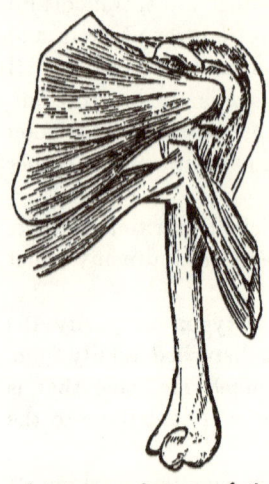

A transverse fracture of the humerus, or arm bone. This also shows the tendency to displacement due to the action of the muscles.

SYMPTOMS OF FRACTURE.

The symptoms of most fractures are characteristic and easily recognized as excessive mobility, deformity and crepitus. The character of the fracture determines the symptoms which will be manifested. If the fracture is transverse there may be no deformity at all; if it is oblique there will be deformity owing to the contraction of the muscles, which will cause the ends of the fractured bone to ride upon one another thus shortening the injured limb. The muscular attachments of a fractured bone often cause characteristic displacement, but in order to understand the peculiar action of the various muscles an extensive knowledge of anatomical surgery is essential.

After a fall or direct violence resulting in fracture, there is usually inability to move the injured limb, but by taking hold of it, it moves in an unusual manner as if supplied with an extra joint. This increased mobility is artificial and can be readily recognized. The movement however causes great pain, and the ends of the bone grate together; this grating sound is a valuable and certain sign of fracture and is known as crepitus.

Many fractures may be recognized by a shortening of the injured limb. After an injury which results in fracture considerable swelling quickly follows. This is caused by injury of the soft parts and the pouring out of serum from the tissues and blood from the numerous small vessels which are ruptured. Comparing the injured limb with the sound one is a valuable means of discovering deformity. It must be remembered by the surgeon that in the bones of young persons there are natural lines of separation known as the epyphyses and violence sometimes causes separation at these points.

Fractures of the bones of the cranium and pelvis are often obscure and may occur without being recognized.

TREATMENT OF FRACTURE.

Much care is required in the examination of a fracture in order not to augment the injury. Repeated examinations are unnecessary and likely to do further harm. When the extent of the injury cannot be made out the patient should be put under the influence of ether in order that the full extent of the injury may be learned. As soon as convenient after a fracture the patient should be attended and the fracture put up or set.

The rule for treating fractures is the most simple of all directions and the most difficult of all to follow. It is as follows : "Bring the fractured ends into perfect apposition and keep them there by splints or suitable appliances." While the treatment is so simple in theory in practice great skill and ingenuity is often required to achieve success. It requires good judgment and considerable experience.

When a person is injured and a bone broken place the limb in a natural position and bind it to a piece of board or stick to prevent movement. In fracture of the lower extremities the injured limb may be bound to the sound one after which the patient may be carried home or to a hospital. If severe bleeding occurs bind a pad over the wound and in addition raise the injured limb above the level of the head. A fracture is set in the following manner. An assistant holds the upper part of the broken limb firmly while extension is made in the opposite direction to overcome muscular contraction, then by means of a little skillful manipulation with the thumb and fingers the broken bones are brought into place or coapted. The parts having been put into the right position must be held there as immovably as possible. For this purpose well-padded splints of felt, sole-leather, wood or metal are made use of. Sandbags sometimes take the place of splints in fracture of the thigh or femur. Serviceable splints are also made of plaster of Paris and a great variety of other appliances have been used.

Plaster of Paris dressings are appropriate after all swelling has subsided, but are not recommended for the first dressing of fractures except in experienced hands. Extension is a valuable remedy in the treatment of fractures, especially of the lower extremities. It is accomplished in different ways, but most commonly by attaching a weight of eight or ten pounds to the foot and leg so as to draw over a pulley at the foot of the bed. Counter extension may be accomplished easily by elevating the foot of the bed about six inches.

Extension counteracts the contraction of the muscles and prevents the broken ends of bone from grinding against each other and from riding upon each other, as they will when one end slips by the other. Without extension there is great danger from shortening and permanent deformity of the limb. Extension also prevents a large amount of suffering from pain. Simple dressings for fractured bones are the best, for extemporized splints and other contrivances invented by the ingenious surgeon often produce better results than costly appliances. Having fixed a fractured limb by extension, sand bags may be placed on both sides of the limb to prevent movement, or they may be bound to the limb by means of plasters. From such simple appliances the author has seen almost perfect results, as well as great comfort experienced by the patient.

When the fracture is compound, that is complicated by an external wound, it must be thoroughly cleansed by a carbolic or corrosive sublimate solution. Over the wound some carbolized or iodoform gauze should be placed. Under the modern method of antiseptic dressing, compound fractures are almost wholly bereft of risk, whereas formerly they were regarded with much concern by the surgeon.

Crushed or smashed limbs may require amputation when the integrity of the nerves and arteries are so injured that life in the injured parts cannot be maintained, but at the present day many limbs are saved and perfectly restored which in former times would have been cut off. As nature possesses great recuperative force, it is often worth while to wait for her to demonstrate whether or not amputation is necessary.

Broken bones repair rapidly in young persons, only about four weeks being required to complete the whole process, but ten weeks may be required for the same process in the case of old people. The best results are obtained when the broken ends are brought into proper position and held there immovably.

It is impossible to fix a fractured rib or a broken collar bone so as to prevent some movement, but this does not prevent a satisfactory result. When a bone has been fractured there seems to be but little activity toward recovery for a few days; from the twelfth day onward, however, recovery progresses quite rapidly, and in a few weeks is complete. When the splints are removed from a fractured limb there is usually considerable stiffness, but rubbing the muscles with oil, and constant use, soon brings about perfect recovery.

It sometimes happens, though rarely, that a fracture fails to unite, owing to debility, or to a separation of the bones, by the intervention of some of the soft tissues. In such cases the surgeon's skill is usually adequate to remedy the difficulty. Time and patience are essential in all instances to the perfect repair of fractured bones.

Of the special fractures only a few of the more common will be noticed. In fractures of the collar bone, or clavicle, the arm should be lifted upward, outward and backward by the application of a suitable bandage. Rest upon the back, in bed, accomplishes this purpose admirably and should be encouraged. Fractures of the radius, or wrist, are common from falls. This fracture is usually dressed with two padded splints, and the forearm is suspended so that the hand rests against the chest with the thumb looking upward toward the face. The splints need to be worn three weeks, and often longer. Fractures of the hip, or femur, are all best treated by means of extension to overcome the contractions of the powerful muscles in these regions, and sandbags may be used to lessen the need of splints. Fractures which involve the joints should be carefully watched, and passive motion employed at the

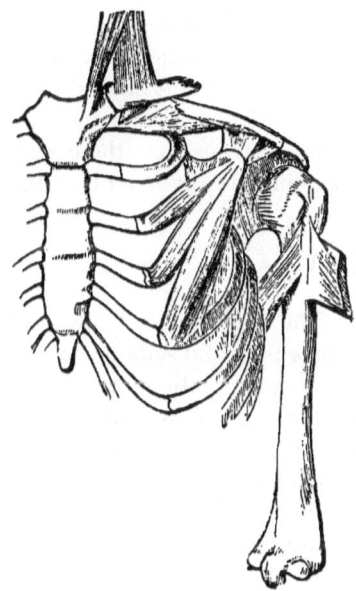

An oblique fracture of the collar bone. The shoulder drops, and there is much displacement of the ends of the broken bones.

right time to insure success and prevent an unfortunate stiffness of the injured joint. For fracture of the spine see injuries of the spine. The repair of fractured bones, if possible should be under the direction of the surgeon.

XIV.—DISLOCATIONS.

Dislocation occurs at some joint and is commonly the result of violence, the head of the bone being wholly or partially forced out of the socket or articulation. In many instances the surrounding ligaments of a joint are torn and injured as well as the muscles and other soft parts. When a dislocation has occurred the sooner the bone is put back into place the better. On account of swelling, it is sometimes difficult to determine whether a bone has been dislocated or not as the result of an injury, but typical cases are readily recognized. Dislocations are sometimes overlooked or mistaken for sprains.

SYMPTOMS.

The prominent symptoms of dislocation are deformity, loss of voluntary motion and limited mobility. There is an absence of crepitus. In cases of doubt it is the best plan to put the patient under ether when the injury can be readily made out and reduction at once accomplished. When a fracture complicates a dislocation there may be considerable trouble experienced in making out the extent of the injury.

TREATMENT.

This should be prompt and efficient. The dislocations of the small joints can be reduced readily by making extension and suitable manipulation; the head of the bone slips into place and natural mobility is restored. In reduction of the hip and other large joints, ether should be used in preference to the employment of any considerable force. The patient when brought under ether is in a state of muscular relaxation and manipulation can be accomplished without pain and the reduction of the dislocation is easily accomplished.

The head of the bone goes back through the rent made in the capsular ligament at the time of injury, if the manipulation is skillful. The after treatment consists in rest and hot packs to reduce the swelling and allay inflammation. Three or four weeks may be required for the recovery of a dislocated joint, although passive movement can be permitted after a couple of weeks and in some cases sooner. Dislocations can be reduced, weeks after they occur, by the aid of ether, but old adhesions have to be broken up by force and the risk is greater than in recent injuries.

SPECIAL DISLOCATIONS.

A few of the more common dislocations will be mentioned in detail but it would be impossible to give directions so that the unskilled could reduce the various dislocations which are liable to occur.

Dislocation of the shoulder is common and there are several varieties of this injury. It can usually be reduced by skillful manipulation without the use of ether. Dislocation at the elbow is less common, the radius and ulna being pushed backward. This gives the elbow a peculiar appearance which having been seen once will be readily recognized. This injury is easily reduced with the patient under ether by making extension upon the forearm bent at the elbow at right angles.

A dislocation of the hip is a grave accident as considerable force is usually required to produce it. There are several varieties of this dislocation. It will require a competent surgeon to treat an injury so serious as dislocation of the hip, and indeed for all the important dislocations the same is true, for no description or plates could give the ability sufficient to do this important branch of surgery. It re-

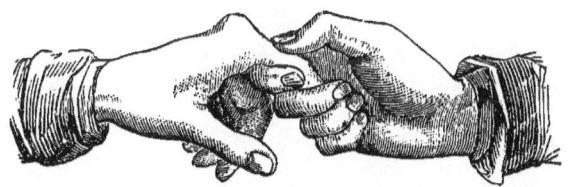

Dislocation of the third bone of the index finger, showing how to reduce it.

quires that skill which alone results from study, observation and experience. Dislocation of a finger, thumb or even the wrist anyone could probably reduce by grasping the forearm with one hand and pulling in a straight direction upon the dislocated member with sufficient force to bring it into place.

Dislocation of the lower jaw sometimes takes place from gaping or opening the mouth too widely. This injury can be reduced by placing the thumb of each hand upon the lower back teeth and making pressure downward and backward; the thumbs should be wrapped with a piece of muslin for protection. A very small amount of skill is sufficient to overcome this dislocation. Dislocation of the vertebræ of the spine is treated of under injuries of the spine. A dislocated knee cap could be brought back into place by straightening out the leg and pushing the patella into place with the thumb and fingers.

CHAPTER IX.

THE BLOOD AND ITS DISEASES.

I.—ANÆMIA. II.—CHLOROSIS. III.—LEUKÆMIA. IV.—SEPTI-
CÆMIA, PYÆMIA, BLOOD POISONING.

THE BLOOD.

THE blood is a crimson fluid which holds in solution a large number of solids. It circulates through the arteries, capillaries and veins, and changes its color from a rich scarlet to a dark red, owing to changes which take place during the circulation. The blood is a complex substance. It contains a colorless nutritive fluid, blood corpuscles, fibrin, albumen, chlorides of soda and potash, phosphates of soda, lime and magnesia. These mineral substances are held in solution and give it a saltish taste.

The blood also contains iron in solution, which gives to it color, and also colors many of the tissues which it nourishes. The blood contains a vast number of disks, called corpuscles. These are of two kinds, red and white. The red are smaller than the white, being $\frac{1}{3500}$ of an inch in diameter, and they are also much more numerous.

In some diseases these corpuscles are very greatly changed, and an examination of them shows their number much increased or diminished and the ratio between the white and red to be much disturbed. Other changes may occur, so that an examination of the blood is often of much importance and aids in ascertaining the proper line of treatment for some obscure diseases.

The red corpuscles in the blood of man differ somewhat from those of other animals. This is of considerable importance in the conviction of criminals and the vindication of the innocent.

An explanation of the appliances for examining the blood and determining the number of corpuscles would be of so little interest to the general reader, that the few interested in such studies are referred to scientific works upon this subject.

The reaction of blood is alkaline. This is determined by litmus paper, an acid fluid turning blue litmus red, while an alkaline fluid turns red litmus blue.

The specific gravity of the blood varies between 1045 and 1075. If you weigh a thousand grains of water the same measure of blood would weigh from forty-five to seventy-five grains more. The quantity of blood is about one-thirteenth of the weight of the entire body.

Blood after being drawn from the veins and standing awhile separates. That part which contains the fibrin solidifies, the fibrin enclosing in its meshes the corpuscles. This part is called the coagulum or clot, while the thin fluid which remains is the serum.

The circulation of the blood is carried on chiefly by the heart which throws or pumps a new quantity out into the arteries at every beat. The arteries diminish in size as they recede from the heart and give off many branches on the way, spreading out like a branching tree.

The capillaries are a fine network of vessels, a continuation of the arteries, and it is while the blood is passing through them that the different organs and parts take from the blood fluid, that nutrition which is required for their maintenance and for the performance of their functions, and return to it the waste products which must either be wrought over into new material or eliminated from the system.

The blood in the arteries is bright red for the reason that before it is pumped out of the left ventricle of the heart, it has just returned from the lungs where it has lost its carbonic acid and received a fresh and bounteous supply of oxygen. The difference between arterial and venous blood is chiefly this, that venous blood is deprived of oxygen and loaded with carbonic acid while arterial blood is deprived of carbonic acid and loaded with oxygen.

The blood corpuscles have great affinity for oxygen and are able to take it from the air through the thin, moist membrane in the lungs which separates the blood from the air; the carbonic acid also passes out through this thin membrane and vitiates the respired air.

The circulation of the blood is fully explained elsewhere. (See chapter on the heart.)

Diseases of the blood are frequent but most of these are somewhat obscure. The most common and important disease of the blood is anæmia.

I.—ANÆMIA.

The name of this disease is derived from the Greek language, and signifies bloodless. This, however, fails to convey the precise meaning of the term. It is a disease due to an impoverished or reduced state of the blood. This fluid becomes thin and watery and does not contain sufficient nutritive elements for sustaining and building up the weakened body.

There is found to be a great reduction, sometimes amounting to one half, in the number of the red blood corpuscles, which are essential to health. The cause of this condition may be a direct loss of blood, as in frequent or profuse hemorrhages. By overtaxing the nervous system with anxiety, care or loss of sleep, as occurs in taking care of the sick, nutrition is impaired and a condition of anæmia is developed.

Living in poorly ventilated or over heated rooms, neglecting outdoor exercise, excess of study, which draws away the blood supply to sustain the activities of the brain; novel reading, which consumes the mental force by trifling with the emotions; unnatural excitements, which use up the nerve force; irregular, unwholesome or insufficient food, or a diet consisting chiefly of pastry, confections and nicknacks; in fact, any mode of life which prevents full compensation for the bodily wastes sooner or later brings on an anæmic condition.

Young women in boarding schools, as a class, are especially liable to suffer from this trouble, on account of monotonous fare, over study, want of exercise or loss of appetite. It is impossible to prolong mental labor and escape anæmia without sufficient, wholesome, nourishing food and good digestion.

There are not a few diseases, as fevers, rheumatism, consumption and dyspepsia, which diminish the nutritive elements contained in the blood and reduce it to a thin and watery condition.

The physician recognizes this disease at a glance, often in passing a person on the street, its symptoms are so well marked and characteristic; whereas the patient's friends are slow to interpret the cause of the pallid countenance. Its approach is so insidious that months are wont to pass before the patient's friends are aware of the situation, hence it will be well to give heed to the following symptoms, which are easily recognized.

SYMPTOMS.

The cheeks, lips, and even the tongue, look pale, the ears are quite transparent, the veins have a dark, empty appearance, the heart beat is weak and rapid. These symptoms are intensified by emotion or exercise, and physical and mental fatigue follow slight exertion. Climbing a hill or ascending a flight of stairs produces rapid breathing, quickened action of the heart and perhaps palpitation. The emotions are easily excited, and such persons are often subject to fainting attacks or symptoms of hysteria, such as laughing or crying without cause. The feet and hands suffer from cold on little exposure and the whole bodily condition is one of debility.

TREATMENT.

This requires the use of varied means. Exercise in the open air and sunlight are valuable aids to recovery. Judicious bathing with friction of the skin, a nutritious diet, rest, change of scene and recreation are helpful and sometimes these simple remedies alone will be sufficient to improve the condition.

Bitter tonics are often indicated to improve the appetite and pepsin to assist digestion. In the most persistent cases of anæmia iron in suitable amount is an agent of great efficiency. Nux vomica is also a valuable remedy to aid the blood-making functions. The following prescription has been thoroughly tried and will benefit a large majority of cases.

℞ Podophyllin one grain
Reduced iron twenty grains
Ext. nux vomica four grains
Ext. gentian twenty grains
Piperine five grains

Mix and make twenty pills. Dose, one three times a day after meals.

If the condition of anæmia is the result of malaria from twenty to forty grains of quinine may be added to the above prescription. When indigestion exists three grains of concentrated pepsin may be taken with each meal. The above doses are intended for adults.

It may be added that chronic constipation is often associated with the worst forms of anæmia and should be remedied before decided improvement can be expected. For its treatment see constipation.

II.—CHLOROSIS.

Chlorosis is an affection of girls at the age of puberty and is sometimes called green sickness. It is closely related to anæmia if not, as held by some authors, identical with it. The blood is in an impoverished condition and there is a deficiency in the number of red blood corpuscles. There is usually lack of nourishment owing to poor appetite or deficient food supply.

SYMPTOMS.

The symptoms are headache, palpitation, shortness of breath, a feeling of fatigue and an inclination to sleep. Other symptoms are loss of appetite, inability to labor either with the hands or mind, cold feet and hands and pallor of the skin.

TREATMENT.

The treatment demands plenty of nourishing food, exposure to the fresh air and sunlight, sea air and sea bathing, light gymnastics and the use of the remedies suggested for anæmia to stimulate the blood-making functions.

III.—LEUKÆMIA.

This is a name given to a disease characterized by a large increase in the white blood corpuscles and a diminution in the red.

The spleen and lymphatic glands are usually enlarged and the color of the blood is more or less diminished.

The symptoms are marked pallor, enlarged spleen and enlargement of the glands in the neck and armpit. Hemorrhage from the nose occurs frequently and is difficult to control.

Unless relief is obtained these symptoms are intensified, the pallor becomes more marked, hemorrhages are more frequent, fever or dropsy may develop, and a fatal debility at length supervenes.

Malaria seems to be in some cases the forerunner of this affection. The treatment demands improvement of the nutrition and strength. The remedies recommended for anæmia are appropriate also for this affection.

IV.—SEPTICÆMIA—PYÆMIA. BLOOD POISONING.

The term blood poisoning has come into such prominence, during the last decade, that a few words upon this important subject will not be out of place in a work upon household medicine.

Blood poisoning refers to a condition of the blood and not to a particular disease. It is the result of some septic or purulent material, the product of inflammation, circulating in the blood. Nature attempts to eliminate these purulent products by absorbing them into the general circulation and then carrying them in the blood current to the different organs to be cast out of the body.

When there is acute inflammation in any part or organ of the body, as the result of disease or injury, more or less poison material is absorbed into the system. When these toxic, or putrid, products are not too numerous they are eliminated from the body with ease, along with the natural wastes of the system, which, if retained, would soon act as violent poisons. When, however, these purulent products are so abundant as to overwhelm and paralyze the nervous system, so that they cannot be removed, the patient at length becomes stupid or comatose and the whole machinery of the body stops. It is in this way that death results from blood poisoning. Sometimes abscesses break out upon the limbs, nature making an effort in this manner to assist in the work of elimination, but when abscesses form in the lungs or other internal organs death invariably results.

Septicæmia and pyæmia are the names of the condition described, but known to the people as blood poisoning.

Septicæmia is the term applied to the milder forms of blood poisoning. Pyæmia is the term applied to those severe conditions in which abscesses are formed in the internal organs or joints ending usually in death. The primary cause of septicæmia is often some injury which is regarded as slight till the symptoms of blood poisoning manifest themselves.

It is well remembered that President Garfield died of pyæmia or blood poisoning. In his case the injured bone was doubtless the cause of the trouble. Nature attempted to remove the dead particles of bone. This purulent material was absorbed into the general circulation but nature was unable to complete the work she had undertaken; for she could not eliminate the poison and abscesses formed in the lungs, and the whole system at last infected and poisoned yielded to the inevitable.

Blood poison follows surgical operations but much less often than formerly, owing to anti-septic dressings. Injuries of the bone are more liable to be followed by these disasters than other injuries.

Severe or malignant blood poisoning is liable to follow diphtheria, scarlet fever, malignant pustule, glanders, childbirth and in mild form all the germ diseases as erysipelas and consumption. In fact nearly all disease is due to waste or toxic material circulating in the system.

SYMPTOMS.

The symptoms of blood poisoning are severe chills, fever, striking variations of temperature, profuse sweating and great depression of the powers of life. Should the symptoms be severe, it indicates that the attack is also severe. The symptoms usually come on in about nine days after an injury. The wound becomes fetid, its discharge is thin and unhealthy. After a severe injury or after capital operations symptoms of blood poisoning are usually absent, but they may supervene after very slight injuries. There is this element of uncertainty, but in recent years the risk has greatly diminished. Every degree of severity may be manifest in the symptoms of blood poisoning. They may be so slight as to last only a few hours, or so severe and prolonged as eventually to produce death.

TREATMENT.

After injuries and surgical operations every effort should be made to prevent blood poisoning, by looking after every detail, as cleanness of the wound, fresh air, nutrition and diet. Sewer gas must not be permitted to enter the patient's apartment. If pus forms arrangements must be made for its escape, and the wound washed thoroughly with anti-septic solutions, as carbolic acid or corrosive sublimate. The proper strength of these solutions is given elsewhere in detail. Cleanliness should be emphasized as the most important of all measures. Sponges are objectionable and should not be used unless thoroughly disinfected and scrupulously clean.

A charcoal poultice will often improve the character of a septic wound. For a high grade of surgical fever give quinine in generous doses combined with phenacetine as follows.

℞ Quinia sulphate   one dram
   Phenacetine   thirty grains

Mix and make in twelve capsules. One of these may be given every four hours if the fever is severe until the temperature is reduced.

The diet should be nutritious. Milk, eggs and animal broths should be used. Stimulants may be required but must always be used with caution. Morphine may be used for pain and chloral or sulphonal to produce rest but always cautiously.

It would be better to confine the term blood poisoning to those septic conditions which follow operations or injuries and where some septic material is inoculated into the system as in malignant pustule, glanders and diseases of similar type. The poison of other diseases as typhoid fever, small pox, scarlet fever, diphtheria, gonorrhea and syphilis should be recognized and treated under their own individual names, and not under the name of blood poisoning.

CHAPTER X.

THE LYMPHATIC SYSTEM AND GLANDULAR DISEASES.

I.—The Lymphatic System. II.—Scrofula. III.—The Pancreas. IV.—Diseases of the Pancreas.

I.—THE LYMPHATIC SYSTEM.

WITHIN the body and found in most of the tissues is a system of delicate vessels which form a minute network converging toward the interior. They are more numerous but of smaller size than the blood vessels. They communicate with glands which are also numerous in certain locations as the neck, the axilla, the bend of the elbow, the groin, under the knee, in the mesentery and in many other situations. These vessels absorb liquid material from the tissues and convey it into the general circulation. The lymphatic vessels are also known as absorbents and lacteals.

The lacteals are more properly the lymphatic vessels of the small intestines, so named because during the process of digestion they contain a milk-colored fluid sometimes known as chyle. Chyle differs from lymph in that it contains a large amount of flat globules in a finely divided or emulsified state. The chyle is absorbed by the villi of the small intestines and is rich in nutritious material. It is mixed with the lymph and enters the circulation through the same channel.

The great central canal which conveys the lymph and chyle into the blood is called the thoracic duct. It is eighteen or twenty inches long and about the size of an ordinary goose quill. To this common duct the lymphatic vessels converge, bearing the products they have absorbed in their course, just as little streams drain the country of a certain region and convey it to the river, which swallows up all its tributaries. The thoracic duct passes up the body in front of the spinal column, carrying this liquid current which is emptied into the left subclavian vein, quite near the heart and it is then mixed with the venous blood.

These lymphatic vessels contain valves to prevent the fluid from flowing in the wrong direction and the opening of the thoracic duct

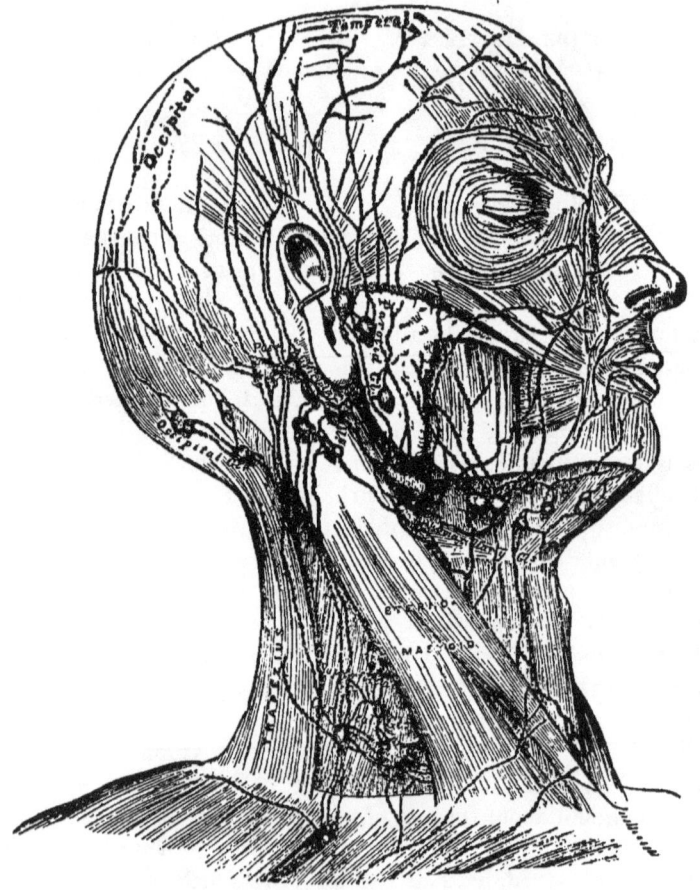

Lymphatic vessels and glands of the head, face and neck.

is also guarded by valves to prevent the venous blood from entering it. The lymphatic vessels are numerous in the cellular tissues beneath the skin and it is owing to this fact that medicines injected beneath the skin are absorbed so quickly and produce characteristic results with such certainty.

II.—SCROFULA, KING'S EVIL.

Scrofula has reference to a peculiar condition or diathesis of the system, in which there is a tendency to develop certain disorders of the glands, joints, bones, skin, and various other tissues and organs. It is concerned in indolent growths of the glandular system, and in slowly progressing inflammations, which are liable to end in the formation and discharge of pus, from a sore showing great unwillingness to heal. It often pursues a tedious and intractable course. It is largely a disease of childhood, and rarely develops after twenty years of age.

CAUSES.

Among the predisposing causes, heredity has always been believed to occupy a strong place. It has been regarded by many as the result of syphilis, manifested in succeeding generations, or several removes from the original source. Others believe it to result from some faulty composition of the blood, whereby it contains morbific or disease producing elements. All agree that it is a disease of faulty nutrition, and whatever disarranges these functions is favorable to its development.

Improper sanitary conditions are found to have a strong place in the development of scrofula, as polluted atmosphere, cold and damp situations, improper foods, unhealthy localities and habits of life.

It has been observed that scrofula is often brought into activity by the injurious effects of certain diseases, as typhoid, and scarlet fever, or measles. Diseases of the eyes, ears, various catarrhs and eczema are often properly regarded as forms of the manifestation of scrofula.

Scrofulous swellings of the glands in the neck, or chronic discharges from the ear, may follow attacks of mumps, diphtheria, measles and scarlet fever. Falls or injuries may appear to be the starting point of cases of this affection, and so slight an operation as vaccination might cause scrofula to develop if already in the system, but in the author's experience this has never occurred, and in the experience of others but rarely. It has been known to result from the severe drain upon the system due to frequent pregnancies and lactation, but this also is rare.

Many have thought tubercular disease and scrofula closely related, or perhaps the same, but the ground for such belief disappeared with the discovery of the bacillus of tubercle. It is possible, however, that those who have manifested the condition of scrofula in early life are more liable to become the victims of tubercular consumption at a later period.

SYMPTOMS.

The symptoms of scrofula may develop in any temperament or condition of early life, owing to the activity of the lymphatic glands at this period. Children who develop scrofula are apt to be pale, have soft, flabby muscles, and a capricious appetite, but to this statement there are frequent exceptions.

Children who are fussy about their food at the table, rejecting hearty articles of diet, and removing every shred of fat from a piece of roast, choosing starchy foods and sweet substances are especially prone to scrofula. Such children always feel the cold, and hover about the register; their teeth show signs of early decay. With them injuries produce unexpected results, abrasions are slow to heal, and their wounds are hard to cure, while pus shows a tendency to form on slight provocation.

Joint troubles, glandular swellings, abscesses slow to form and loth to heal, a discharge from the ear and a tendency for such ailments to become chronic, these and similar symptoms, indicate that condition to which the term scrofula has been given.

TREATMENT.

Preventive measures must consider the marriage of persons who are unlike in physical temperament, or, in other words, who are physically compatible. Two persons who have had the scrofulous tendency in early life should not marry each other. Families afflicted with the scrofula diathesis, and related, should not for a moment consider the thought of intermarriage, for the result would be puny, scrofulous children, liable to die at an early age.

Children should not sleep in the same bed with their parents. Children and young persons must not sleep in bed with old people. This is a law that ought not to be violated.

Pure air and constant attention to the subject of ventilation will do something to prevent the development of this struma.

School-rooms should be looked after to prevent over crowding, and to see that pure air, pure water, and thorough ventilation are supplied. Good appetite, good digestion, nutritious food and systematic bathing are all in the line of the best preventive remedies.

Artificially fed babies need close attention, for they are especially liable to develop scrofulous affections.

As regards medical treatment, the syrup of the iodide of iron is a valuable remedy. It may be given in doses of from ten to thirty drops to children under five years of age, and to older persons one teaspoonful three or four times a day. The teeth must be protected from its injurious effects. Cod liver oil is beneficial in thin, scrawny children, who are destitute of fat tissue.

The following is a good prescription:

℞ Lacto-phosphate of lime	four ounces
Pulverized acacia	two drams
Oil of bitter almond	six drops
Cod liver oil	four ounces

Mix. The dose is from one teaspoonful to a tablespoonful, according to the age.

III.—THE PANCREAS.

The pancreas is a glandular structure situated behind the stomach. It extends from the spleen on the left to the duodenum on the right, a distance of six or eight inches. Its shape is compared to a dog's tongue, the pointed end of which touches the spleen. It is an inch or more in thickness and an inch and a half in width and weighs two or three ounces.

The right end is broader and curved downwards fitting into a curve in the duodenum. It contains a duct about the size of a goose quill which empties into the duodenum. In structure the pancreas resembles the salivary glands. It secretes a fluid which is conveyed by the duct already mentioned into the duodenum or small intestine. This secretion mingles with the substances that have been acted upon by the gastric juice in the stomach. Its principal ingredient is called pancreatin and except for this the secretion almost completely resembles saliva. The pancreatin forms about ten per cent. of the whole secretion and renders the fluid thick and viscid.

The secretion of the pancreas is alkaline in reaction and unites with fats and oils to form an emulsion. It together with the secretion of the liver is the great factor in the digestion of fats and oils. It also converts starch into glucose or sugar at the bodily temperature with great rapidity. Fatty substances are not acted upon in the stomach but their digestion follows the passage of food into the small intestines. The action of the secretion of the pancreas is of great importance in the digestion of food which always contains a greater or less amount of fatty material.

The emulsified food is known as chyle.

The pancreas is active during the process of digestion and pours out a large amount of fluid and after the process is over it returns to a state of quiescence.

It should then be remembered that fatty substances are digested in the small intestines and that the chief agent in this process is the

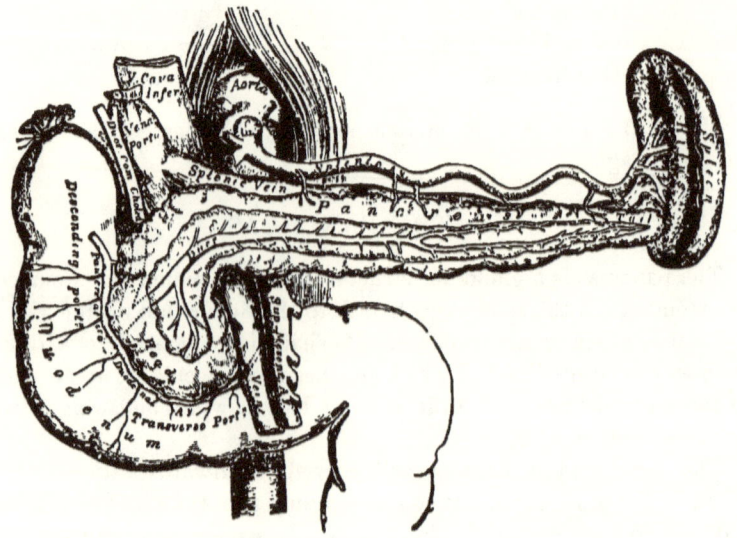

THE PANCREAS AND SPLEEN.

pancreatic juice which emulsifies them. Emulsified fats form a thick white fluid, chyle, which in appearance resembles milk. This process will be referred to later when the functions of the intestines are considered.

IV.—DISEASES OF THE PANCREAS.

Diseases of the pancreas are neither numerous nor common. Inflammation of the pancreas may take place but it is rarely recognized as the symptoms are few and similar to bilious colic and neuralgia of the stomach.

The only common affection of the pancreas about which much is known is cancer. The earliest symptom is persistent pain in the epigastric region and at length fat globules appear abundantly in the stools, jaundice and dropsy usually appear but those symptoms are confusing. Digestion is also disturbed. Other symptoms may arise from pressure by the growth upon neighboring vessels and organs.

There is the same peculiar waxy look as seen in those suffering from cancer of the stomach. The same internal treatment is applicable as in cancer of the stomach or other internal organs.

The progress of the disease is onward, and terminates fatally in one or two years. This gland may undergo fatty degeneration, but as diseases of the pancreas are more or less obscure till after death, an extended discussion would be out of place in a hand book of domestic practice.

CHAPTER XI.

THE SKIN — ITS ANATOMY, FUNCTIONS, AND DISEASES.

I.—The Skin. II—Management of the Skin. III—Cosmetics. IV.—General Observations on Diseases of the Skin. V.—Disorders of the Sweat Glands. VI.—Disorders of the Sebaceous Glands: *a*, Seborrhea or Dandruff; *b*, Wens or Tumors of the Scalp; *c*, Baldness or Alopecia. VII.—Acne and Comedo. VIII.—Milium. IX.—Prurigo, Itching or Pruritus. X.—Shingles or Herpes Zoster. XI.—Eczema, Tetter, Milk Crust or Salt Rheum. XII.—Urticaria, Hives or Nettle Rash. XIII.—Psoriasis. XIV.—Leprosy. XV.—Lice or Pediculosis. XVI.—Itch or Scabies. XVII.—Ring Worm or Tinea. XVIII.—Favus. XIX.—Freckles or Lentigo. XX.—Moles. XXI.—Warts. XXII.—Corns or Clavus. XXIII.—Bunions. XXIV.—Scurvy.

I.—THE SKIN.

IN order to explain the functions of the skin it is necessary to give a general description of its anatomy. It will be sufficient to say that the skin is made up of two layers although others are sometimes given. The derma or true skin and the epidermis or scarfskin, also called the cuticle.

The epidermis or scarfskin is a tough layer upon the outside of the body varying in thickness in different places, conspicuously upon the hands and soles of the feet. It is composed of flattened cells which are constantly exfoliated and renewed by the growth of the parts underneath. It forms a covering for the true skin, it limits the evaporation of fluids from the body, prevents the absorption of poisons and protects from other injury.

The epidermis is rendered thick by the sunlight and rough usage but is soft, thin and smooth where the body is protected by clothing or otherwise from exposure. While the outside is dry and tough and constantly becoming waste to be cast off, the inner surface is soft, moist and more like living tissue.

The scarfskin contains a substance called keratin which neither water nor alcohol will dissolve. The microscope is essential to aid in studying and understanding the anatomy of the skin. The color of the skin is due to a pigment deposited in the lower layer of the epidermis. The amount of pigment is influenced by the rays of the sun. In hot or tropical countries people have yellow, brown or black skins.

The dermis or true skin lies beneath and in contact with the epidermis. It is composed of strong, dense, tough fibers which interlace each other, some of which possess elastic properties. It also contains nerves and lymph vessels while the whole is traversed by a network of small blood vessels which make it appear red wherever the scarfskin is removed. It varies in thickness in different places. The skin rests upon a layer of connective tissue and fat.

The skin has a variety of appendages as hair, nails, sudoriferous and sebaceous glands.

The roots of the hair or hair bulbs are deeply implanted in the derma or true skin and in close contact with a little papillary elevation which contains a blood vessel that supplies nutrition. Each hair is composed of a shaft outside a central pith.

The nails are similar in composition to the epidermis of which they are a modification. They are firmly attached to the skin and seem to be chiefly designed to protect the ends of the fingers and toes. The main portion is called the body and the lower portion from whence growth takes place is called the matrix.

The sebaceous glands are little bodies imbedded in the lower strata of the true skin, where they secrete an oily liquid. They are more numerous in the scalp and face than in other parts of the body. About the face and nose they are often large and become congested, containing a thick, oily secretion, which, when pressed out, resembles very much a small worm.

The sebaceous glands open usually by means of a little duct into the hair follicles close beside the hair bulb, and the secretion lubricates the hair and prevents it from becoming dry and brittle. On the face the sebaceous glands open mostly upon the surface of the skin, and prevent it from becoming parched and chapped by the sun's rays. In hot countries these glands do not secrete sufficient material to protect the face and hands, and oil is used to supply the deficiency and prevent the exposed parts from chapping.

The sudoriferous, or sweat glands, are very numerous, and are found throughout the entire surface of the body. They present little, valve-like openings upon the surface, which are connected by spiral tubes, or ducts, with little yellow globular glands, situated on the under surface of the true skin. These tubes, or ducts, which lead to the surface are presided over by delicate little sensitive nerves, which

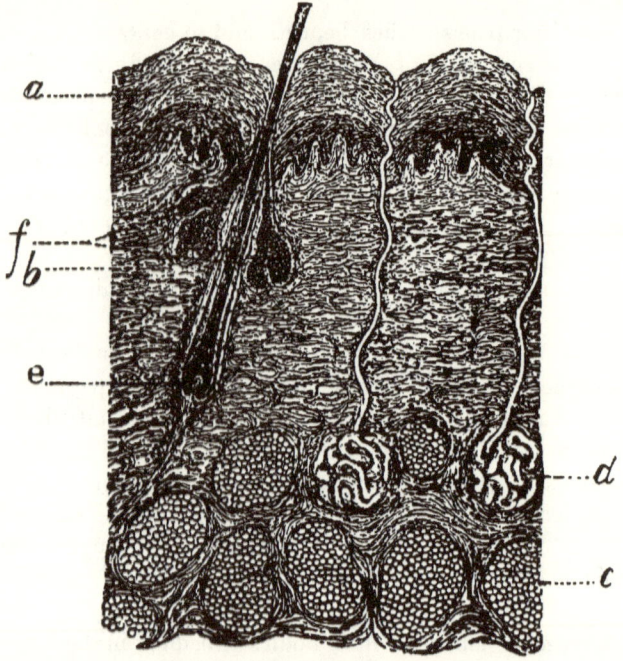

A SECTION OF HUMAN SKIN MAGNIFIED.

a, the epidermis, or scarfskin; *b*, the true skin, or dermis; *c*, fat cells under the skin; *d*, a sweat gland with a duct, or canal, leading to the surface; *e*, a hair bulb with a shaft leading to the surface; *f*, sebaceous glands near the hair shaft.

respond to the influence of heat and cold. The latter contracts and the former expands these tubes. This is an arrangement for regulating the temperature of the body.

These tubes, which convey the moisture to the surface, are large, and exist in great numbers in the armpits and groins, and hence in these places free perspiration takes place. In the palms of the hands the sweat glands are very numerous, but much smaller usually than in the armpits, otherwise the moisture of the hands would be quite annoying in summer. It is estimated that there are between two and three millions of these sudoriferous, or sweat glands, in the human body, every one connected with the surface by a spiral canal and valve-like orifice, and if all these tubes were stretched into one connected line it would measure over eight miles.

The body is always perspiring, but when the amount is unobservable it is called insensible perspiration. When the body becomes over heated by hot weather, by exertion, or artificial heat, these tubes dilate and the activity of the sweat glands is greatly increased, so that drops of moisture are seen trickling down from the face. Men in the hay field, or those working upon the railroad track, and elsewhere, often sweat profusely, and are obliged to drink large and copious draughts of water to replace that lost by the evaporation going on at the surface of the body.

With this moisture a large amount of waste material is carried out, which amounts in an active person to over two pounds daily. Work always means destruction of tissue, and the debris must be removed; for it is charged with carbonic acid gas. It will be seen that a process quite similar in some respects to respiration goes on in the skin by means of the sweat glands. Not only does carbonic acid gas pass off through the pores, but a small amount of oxygen is absorbed. This process of absorbing and expelling gases is essential to the maintenance of animal heat. Animals that have been varnished over soon die and the blood is found to be deficient in oxygen.

The process of sweating performs two main objects; the elimination of waste and the increase of evaporation whereby the animal heat is reduced and prevented from becoming excessive. Hence it is that we can be exposed to high ranges of temperature without serious injury and that the skin is able to assist the kidneys in eliminating waste products from the system.

The odor of assafœtida, musk, garlic and sulphur can be detected in the perspiration soon after being taken in considerable quantity into the stomach. It is also probable that every human being exhales a peculiar odor in his perspiration which enables a dog whose sense of smell is very acute to distinguish one person from another and several hours after to recognize the track of his master. The dog probably recognizes as great difference in the odors of two persons as we do in their form and features.

The blood vessels of the skin are very minute arteries and capillaries growing smaller and smaller as they extend upward toward the surface. They are very numerous, forming a complete network throughout the true skin and so dense are they that the prick of the finest cambric needle wounds several of them. The fibers of the skin cross each other obliquely thus leaving small openings through which the blood vessels and nerves pass and form a terminal network, which are finally gathered together in little elevations under the epidermis. These elevations can be plainly seen in the palm of the hand and inner side of the fingers. When these blood vessels have reached their highest point and smallest size they terminate in returning veins which pass back through the openings already described.

The blood vessels of the skin supply the glands, the hair follicles and all the other tissues connected with it with that abundant nutrition which is essential for their warmth and development. So small are they that they measure less than a thousandth part of an inch in diameter, but they are capable of a large amount of expansion should the sensitive little nerves which preside over them be temporarily paralyzed or suffer shock as is the case in the familiar act of blushing.

After intense cold is experienced and before the nerves have recovered their activity marked congestion of the skin is noticed. Belladonna or atropia in full or repeated doses temporarily disables or paralyzes the terminal nerves and allows a large amount of blood to be thrown into the superficial blood vessels. Sometimes such a course is pursued in giving medicine in order to congest the blood vessels of the skin and relieve congestion of the lungs and other internal organs. The ease with which the superficial blood vessels dilate is sometimes a great relief to the delicate and sensitive organs within.

The nerves of the skin are numerous forming a delicate network of fibers. The greater part of these are acutely sensitive and supply us with the delicate sense of touch. Others preside over the blood supply and nutrition and regulate all the various functions of the skin, including absorption and secretion of the glands. Various sensations as of pressure and pain, heat and cold, soft and hard, smooth and rough, are transmitted to the brain by means of these terminal nerves whose sense of touch is exceedingly delicate.

These nerves of touch are gathered together in masses with the terminal blood vessels and form papillæ or little elevations in the palm of the hands and the fingers and also in the lips where the sense of touch is exceedingly delicate. Blind persons are taught to read by passing their fingers over raised letters. Owing to the absence of sight the sense of touch becomes more highly developed so that they can distinguish coins, transact business and do many kinds of work which would seem impossible without sight.

The lymphatic vessels are abundant in the skin; they absorb a certain portion of waste liquid material and convey it back to the circulation. Here nature shows her economy by casting off that which is poisonous and for which she has no further service and re-using all that can be of any further aid to the system.

The skin, upon close inspection, as we have already seen, is found to contain little lines or furrows and elevations, which are composed of a minute artery and vein, or blood points, and the meshes of the nerves of touch already referred to. These elevations are called papillæ, and are very minute and abundant, the tip of the finger containing several hundred. On account of the existence of these papillæ in the external portion of the true skin, that portion is sometimes called the papillary layer.

The study of the skin in general is of great interest. It forms a wonderfully efficient, intricate and beautiful covering for the body, without which man would be incapable of communicating with the world about him. So necessary is the scarfskin to our existence and to the well being of the structures beneath it, that existence could be maintained only a few hours without it. The skin regulates all the impressions made upon the body by the world around us, and in health enables us to receive these impressions without distress and transmits them to the brain. Thus we become conscious of the world around us and the properties of material things.

The millions of pores of the skin stand ever ready to do their important work in the elimination of effete material and the regulation of the temperature of the body. The skin is in full sympathy with the lungs, the kidneys and other organs of the body, and aids as is necessary in the performance of their work. In fevers, almost the first sign of improvement is manifested by the activity of the skin.

The skin is subject to a great variety of diseases, some of which are of serious import. These we will consider as their importance requires. Every intelligent person should be interested in this subject. If ladies would give more attention to this complex organ they would be unwilling to cover the face with injurious lotions and powders, which in the end can only harm the delicate bloom of the complexion they are so anxious to preserve.

Not only is the skin subject to a great variety of diseases, but it shares in all the disarrangements of the system. Fever disturbs its functions, also indigestion, congestion of the liver, the eating of certain unwholesome foods, and the use of certain medicines. Before entering upon the special diseases of the skin some general remarks will enable us to comprehend the subject more fully and render the consideration of skin diseases more satisfactory.

II.—MANAGEMENT OF THE SKIN.

The skin requires considerable attention to preserve it in a healthy condition. Its structure is complex as we have seen, its functions are various hence it is liable to become disordered by a great variety of causes. Many diseases of the skin if not caused are certainly augmented by an improper diet and in the management of the skin the question of food in its relation to health stands first.

There are many conflicting ideas with respect to diet which we shall not attempt to discuss. It is sufficient to say that food should be adequate in quantity and of suitable variety and quality. It seems probable that in this country at least more persons are over than underfed and that on the whole too much meat and heating food is consumed. Those afflicted with skin affections should pay particular attention to the diet and avoid greasy food, rich gravies and pastry. Moderation is as essential in eating and drinking as in labor either of body or mind.

It is possible to eat too much meat thereby clogging the portal circulation and obstructing the various outlets of the eliminative system. This acts unfavorably upon the skin and gives it a muddy appearance if it does not contribute to more marked disturbances.

Tea and coffee do not improve the complexion, and if used should be of good quality and employed moderately. Vegetables are essential to health as they contain various chemical properties which are required to keep the system and especially the skin in a healthy condition. Scurvy never breaks out unless the diet is deficient in this respect.

A variety of ripe fruits may be regarded as conducive to health.

Beer drinking is unfavorable and will certainly injure the complexion if persisted in. Alcoholic spirits cause congestion of the capillary blood vessels of the face, and unduly stimulate the sweat glands, and are objectionable on this score as well as on many others.

Avoid especially over indulgence at night. Do not eat heartily enough to spoil the appetite for breakfast. A poached egg or two, or a slice of lean cold roast, with a baked potato, a slice of stale bread or toast or fruit sauce, ought to be a sufficient meal for the close of the day. More than this overtasks the eliminative organs and works detrimentally.

There is one other important matter associated with the care of the skin, and that is cleanliness. The surface of the body is not only exposed to dust and dirt, but the evaporation of the perspiration leaves upon it a residum of salts and fatty matter which requires frequent removal to prevent an offensive odor from the person. In addition to this, scales of epidermis are being constantly exfoliated; and all such dead and waste material should be removed. Cleansing requires the addition of a small amount of soap to the water, as the alkali acts upon the fatty waste material and accomplishes its removal.

After this is removed, rinse the face, hands or body in pure water and rub till thoroughly dry. Friction is a valuable promoter of a healthy skin. Hot water is, for many reasons, preferable to cold for sponging the skin. It is beneficial to the complexion of the face. In some diseases, as acne and eczema, it also possesses curative properties.

Outdoor exercise is beneficial to the skin. Do not be afraid of tan or freckles.

The scalps of children should be kept clean. Do not allow scurf and dirt to accumulate. Water to which a little pulverized borax has been added will be found serviceable for removing dandruff; do not use the costly washes advertised for sale, for they are no better than water to which a little alcohol has been added.

When skin diseases exist they should always be cured if possible. Health is always preferable to disease. There is no more danger in curing diseases of the skin than there is in curing disease in any other part or organ of the body.

Children of low vitality should not be bathed or immersed in cold water. A warm sponge or towel bath is much preferable. The parts liable to chafe may be dusted, after bathing and drying, with rice or talc powder.

III.—COSMETICS.

If these were essential to health or even good looks there would be some excuse for their use. It is known that they do not make the skin fair nor improve its condition in any respect but do just the opposite, for they extract from it oil, rendering it faded, wrinkled, dry, chapped, sallow and unhealthy, and hence after awhile injure the complexion and it would seem as though no one could be induced to make use of them.

Those which contain lead or mercury are poisonous because these minerals cannot be used without being absorbed into the system more or less and without doing injury to the skin and destroying its natural qualities. It is impossible to use cosmetics and conceal the fact from the eye of any person who has any keenness of perception. This last fact should deter any sensible person from their employment.

The following is a non-poisonous mixture which can be prepared by any good druggist, and when the use of cosmetics is considered necessary to cover over some natural blemish is recommended on account of its being safe and free from deleterious substances.

  ℞ Wheat starch   four drams
     Zinc oxide   half a dram
     Magnesia carbonate   four grains
     Red carmine   one grain
     Ol rose   three drops

Mix. Apply as needed.

It should be remembered that beauty does not consist in a painted face. Beauty has been defined by a recent writer as intelligent expression combined with refined manners, pure skin, healthy bloom, sparkling eye, pearly teeth and smiling lips.

IV.—GENERAL OBSERVATIONS ON DISEASES OF THE SKIN.

There are in all about sixty distinct diseases of the skin enumerated, a few of which are important from their frequent occurrence. Others are less important because rare, and in this work deserve only a passing mention, while many others are more properly omitted.

Some skin diseases are well known and easily recognized by any experienced person. Still a greater number are so rare that the busy practitioner, outside of the large cities, scarcely ever sees them. Many diseases of the skin, as might be supposed, are so mild as to cause but little disturbance, and are without danger, while others may be formidable, obstinate or perhaps malignant.

In nearly all acute diseases and inflammations the skin manifests sympathetic symptoms of the affection to a greater or less extent. In the acute stage of scarlet fever the skin is hot, dry, red and itchy, and the exfoliation which takes place after recovery proves how great was the disturbance of this organ.

As we have seen, the skin is very liberally supplied with sensitive nerves. It is owing to this fact that injuries like burns and scalds even though superficial, when a large extent of the surface is involved, often prove fatal. The nervous system is liable to suffer from shock when any powerful impression is suddenly made upon it.

When a person is overheated and all the pores of the skin are dilated or relaxed, a cold current of air striking the body produces a violent impression upon the cutaneous nerves and perhaps temporarily paralyzes them, or else the shock is transmitted to the great nerve centers which control the processes of organic life. A cold, a fever or congestion of some internal organ may result. Many a fatal sickness has had its beginning in a current of air after the manner described.

In a similar way the nervous system may be shocked by the excessive drinking of ice water when overheated and occasionally the shock is said to have been sufficient to produce death. Fatal results have sometimes followed a blow upon the abdomen, apparently of insignificant force but sufficient to startle and paralyze the nerve centers.

Sudden checking of the perspiration, apparently trivial, often powerfully impresses the nervous system, throws it into a state of shock and it is in this manner that those grave results are brought about which are attributed to catching cold. An entire arrest of the functions of the skin would prove speedily fatal. In reality this never occurs but to a partial arrest of these functions a vast number of serious complaints as catarrh, pleurisy, bronchitis, croup and many others can often be attributed.

When the secretions of the skin are partially arrested extra labor has to be performed by the lungs, the kidneys and all the eliminative organs. If at such a time there is weakness or disease of these compensating organs the danger is much increased.

It is an old notion that skin diseases are due to impurities of the blood; this notion though false is so strongly intrenched in the minds of the people that a statement of the truth stands little chance of being believed. Another old fallacy is that eruptions upon the skin should not be too speedily cured. Effort should be made to cure eruptions upon the skin with as much promptness as disease of any other part or organ.

Before entering upon a description of particular skin diseases, a few general observations will assist much in a complete understanding of what follows, and render it possible for the uninitiated to diagnose the more common skin affections.

A red spot, or blush, upon the skin is due to an excessive blood supply in the capillaries; it may be temporary or permanent. Blushing is temporary, and due to a slight shock of the vasomotor nerves of the face, by means of which shock or temporary paralysis the blood supply of the capillaries is momentarily increased and the blood rushes in and distends them to the extent of their capacity. Belladonna may be given in sufficient doses to paralyze for the time being the cutaneous nerves which regulate the blood supply of the capillaries and produce a pink blush upon the skin.

In scarlet fever the poison of the disease probably paralyzes the tropic cutaneous nerves, hence the skin is hot, dry and flushed from an excessive blood supply.

A red spot upon the skin, due to hyperæmia, is known as erythema, but when the spots are small they are sometimes called roseola.

The term papule (a pimple) is applied to small, inflammatory elevations of the skin the size of a pin head, and sometimes a little larger. When the diameter of a papule is about one-third of an inch or more it is then known as a tubercle. A tubercle is smaller than a tumor.

Vesicles are little cone-shaped elevations which contain a straw-colored fluid; they usually cause itching.

Pustules are small elevations which contain pus or matter. A vesicle may become a pustule at a later stage.

Tumors vary in size from a hickory nut to a goose egg. A tumor is a general term which is applied to any swelling or growth, as a wen or cancer.

Scales are flakes of dried epidermis. In some inflammatory affections, especially after scarlet fever, their proliferation is abundant.

Excoriations are portions of the skin denuded of epidermis by scratching, friction, some slight injury or otherwise.

Crusts are composed of fluids which dry and harden after exuding from an inflamed surface. In infantile eczema such crusts are abundant, hence the name milk crust. They vary in size and shape and their contents are serum, pus and blood. When they are composed of blood they are dark colored, when of serum alone they are yellow.

Fissures are cracks in the skin which vary in length and depth, situated about the corners of the mouth, nose, ear, neck, tips of the fingers, soles of the feet, bends of joints, and in folds of the skin subject to motion and tension. They are often quite troublesome and painful, and interfere with the natural movements of the parts to a greater or less degree.

Ulcers are destructions of a portion of the skin due to suppuration or the formation of pus. They vary in size, depth and appearance. They result from various causes, as diseases or injuries. A simple ulcer tends to heal readily. Chronic or indolent ulcers are more difficult to heal. Malignant ulcers possess a sloughing and gangrenous character, and the destruction of the diseased tissue is essential to the healing process. Unless this can be accomplished the destructive process continues till vital organs are involved.

Scars are new tissues resulting from burns, scalds, wounds, ulcers and numerous injuries. They are usually painless and they vary as much as do the injuries by which they are caused.

Skin diseases are usually classified by authors, and such classifications are numerous. If simple, they are an aid to the student, but no classification would help the readers of household medicine, since so many affections treated in technical works are here omitted.

It is well, however, to bear in mind that certain affections of the skin are due to disorders of the glands, others are due to inflammatory action, while others are due to vegetable or animal parasites.

It is well to bear in mind that syphilis causes disturbances of the skin to a remarkable degree.

V.—DISORDERS OF THE SWEAT GLANDS.

There may be lack or excess of perspiration, or there may be offensive odor to the perspiration and these may exist to such an extent as to require treatment.

Absence of perspiration causes a dry and unnatural condition of the skin which is greatly relieved by the application of olive oil or vaseline to the surface. This is liable to occur in the early or hot stages of fevers in diabetes and albuminuria. Suitable for absence of perspiration are vapor or hot baths followed by the application of oil to the surface of the body.

Excessive perspiration may cause weakness and exhaustion. It is very rarely that death is caused by the exhaustion from excessive perspiration. Excessive perspiration often occurs in rheumatic and malarial fevers, in pyæmia, consumption and at times in some other affections. When this condition exists much relief is obtained by sponging over the body with alcohol and water and a complete change of clothing.

The excessive perspiration of certain portions of the body as the palms of the hands, soles of the feet, the armpits and groins is often troublesome. This condition is rendered especially annoying when attended by offensive odors.

The treatment consists in frequent bathing of the parts with cleansing lotions, as for instance water to which a small amount of permanganate of potash sufficient to give to it a crimson tinge has been added. Frequent ablutions of the feet are needful and when this does not prevent the detection of unpleasant odors a little borax, two teaspoonfuls, may be used in the foot bath and a little boric acid dusted into the stockings which are to be worn only for a single day without change. For offensive perspiration sulphur taken internally is highly recommended. The following is reliable.

   ℞ Pulv. sulphur precip.   two drams
    Pulv. chalk comp.   four drams
    Pulv. cumin comp.   two drams

Mix. Take a level teaspoonful in water each night and morning.

Where the perspiration is general instead of being confined to some local region atropia sulphate is an excellent remedy. A tablet containing $\frac{1}{100}$ of a grain should be taken each night and morning, the dose being increased, as toleration is established, to $\frac{1}{50}$ of a grain, or perhaps more.

A wash, containing astringents, as alum and tannin, is harmless, and may be used to check temporarily excessive sweating of the armpits. For the most part disorders of the sweat glands are due to diseases of internal organs, which should receive appropriate treatment.

Excessive perspiration may cause in infants a condition known as prickly heat. It is the result of hot weather, combined with an excess of clothing. The body should be sponged over with soda or borax water; two teaspoonfuls of borax or soda is sufficient for a bath, and heavy clothing exchanged for that of a lighter character.

What is called the red gum of infants is of the same nature as prickly heat, and requires similar treatment, viz.: a light, bland diet, light clothing and cooling or saline drinks, as citrate of magnesia, occasionally, until quite free action of the bowels is secured.

A bland dusting powder, as the following, is beneficial: Oxide of zinc and starch, equal parts, dusted over the surface, or the stearate of zinc with boric acid.

VI.—DISORDERS OF THE SEBACEOUS GLANDS.

1. SEBORRHEA, OR DANDRUFF. 2. WENS OR TUMORS OF THE SCALP. 3. BALDNESS OR ALOPECIA.

Seborrhea.—Seborrhea is an affection which may occur on all parts of the body supplied with sebaceous glands. The cause of seborrhea is unknown, but it is supposed to be due either to an excessive or an altered secretion of sebaceous matter. There are two general varieties of this affection, one dry and the other moist, but both contain the evidence of oil either in fluid or solid form. Moist seborrhea is common on the face of young persons, especially those of dark complexion, to whom it gives a glossy or greasy look.

Dry seborrhea is a very common affection of the scalp known as dandruff, the hair being filled with immense numbers of fine epithelial flakes, apparently dry, but always oily. Moist seborrhea of the scalp is often seen in infants, if bathing is imperfectly performed. It appears as crusts upon the top of the head, upon which dust collects, giving to the scalp a dirty, scabby appearance and a rancid odor.

Dry seborrhea, of which there are several varieties, requires the more especial attention, on account of its liability to injure the lustre and nutrition of the hair and cause it to fall out. It is one of the most frequent causes of premature baldness.

Dry seborrhea of the scalp and loss of hair are frequently caused by acute diseases, as fevers, and such loss of hair may be temporary or permanent. Dry seborrh'ea of the scalp often causes a mild grade of itching, but usually there is no inflammation of the skin which is found to be quite healthy beneath the dandruff. Unless the fine scales are very abundant or the hair falls out freely but little attention is given to this common affection.

TREATMENT.

This is apt to be tedious, the affection frequently lasting for years. Sometimes there exists a debilitated condition of the general system which requires appropriate treatment. Gastric troubles should be remedied and tonics administered according to the needs of each particular case.

For seborrhea of infants it is necessary to soften up the crusts by the application of sweet oil or vaseline and then to wash the head thoroughly with castile soap and warm water, or with a solution of glycerine, borax and water or buttermilk may be used.

External remedies are beneficial to soften the secretions and aid in their removal, to improve the general condition of the skin and to prevent the reappearance of the affection. Dry seborrhea will be benefited by the following:

℞	Sulphur sublimed	twenty grains
	Thymol	fifteen grains
	Vaseline	one ounce
	Oil bergamot	one-fourth of a dram

Mix. Rub some into the scalp each night.

After washing and cleansing the head thoroughly with soap and water or the borax and glycerine lotion the following may be used:

℞	Corrosive sublimate	one grain
	Rose water	one dram
	Vaseline	four drams
	Oil of sweet almonds	two drams

Mix, and rub a little into the scalp every night.

This affection is apt to recur.

Wens or Tumors of the Scalp.—A wen is a sebaceous tumor, occurring most frequently upon the head. A wen may be due to obstruction of the outlet of a sebaceous gland, and its secretion being retained forms a tumor of varying size.

The contents of a sebaceous tumor may vary. It is sometimes

solid and sometimes fluid. A degeneration may occur when the tumor softens and suppurates, the contents finally escaping by ulceration. These growths are sometimes mistaken for cancers.

TREATMENT.

This consists in removal. An incision should be made into the tumor and the accumulated material removed together with the sack which surrounds it. A small wen can sometimes be squeezed out by the thumb and finger, using sufficient pressure. The risk of removing a sebaceous tumor is very slight. Cancerous tumors of the skin are included under the general subject of cancer.

Baldness or Alopecia.—Baldness of a whole or even a small part of the head is never desirable. It is usually regarded as a sign of approaching age, but this is not necessarily so, for many persons are more or less bald before reaching forty years. In some families baldness comes on at an early period. It may occur in persons otherwise healthy, and in such cases it is often due to hereditary tendency.

There are several varieties of baldness, as congenital, presenile or premature, and baldness due to some affection or mismanagement of the scalp.

Congenital baldness is usually unimportant, as in most cases it exists only for a limited time, and does not require treatment. Children born without hair usually develop a growth of it in at least one or two years without treatment.

Senile baldness, or that of old age, is another form about which but little is necessary to be said. After forty-five or fifty it may be expected that the hair will get thinner and baldness appear on the dome or crown of the head. Senile baldness cannot be remedied to any great extent. It may in some instances be delayed by treatment, but a cure cannot be expected.

Premature baldness may be regarded as that which occurs prior to forty years of age. It is much more common in civilized than in savage or primitive life and is also much more frequent in men than women.

Naturally the hair falls out and is renewed quite frequently, as often as two or three times a year, and unless sufficient renewal takes place baldness will finally ensue. Premature baldness may be due to a variety or a combination of causes.

Among the prominent causes of this affection heredity is regarded as taking foremost rank. It is not uncommon to find families from father to son manifesting this tendency in a marked degree, and that such a tendency should exist is no more strange than a similarity in other respects as looks, voice, gesture, build, etc.

Another cause of premature baldness is atrophy or disease of the hair bulbs resulting perhaps from acute fevers of a severe type, erysipelas, gout, leprosy, syphilis and seborrhea. When syphilis is the cause of alopecia proper treatment usually succeeds in the restoration of the hair. The treatment in every case depends to a large degree upon the cause which produces the affection and upon the management of the scalp.

Preventive treatment is much more successful than curative and hence it is that the care of the hair is of special importance.

The hair needs for luxuriant growth light and air; the wearing of stiff, unventilated hats is detrimental to its health. The hats of women are less injurious than those of men, they do not press heavily upon the head, but being light and small admit the air and sunlight. This accounts also to some extent for the difference between civilized and primitive life.

It is said that hot curling irons and crimping the hair upon papers is not a harmless process, as it usually in time injures the hair.

Constant mental strain and worry are said to cause baldness. Working under artificial lights which emit a perceptible amount of heat is said to be detrimental. Too much wetting of the hair is also injurious.

When the head needs cleaning a borax solution does its work well but should not be repeated too often. After washing the scalp it should be thoroughly dried and if necessary oiled with a small amount of vaseline or almond oil. When the hair is properly brushed it will require but little oil to keep it in a healthy condition. The hair should be exposed to the air and sunlight for they are the natural stimulants of the scalp. Hair restoratives containing lead are poisonous and should not be used.

Of all the causes of premature baldness dandruff occupies a prominent place; it does not always occasion baldness but does in a large number of cases. The scalp is itchy, there are a large number of scales which fall upon the clothing, the hair is dry and falls easily and rapidly. It is noticed that the hair gets thinner, especially upon the top of the head and crown. For premature baldness caused by dandruff sulphur is regarded as the most important remedy. No satisfactory domestic line of treatment can be well detailed for these affections, as many remedies are suggested by eminent authority and the skill of the practitioner is usually required to select the appropriate means for individual cases. A few only of the more efficient and usual remedies can be suggested at this point.

For the prevention of baldness the following claims high sanction:

℞ Sulphur precip.   thirty to sixty grains
   Vaseline   one ounce
   Oil bergamot   one-fourth of a dram

Mix, and apply to the scalp every night for three weeks, then give the scalp a thorough washing, after which apply every other night for three weeks more, and then gradually taper off its use as suggested by the progress of recovery. If the sulphur irritates the scalp use olive or almond oil in its place till the irritation subsides. Only a small quantity of the above prescription should be used at one time, and the treatment often needs to last for several months or a year.

In the same line of cases and to be used in about the same manner is the following: It is said to be an excellent formula, to be used preventively, in mild forms of dandruff, before baldness becomes an actual fact:

℞ Ammoniated mercury   twenty grains
   Mild chloride of mercury forty grains
   Vaseline   one ounce

Mix, and apply two or three times a day.

The following lotion has been used with success:

℞ Quinine   one half dram
   Acid sulphuric aromat.   one half dram
   Tinct. cantharides   one half ounce
   Myroxylon   one dram
   Cologne water   eight ounces

Mix, and apply three times a day to the scalp.

The following is a lotion of a more stimulating character, and works well in selected cases:

℞	Alcohol	one ounce
	Tinct. cantharides	two drams
	Tinct. capsicum	two drams
	Spirits rosemary	one ounce
	Strong spts. of ammonia	one ounce

Mix, and apply twice a day.

VII.—ACNE AND COMEDO,
OR FACE PIMPLES AND BLACKHEADS.

Acne is a very common disease of the skin especially annoying to young persons after the fourteenth year. It exists in several forms upon the face, neck and chest. The most common form is an eruption of pimples varying in size which are succeeded by renewals of the affection so that its duration is uncertain. The pimples may or may not contain pus. The pus may be superficial or deeply seated. When the latter condition exists the swelling is often quite large and the amount of inflammation considerably increased.

Comedo or blackhead is the name applied to acne when there is no inflammation, redness and swelling. In this form the sebaceous glands are filled with a semi-solid cheesy substance and dust lodging in the depression at the opening of the sack causes the resemblance to a worm or grub. This resemblance is very striking when the contents of the gland is pressed out. In addition to pimples whiskey drinking causes a dilation and congestion of the capillary blood vessels about the nose and this disorder is called acne rosacea.

CAUSES.

The sebaceous glands have been described elsewhere. They open by a little duct into the hair follicles close to a bulb or root of the hair. This secretion prevents the hair from getting dry. Upon the face these glands open upon the surface of the skin and prevent dryness or chapping. When the sebaceous glands are active the fluid they secrete is constantly poured out in a normal manner. There is then no formation of pimples but when the secretion is retained in the sack or becomes hardened, the sack becomes distended and in order to get rid of it nature sets up an inflammation about the gland. Comedo is the name of the retained secretion before it has excited inflammatory action hence it is really but one stage of the affection.

The cause of acne then must be due to an altered condition of the sebaceous glands so that their functions are disturbed. This altered condition results either in an excessive secretion of sebaceous matter or else in its being hardened and retained in the sack until it excites some inflammatory action.

The causes of acne must be sought for back of the inflammation which results in pimples, swellings and the formation of pus. These causes are somewhat obscure but among them are a sluggish circulation, a disordered liver and constipation. Alcoholic excesses, disorder of the sexual organs and nervous changes taking place in the system at puberty, errors in diet as overeating, the eating not only of too much but too rich food, especially the consumption of fatty foods, close habits of study causing too much indoor confinement, bad hygienic surroundings in general and a sluggish condition of the eliminating organs. Several of the above causes probably combine in every case of this affection to produce the changes in the functions of the skin which are characteristic.

TREATMENT.

The treatment is often unsatisfactory and ought to be carried on for some time. When the cause of the disorder can be ascertained it should be removed, if possible, by appropriate measures. Improve the general condition by hygienic measures, as exercise and bathing. Regulate the digestive functions and correct derangements of the nervous system. Avoid highly seasoned and indigestible articles of food, also stimulants, as beer and alcoholic drinks. Tonics containing iron, nux vomica and arsenic may be essential. The following pill may be used with benefit. As it contains active poisons care should attend its use :

℞	Reduced iron	ten grains
	Strychnia	one-fifth grain
	Arsenious acid	one-fifth grain

Mix, and divide into twenty pills. Take one pill three times a day, after meals. At the same time local treatment must be made use of, and chief reliance must be placed upon it. It is necessary to squeeze out the black heads with the fingers or a watch key, and a little practice will render the process rapid and almost painless. Pimples that have festered should be pricked with a clean steel needle and their contents pressed out with the fingers. Bathe the face every night and morning with hot water, as hot as can be used without burning it. This is of great benefit in bringing about a healthy condition of the glands.

The following are some of the best prescriptions known to the profession, and either of them can be selected and used according to directions:

℞	Naphthol	one dram
	Sulphur precipitate	five drams
	Vaseline	two and one-half drams
	Green soap (German)	two and one-half drams

Mix, and spread some of this on the skin daily for ten minutes, then cleanse the face and dust on talc powder.

℞	Sulphur sublimed	thirty grains
	Thymol	three grains
	Zinc. oleate	one scruple
	Vaseline	one-half ounce

Mix, and apply to the face each night, cleansing the face thoroughly in the morning. If the remedy inflames the skin, it must be omitted for a few days and then its use again commenced.

The following is a stimulating lotion recommended by high authority:

℞	Green soap (German)	two ounces
	Rectified spirits of wine	one ounce

Dissolve the soap in the spirits then strain through a muslin cloth and add:

	Spirits of lavender	two drams

Mix, and bathe the face with this each night and morning.

The following prescription is much used in Germany:

℞	Sulphur precipitate	two drams
	Camphor	ten grains
	Gum arabic	twenty grains
	Lime water	two ounces
	Rose water	two ounces

Mix, shake the bottle well and apply to the face at bed time; in the morning remove the sulphur without wetting the skin.

Other remedies are made use of by the surgeon in stubborn cases.

VIII.—MILIUM.

Milium is the name applied to certain small white points or tumors seen imbedded in the skin of the face especially about the angles of the eyes.

They vary in size from a pin point to a pin head and get their name from their resemblance to a millet seed. These little tumors are similar to those larger ones which sometimes appear in the Meibomian glands of the eyelids.

The treatment of these little tumors is simple and consists in their removal. This is accomplished by means of a small incision and by the application of sufficient pressure to force out the little hard, white globular substance.

IX.—PRURIGO, ITCHING OR PRURITUS.

Itching is a symptom of several skin diseases but it may exist as a separate affection and is often an important and troublesome condition. It is often worse at night when the patient gets warm in bed and may be so severe as to disturb or even prevent sleep. It may be general and extend over the whole surface of the body or local and confined to some particular area. It is frequently very annoying about the anus or genital organs and so obstinate as to resist for a long time the best directed treatment. This affection is augmented by scratching and the skin is liable to become thickened or take on a chronic condition resembling eczema.

In order to treat pruritus successfully it is necessary if possible to ascertain the cause on which it depends. Unless the cause can be ascertained the treatment is likely to fail altogether. It is sometimes due to the change from warm to cold weather or to wearing woolen underwear. It may result from certain diseases of the liver, kidneys or nervous system or from constipation or piles. Disorders of menstruation and the condition of pregnancy sometimes favor the development of this affection. It is sometimes due to disorders of digestion, to intestinal worms or to some disturbance of the nervous system.

TREATMENT.

Whenever pruritus is due to any of the above causes they should receive appropriate attention. The diet should be regulated; strong tea, coffee, highly seasoned dishes and alcoholic stimulants should be avoided. Easily digested, wholesome food, a proper amount of excise in the open air and soft underwear should be prescribed. Local treatment consists in hot water baths containing borax, carbolized lotions and ointments. A lotion made by pouring a pint of boiling water upon two drams of leaf tobacco is said to be of considerable virtue.

The following is an excellent lotion:

℞	Acid carbolic	one or two drams
	Alcohol	one or two ounces
	Aquæ	one pint

Mix. This makes an excellent external application.

The following will often give prompt and decided relief:

| ℞ | Menthol | thirty grains |
| | Alcohol | one ounce |

Mix, and apply externally as needed.

The following ointments may be used:

| ℞ | Naphthol | one dram |
| | Vaseline | one ounce |

Mix, and apply externally, or:

| ℞ | Menthol | thirty grains |
| | Vaseline | one ounce |

Mix, and apply externally as needed.

The following ointment containing cocaine is said to afford marked relief:

| ℞ | Cocaine | fifteen grains |
| | Vaseline | one ounce |

Mix, and apply as needed.

For internal treatment a tablet containing $\frac{1}{100}$ grain of atropia sulphate may be taken twice a day. Many other remedies have been used, but for ordinary cases no better remedies can be prescribed than those already suggested. When the trouble does not yield to these remedies it will be necessary to consult some one who gives especial attention to disorders of the skin.

X.—SHINGLES OR HERPES ZOSTER.

This is an acute disease characterized by neuralgia pain and the formation on the surface of groups of vesicles over the line of certain nerves.

CAUSES.

The following are regarded as the usual causes : exposure to cold, the sudden checking of the perspiration and the irritation, compression or injury of a nerve ganglion or nerve tract. The injudicious use of arsenic medicinally has been thought to give rise to this affection and there are probably other obscure causes.

SYMPTOMS.

Pain either mild or severe is the first symptom. The pain is of a neuralgic character accompanied by a sensation of smarting, burning or throbbing and sometimes persistent itching. The next symptom is an inflamed condition of the skin in patches on one side or half of the body, following the line of some nerve, commonly the intercostal, extending from the spine along the line of the ribs to the median line in front. Upon this inflamed and reddened surface groups of vesicles begin to form about the size of a pin's head which increase in size until they are as large as a pea. This process goes on for five or six days. Within these vesicles is a yellow fluid which at length dries away. This affection usually appears but once during a lifetime and is especially troublesome when it attacks aged persons. Its duration is indefinite varying from ten to twenty days or more. Vesicles which form about the lips, nose, forehead or face after fevers and attacks of malaria are forms of this disease. They are known as fever sores or cold sores and receive different names depending upon their locality. They sometimes attack the genitals.

TREATMENT.

Internal remedies seem to do but little good. Herpes about the lips can often be aborted by applying to them in their beginning strong camphor, pure cologne water, or a solution of carbolized water or vaseline. It is necessary to abstain from rubbing them, which hastens and favors their development.

The strength of the carbolic solution should be twenty grains of the acid to the ounce of water or vaseline.

For herpes upon the body oxide of zinc ointment makes a good dressing. To an ounce of this may be added cocaine, ten grains, or menthol fifteen grains. Or the following may be used and relieve the pain and itching, and its application is soon followed by a cool sensation:

℞ Menthol — one dram
Alcohol — one ounce

Mix, and apply as needed for relief.

If a more soothing application is needed use the following:

℞ Extract belladonna — ten grains
Extract stramonium — ten grains
Extract opium — ten grains
Vaseline — one ounce

Mix, and apply as needed.

Warm poultices, containing poppy heads or belladonna leaves are said to afford relief. A Dover's powder may be needed to relieve pain; five or ten grains at night.

XI.—ECZEMA, TETTER, MILK CRUST OR SALT RHEUM.

Eczema is the most common of all skin diseases. It is an acute inflammatory affection much inclined to take on a chronic condition. It presents many stages and varieties and for this reason is sometimes difficult to diagnose. It may appear upon any part of the body, but is more common about some portion of the face or scalp.

The skin is somewhat reddened and an eruption of vesicles appear from which there is a copious flow of serum or weeping. The drying of this serum forms crusts, which cause sometimes an unsightly appearance. The disease is accompanied by intense itching, and if the patient scratches the eruption the affection is aggravated and scabs form composed of serum, pus and blood. The skin becomes thickened if it lasts for some time and the disease takes on the chronic forms.

Infantile eczema, also called milk crust, is one of the most common affections of infants. It is often obstinate and yields reluctantly to treatment. In some cases it covers a large portion of the face or scalp. It has a preference for the region about the ears and nose, but may appear anywhere. Those cases in which the eruption covers the whole body are formidable, and in a few cases have proved fatal. Certain irritating substances favor its development.

CAUSES.

Teething is sometimes regarded as the cause of infantile eczema. It appears often to result from some fault in the process of digestion or nutrition. In adults certain occupations appear to favor its development. Washerwomen, grocers, masons and bakers are more prone to its development than others. Yet in many cases no assignable cause can be perceived.

TREATMENT.

The treatment of eczema often requires great care and patience and depends much upon the age of the patient, the stage of the eruption and its locality. In general, constitutional irregularities should be remedied; dyspepsia, constipation and similar disturbing conditions should be relieved.

In some cases internal remedies are necessary while in others local treatment may be sufficient. The oxide of zinc ointment is a mild and efficient remedy in mild cases; it should be carbolized to allay itching.

℞ Oxide of zinc ointment   one ounce
   Acid carbolic   ten grains

Mix and apply externally three times a day.

The following local application is efficient:

℞ Ungt. hydrarg. nitrate   one dram
   Naphthol   one-half dram
   Vaseline   one ounce

Mix and apply externally two or three times a day.

In cases of long standing much benefit often follows the administration of Fowler's solution in connection with the above local remedies. Three or four drops after meals should be given to an adult. It should be diluted sufficiently with water.

The following is a good formula for the administration of this valuable tonic for the skin.

℞ Fowler's solution   one and one-half drams
   Elix. calisaya   two ounces
   Comp. spts. of lavender   two ounces

Mix. Dose one teaspoonful after meals in a little water.

XII.—URTICARIA, HIVES OR NETTLE RASH.

This is a common but mild inflammatory affection of the skin, characterized by the appearance of circular elevations known as wheals. They resemble the eruption caused by the bite of the mosquito and other insects, or the sting of nettles. Itching is usually severe. This affection is very common with children, especially when taken to the seashore for the first time. In addition to the elevated circle and eruption, itching, tingling, burning and pricking are usually troublesome, while scratching aggravates the affection.

It is usually worse at night, and a person troubled with urticaria is restless, and the sleep is much disturbed. In a sensitive skin slight irritation will often cause urticaria. It may be extensive, covering large portions of the body, disappearing and reappearing again for an indefinite period. Stomach disorders are often noticed in connection with this affection, such as indigestion, and sometimes a mild grade of fever. In severe cases delirium, congestion, bounding pulse and high fever have occurred, suggesting meningitis or some brain trouble. These symptoms are temporary, and readily subside.

CAUSES.

It has been noticed that bottle-fed children, who are poorly nourished and who suffer from indigestion, are especially liable to attacks of urticaria. The causes of this affection may come from without or from within. Among the common external causes may be mentioned nettles, insect bites, friction of the skin, irritating clothing, chemical irritants, changes of temperature, the sea air and sea water. Among internal causes may be mentioned the use of the following articles of food: Muscles, shellfish, pork, canned meats, cheese, and certain fruits, as strawberries. There are a number of medicinal substances which may produce a rash upon the skin resembling urticaria.

TREATMENT.

The digestion should be looked after and constipation remedied. Local treatment consists in hot alkaline baths, using soda or borax in the water. The sopping upon the surface of alcohol and water, or alcohol, vinegar and water are recommended. Lemon juice may be rubbed over the eruption. Equal parts of linseed oil and lime water make a soothing application, and will be found very beneficial.

Either of the following prescriptions may be used to advantage:

R. Soda bicarbonate   two drams
Acid carbolic   half a dram
Camphor water   ten ounces

Mix, and apply freely to the surface.

R. Zinci oxide   two drams
Spts. camphor   three drams
Goulard's extract   one and a half drams
Glycerine   one-half ounce
Water   eight ounces

Mix, and apply externally as needed.

Internal treatment may require some mild laxative as the milk or citrate of magnesia, the former in teaspoonful doses.

The following prescription is excellent:

R. Sulphur præcip.   one dram
Cream of tartar   twelve grains

Mix. Divide into twelve powders. Dose, one three times a day. This can be obtained in tablet form and is more convenient to use.

XIII.—PSORIASIS.

Psoriasis is one of the less common inflammatory affections of the skin, characterized by fine scales. Its cause is unknown. It has a great variety of manifestations, but usually begins as a red point, which increases in size, and becomes covered with a multitude of scales. The spot itself is usually circular in form and surrounded by a red marginal line. Under the scales the skin is red and unnatural. Its favorite locality appears to be about the elbow or knee; it does not itch like eczema. Psoriasis is a chronic affection and likely to resist treatment.

The skin under the scales usually becomes more or less thickened. When it attacks the palms of the hands and soles of the feet it is persistent and occasions considerable inconvenience from cracks or fissures. Spring and fall are seasons of the year which appear to favor its development.

TREATMENT.

The internal use of Fowler's solution in three drop doses, taken in water after meals, has a more favorable influence upon psoriasis than any and all other remedies. Instead of this the sulphide of arsenic may be taken in doses of $\frac{1}{100}$ of a grain in pill form. Cod liver oil and the compound syrup of hypophosphites are also helpful in many cases. The following may be used externally with good effect:

℞	Oil of cade	one ounce
	Glycerine	one ounce
	Alcohol	one ounce

Mix, and apply once or twice a day.

℞	Sulphur sublimed	four drams
	Oil of cade	four drams
	German green soap	one ounce
	Vaseline	one ounce
	Precipitated chalk	two and one-half drams
	Oil of lavender	one-half dram

Mix, and apply on a piece of lint.

Many other remedies have been suggested and recommended, and in the hands of physicians are used as occasion requires for the treatment of psoriasis. Whatever remedies are made use of they must be persisted in for a long time. The following prescription is said by foreign authority to have cured when all other remedies have failed.

℞	Bromide of arsenic	one grain
	Alcohol	two ounces
	Simple syrup	eight ounces

Mix. The dose is one teaspoonful two or three times a day.

Bromide of arsenic may be obtained in tablet form in doses of $\frac{1}{20}$ of a grain. These are very convenient.

XIV.—LEPROSY.

Leprosy is a chronic, contagious and incurable disease, somewhat resembling syphilis in its effects upon the skin, but, unlike syphilis, it does not yield to treatment. It is characterized by marked deformities, unsightly growths, painful disturbances, and at last ends in death.

It affects not only the skin, but the nervous and lymphatic system and other tissues, in all of which it develops morbid processes.

It is believed to be due to bacilli or rod-shaped germs, but its method and law of development have not been discovered. It is not actively contagious, so that all danger of contagion can be averted by timely means. It originates in Eastern countries, and appears to thrive best in warm climates. Three forms of this disease are noticed but they all merge into each other. Leprosy can be stamped out by separating those having the disease from others. It is so rare an affection that a complete description of it is not essential. No treatment avails for its cure.

XV.—LICE OR PEDICULOSIS.

Three distinct species of lice find a habitation on the human body, head lice, body lice and crab, or pubic lice. The head louse is found only in the scalp. Its eggs are attached to the hair and are visible to the unaided eye. These eggs are popularly known as nits. Lice multiply rapidly and produce considerable itching, due to irritation of the scalp. Lice are often found in the heads of the untidy, and at school are liable to pass from one head to another. It is not unusual for them in this way to gain access to tidy families and to become a source of no little annoyance.

TREATMENT.

In children the hair may be cut short, the scalp thoroughly cleansed with soap and water, after which apply crude petroleum or kerosene oil; two or three applications are sufficient.

Mercurial ointment may be used thus:

℞	Ammoniated mercury	one dram
	Simple ointment or vaseline	one ounce

Mix, and apply externally a few times.

The ammoniated mercury ointment is popularly known as white precipitate ointment.

The following is efficient:

℞	Beta naphthol	one dram
	Vaseline	one ounce

Mix, and apply externally.

A lotion of alcohol will loosen the nits so that they can be removed by combing. The tincture of staphisagria applied thoroughly will effectually kill any kind of lice. This is a very simple and convenient method.

For body lice apply a lotion as follows:

℞ Acid carbolic — one dram
Water — one pint

The clothing should be put in boiling hot water or subjected to a high temperature. The eggs of the body louse are deposited in the seams of the clothing, where they may seen. Heating the outside garments and pressing the seams with a hot flat are among the successful means of getting rid of these troublesome parasites.

The crab, or pubic louse, may be destroyed by applications of crude petroleum, kerosene oil or mercurial ointment. The nicest remedy is a lotion of corrosive sublimate with cologne, thus:

℞ Corrosive sublimate — four grains
Aqua cologne — two drams
Aqua — four ounces

Mix, and apply a few times externally.

An ointment is made of staphisagria, or stavesacre, which is said to be very efficient for the destruction of lice and the itch-mite. It is used for other cutaneous diseases. It is not irritating, but this caution is essential, that it be applied only to the unbroken skin.

XVI.—ITCH OR SCABIES.

This is a contagious disease of an inflammatory character, due to a parasite, the acarus, also known as the itch-mite. This animal parasite is so small as to be hardly visible to the naked eye. The female itch-mite when transferred to a healthy person works her way down through the epidermis and burrows along forming a canal in which are deposited a number of eggs, and in a short time a new crop hatch out from these eggs. The disease in this way spreads, and more and more territory is successively involved. By means of the fingers and clothing the disease may be carried to other parts until, in neglected cases, nearly the whole body may be involved.

The disease always lasts until the parasites causing it are destroyed. The itch is chiefly a disease of the unclean poor, but may be contracted by any one. It is often troublesome in armies and on ship board, or where large numbers are congregated together with unfavorable surroundings.

This affection usually begins in some sensitive part, especially between the fingers. The first thing to arrest attention is the persistent itching which characterizes the disease and gives it a name. Sometimes considerable irritation of the skin is noticed and, further irritated by scratching, papules and vesicles may form. The itching is worse at night, especially when the patient is in bed.

TREATMENT.

The disease may spread through an entire family before it is suspected, but fortunately it yields readily to treatment.

It is necessary to destroy the parasite without injuring the skin. Sulphur has always been considered a specific for this affection, and it does not injure the skin in any way.

The following is a good prescription unless the skin is very sensitive:

℞	Sulphur pulverized	two drams
	Potassa sub-carbonate	one dram
	Lard	one ounce

Mix, and make into an ointment. This should be rubbed in at night over the whole portion of the body affected; wash with soap and water in the morning. This treatment pursued for five or six nights will generally effect a cure.

The following may be used in the same manner, and is more suitable for a sensitive skin:

℞	Sulphur flor.	three drams
	Naphthol	three drams
	Bals. Peru	three drams
	Vaseline	three ounces

Mix, and make ointment.

Out of the many prescriptions suggested these will prove satisfactory, and if directions are followed will effect a cure.

In using these ointments for infants or persons of unusually delicate skin they may be reduced in strength by the addition of more lard or vaseline.

The clothing worn by an itch patient should be destroyed or else disinfected by heat to destroy the itch-mite, also the under linen and bed clothes should be treated in the same manner.

XVII.—RINGWORM OR TINEA.

There are three diseases usually described as due to ringworm, depending upon the location of the affection. Ringworm of the scalp is known as tinea tonsurans; ringworm of the beard is otherwise called tinea sycosis or barber's itch, and ringworm of the body is known as tinea circinata. These affections are due to a vegetable parasite which multiplies within the tissues of the human body.

Tinia sycosis or barber's itch is an affection of the hair follicles of the beard and face, not only the hair follicles becoming inflamed but also the surrounding tissues. It begins in small red spots, accompanied by burning and itching. It is contagious and may be communicated by the lather brush of the barber if the brush has been used upon the face of some person suffering from barber's itch.

The hair becomes dull and dry and is easily pulled out or broken off. This disease does not get well without treatment.

TREATMENT.

The infected hairs may be removed and the following ointment applied night and morning:

℞	Oil cade	one dram
	Ungt. hydrarg nitrate	two drams
	Ungt. aqua rose	one ounce

Mix, and apply two or three times a day.

In ringworm of the beard the inflammatory action is much more marked than in ringworm of the body, owing to the tendency to the formation of pus and the escape of fluid from the hair follicles, which dries and forms crusts. When crusts form they should be removed by first saturating them with sweet oil and then washing with soap and hot water. Then apply the ointment above as directed.

Tinea tonsurans or ringworm of the scalp also requires thorough treatment. The hair should be cut short and the head thoroughly washed with a lotion of carbolic acid, one dram to a pint of water.

After thorough cleansing the diseased hairs should be removed; this treatment should be continued daily, followed by the application of some suitable ointment, as the following:

R   Ungt. hydrarg nitrate   one dram
    Beta naphthol   one dram
    Vaseline   one ounce

Mix, and apply externally three times a day.

Ringworm may be contracted from several of the domestic animals, when afflicted with the *mange*, as the horse, cow and cat.

The treatment for these affections should not be discontinued until certainty of cure is established.

XVIII.—FAVUS.

This is a contagious disease, caused by a vegetable parasite derived from the cat and other animals. It is characterized by dirty looking, cup-shaped patches or crusts, of a yellowish color, and emitting a peculiar musty or mousy odor.

It usually occurs in the scalp and involves the health of the hair. It is not common in this country. The cause of this disease being known, such remedies must be used as will destroy or remove the parasite, when the diseased parts will be speedily restored.

Mercurial ointments or lotions are generally used to accomplish this end, and ointments containing sulphur and tar are successfully used.

This affection is so rare that the details of treatment are not considered essential. Cleanliness is preventive of this as well as of many other disagreeable affections of the skin.

XIX.—FRECKLES OR LENTIGO.

Freckles are usually a slight disfiguration of the skin. They are especially likely to occur on persons who have light hair and complexion.

Freckles are little circular spots, of small size, on the face and back of the hands. They are due to some disturbance in the even deposit of pigment. All skin is colored by pigment, which causes the hue known as flesh color. This color is considerably removed from white. Dark skinned persons have a more liberal deposit of pigment in the skin than light persons. The color of the hair and eyes are due to special deposits of pigment. Pigment is excessively abundant in the skin of the negro race.

Freckles are influenced by the sun's rays and are more noticeable in summer than in winter, and in cold weather they tend to disappear altogether. Freckles are very annoying to young ladies, if we may judge from the frequent demand from ladies' journals of recipes for their removal. The following lotion is harmless and useful:

℞	Carbonate of potash	three drams
	Common salt	two drams
	Rose water	eight ounces
	Orange flower water	two ounces

Mix, and apply externally two or three times a day.

Also the following:

℞	Corrosive sublimate	eight grains
	Zinc sulphate	thirty grains
	Lead acetate	thirty grains
	Water	four ounces

Mix. Apply for five or ten minutes thrice daily. (See Cosmetics.)

XX.—MOLES.

Moles are dark spots of discolored skin, which vary considerably in size. They are quite common, as but few persons escape the existence of one or more upon the surface of the body.

Their color is due to an excessive deposit of pigment, and they are often the site of an unnatural growth of hair. They derive importance when situated upon the face, in consequence of its disfigurement. Their removal is easily accomplished.

When a mole shows a tendency to enlarge or to become unnatural its removal should be contemplated. Soft cancers of the melanotic variety have been known to develop upon the site of a mole, and hence any change in the appearance of a mole should be regarded with apprehension.

The melanotic cancer when once established multiplies rapidly, spreading and becoming virulent. A mole may be removed by a caustic plaster, the same as an epithelial cancer or by the knife.

XXI.—WARTS OR VERRUCA.

Warts result from an abnormal growth in the skin or a hypertrophy, due to unknown causes. They are sometimes very numerous upon the hands. There are several varieties; they vary in size, and there are certain persons and families which appear to be especially subject to their development. From general familiarity with these growths further description is deemed unnecessary.

TREATMENT.

It is to be observed that they often disappear without any treatment. Sometimes they may be removed by tying a silk cord about the base or pedicle and cutting off the sources of nutrition. This method answers well in those cases where the pedicle is small, but when the base of the wart is extensive other means must be used.

The usual method is to pare off the upper surface of the wart with a sharp knife down to the bleeding point. Then apply some oil or vaseline about the circumference of the base to prevent injury to the healthy tissues. With a pine stick which has been dipped in strong, fuming nitric acid rub over the wart thoroughly. Its caustic effect will turn the touched surface yellow. After a few days pare off the destroyed surface and repeat the operation precisely as before if the wart does not appear to be destroyed thoroughly. Several applications may be necessary, though two or three usually suffice.

Instead of nitric acid, caustic potash may be used. This burns more deeply and one application, if properly applied, will be sufficient. Nitrate of silver can be used, but its caustic action is so mild that too many repetitions might be required. Chromic acid is an efficient caustic, and one application would be sufficient.

Warts that tend to rapid enlargement and have a suspicious appearance should be removed, especially upon the face, lips and some other portions of the body, as epithelial cancers have sometimes had their origin in such warts.

XXII.—CORNS OR CLAVUS.

Nearly everyone is familiar with what are known as corns, and many have had actual experience. They are due to a thickening or hypertrophy of the skin, which becomes hard, almost like a piece of bone. They are usually about the size of a small split pea, but they vary considerably both as to size and form.

Corns are of two kinds, hard and soft, depending upon their situation. Between the toes soft corns are developed, and these are subject to inflammation. They may cause but slight disturbance, or they may become so inflamed as to be not only sensitive and painful, but also interfere with ease in walking, and give one a limping gait. They sometimes occur upon the soles of the feet, though not as commonly as upon the toes and sides of the foot.

CAUSE.

They are caused by hard pressure and the friction of the boot or shoe; hence they are often much more troublesome in warm than in cold weather. A loose or badly fitting shoe will cause corns as well as those which pinch and squeeze the feet.

TREATMENT.

Prevention here, as in thousands of other cases, is more satisfactory than cure. Wear well-fitting shoes, made of soft, pliable material, neither too loose nor too tight. The heel should not be too small nor too high. The fashionable French heel which brings the weight of the body upon the hollow of the foot is an abomination.

The feet require especial care, yet no part of the body is so neglected or abused, or suffers more from vanity or silly fashions.

The feet need frequent, and, if possible, daily bathing; and the nails should be carefully and closely cut and the dead skin removed. Such careful treatment prevents corns and other callosities.

When corns exist soften them by soaking in hot water, pare off the thickened skin down to where it is soft and pliable, but do not draw blood. Then apply the tincture of iodine every night and morning, forgetting not the importance of the daily bath. Make the same application to soft corns. A ring of felt with an opening in the center may be worn to lessen pressure and friction. Such a method of treatment will prove satisfactory and afford relief. The following treatment may be used instead if for any reason preferred:

After soaking and paring the corns as directed above, paint them over each night and morning with the following mixture:

℞ Salicylic acid   thirty grains
    Ext. Indian hemp   ten grains
    Collodion   one and one-half ounces

In a few days the hardened mass of epidermis can be easily removed after soaking the feet in warm water.

The only medicine which has any effect upon the removal of corns when taken internally is arsenic, but the more natural and simple methods here recommended should certainly be preferred.

XXIII.—BUNIONS.

These are common and well known enlargements of the joint of the great toe.

CAUSES.

They are usually caused by shoes which taper too much and which press the end of the toe inward, leaving the joint so prominent as to be irritated by friction and pressure. Various occupations may have some relation to the production of these deformities, especially those which require constant standing and thus bring the weight of the body continually upon the feet. Sometimes they become very painful, or very much inflamed, and troublesome sores may be formed which discharge pus and manifest considerable obstinacy in healing.

TREATMENT.

Preventive treatment in the way of properly fitting shoes is first and best of all. Tight fitting shoes with narrow toes should not be tolerated. Painting the enlarged joints with iodine is in the line of preventive treatment, and will do much good without doing harm. Cup-shaped plasters may be placed over the enlarged joints with good results and will give relief by relieving the pressure upon the enlarged bursa. The biniodide of mercury, two grains to an ounce of water, may be applied externally, and this treatment is recommended by high authority.

Many other applications have been suggested, and even surgical operations for the relief of bunions, but they are too complex or difficult to introduce with any profit here. When the measures above proposed do not afford relief, and easy fitting shoes and rest do not avail, the case should be submitted to some one who is skillful in their treatment.

XXIV.—SCURVY.

Scurvy is a condition of the body due to the prolonged employment of foods deficient in acids and vegetable matter. It breaks out as the result of a diet consisting exclusively of salt meats, smoked and dried fish or flesh; hence in famine stricken regions, among those shut in by siege, and on board of ships in long voyages, this disease in the past has often been of serious import. Since the modern method of preserving fruits and vegetables by canning, it has almost become unknown.

SYMPTOMS.

These may be briefly stated as dull complexion, headache, dizziness, loss of strength and vigor, or muscular debility, despondency, short breath, and finally effusion of blood into the skin, causing blotches, spots, ulcers and spongy gums which bleed easily. At length the prostration is extreme, the heart is slow and feeble, the mental powers are impaired, the face looks haggard, the sleep is broken, the glands become enlarged and swollen, and the hair falls off. Pains, mistaken for rheumatism, are felt in the limbs, joints and loins, and hemorrhage from the nose is common.

The victim at length sinks into a condition of apathy. The blotches on the skin give name to the disorder. They are from the size of the finger nail to two or three inches in diameter. These spots are at first reddish, but later become darker colored or bluish.

TREATMENT.

Medicines are of little avail in this disease, for fruits and succulent vegetables are what the system craves. Lime juice has great reputation.

Those suffering from this disease, unless beyond the reach of help, recover rapidly on a change of diet. Onions, garlic, mustard, sorrel, dandelion, potatoes, beets, radishes, together with various fruits and lemons are among the best means of warding off and curing the scurvy.

It is often observed how greedy city children are especially for green apples, pickles and unripe fruits, and how seldom they are injured by eating them. They are simply satisfying the system with what it craves.

CHAPTER XII

THE BRAIN, CRANIAL NERVES, SPINAL CORD, NERVES, SYMPATHETIC NERVES, AND THEIR DISEASES.

I.—The Brain and Cranial Nerves. II.—The Nerves and Spinal Cord. III.—Hydrocephalus or Dropsy of the Brain. IV.—Meningitis or Inflammation of the Brain. V.—Neuralgia. VI.—Headache. VII.—Vertigo or Dizziness. VIII.—Insomnia. IX.—Insanity. X.—Apoplexy. XI.—Various Other Disorders of the Brain. 1, Abscess of the Brain; 2, Tumors of the Brain; 3, Aphasia; 4, Amnesia; 5, Numbness; 6, Hemiplegia; 7, Paraplegia; 8, Locomotor Ataxia; 9, Facial Paralysis; 10, Congenital Defects.

I.—THE BRAIN AND CRANIAL NERVES.

> "What a piece of work is man!
> How noble in reason!
> How infinite in faculty!"

THE brain is a large and important organ consisting of an aggregation of nerve centers, together with the vessels by which they are nourished, and the coverings by which they are held in position.

Coverings or Membranes.—The brain has three external coverings, the dura mater, the arachnoid and the pia mater.

The Dura Mater.—The inside of the skull is covered over with a dense white membrane composed of fibers, called the dura mater. It is the periosteum of the skull, and surrounds the brain with a smooth covering, and its fibers hold the brain in position. The dura mater not only covers the interior of the skull, but it extends into the numerous openings of the bones and forms a lining so that the numerous nerves and blood vessels which pass through the openings in the bones are surrounded by a smooth surface. The dura mater is attached to the sutures and its reflections form the sinuses which receive and transport the venous blood.

It holds the lobes of the brain in place, and prevents them from pressing upon each other in the different positions assumed by the body.

The Arachnoid.—Next to the dura mater is the arachnoid membrane, a thin, delicate tissue, which secretes a fluid known as the cerebro spinal or arachnoid fluid. When the base of the skull is fractured the arachnoid fluid is liable to escape slowly through the ear. This fluid helps to maintain the positions of the various portions of the brain; it equalizes the pressure and so prevents injury from concussion.

The Pia Mater.—The pia mater is a thin tissue which forms the outside covering of the brain substance. It contains a large number of blood vessels which transport the arterial blood for nourishment and gather up the venous blood and empty it into the great sinuses. It dips down into the deep fissures of the brain and forms a covering for all the lobes.

The brain, though contained within the skull, is connected by means of the spinal cord and its branches with every other organ and tissue of the body.

The main divisions of the brain are the cerebrum, the cerebellum, the pons Varolii and the medulla oblongata.

The brain substance which fills the entire cavity of the skull and conforms to its shape is quite soft, of a white and gray color, known as the white and gray matter, the latter being external and gathered into numerous convolutions which add greatly to its extent, and several deep fissures increase its surface. The gray matter is the seat of the intellectual faculties, and the character of the intellect depends less upon the size of the brain than upon the amount of the gray matter. The average weight of the male brain is forty-nine ounces, and that of the female forty-four ounces. The brain contains the great nerve centers which recognize sensation and originate motion. It contains also the nerve centers of the special senses.

The Cerebrum.—Four-fifths of the space within the skull is occupied by the cerebrum. It extends from the forehead to the occiput and overlies all the other portions of the brain, occupying the whole upper part of the cavity of the skull. A large fissure running from before backwards divides the cerebrum into two nearly equal halves or hemispheres. It is further divided by deep fissures which separate each hemisphere into three lobes known as the anterior, middle and posterior lobes of the brain. The cerebrum is separated from the cerebellum by folds of the dura mater called the tentorium. The two hemispheres are united at the bottom by a band of white transverse fibers known as the commissure, or the corpus callosum.

The Cerebellum.—The cerebellum is situated in the occipital chamber of the skull, and is also divided into two hemispheres, joined together in the central portion. The cerebellum controls the co-ordination of muscular movements. It is connected with the medulla oblongata by means of fibers.

The Pons Varolii—The pons Varolii is the name given to the upper and bulbous portion of the medulla oblongata. It is composed of white fibers which connect the medulla to the cerebellum and the gray matter which is deposited among them.

The Medulla Oblongata.—The medulla oblongata is the expanded and upper end of the spinal cord. It conveys impressions to and from the brain. The nerve fibers in the medulla cross each other from side to side so that an injury to one hemisphere of the brain is followed by paralysis in the opposite side of the body.

The brain is very liberally supplied with arterial blood, which enables it to prosecute with energy its manifold labors. The arteries of the brain pursue a tortuous course so that the impulse given to the blood by the powerful stroke of the heart is not felt as a disturbing force. The arrangement which is made in the great venous sinuses for receiving and disposing of the venous blood, prevents too great blood pressure upon the brain, which would prove injurious in many ways.

A more complete description of the brain would involve such a large number of technical terms as to weary the patience of the general reader and is omitted.

The Cranial Nerves.—(For origin see plate.)—Twelve pairs of nerves have their origin in the base of the brain near the fourth ventricle.

The first pair, the olfactory, give off about twenty branches on each side which are distributed to the mucous membrane or lining of the nose. These are the nerves by which we take cognizance of different odors and they convey the impressions of odor to the brain. The olfactory bulbs lie in front of the optic commissure.

The second pair, the optic nerves, pass from the optic commissure to the back part of the eyeballs and are spread out upon the retina. These are the nerves of sight and convey the impressions of objects to the brain.

The third pair, or the motor oculi, are the nerves which control the movements of the muscles of the eye as their name implies. They originate in front of the pons Varolii and extend to the muscles of the eyeball.

The fourth pair extend to the muscles of the eyeball. They arise near the origin of the third pair and extend to the superior oblique muscles of the eye which are not reached by the third pair. The fourth pair are also known as the patheticus or trochlear nerves. They act in harmony with the third pair.

The fifth pair, trigeminous or trifacial, arise from the vicinity of the pons Varolii. They are the largest of the cranial nerves and are widely distributed to the regions of the face. They are all mixed nerves, possessing functions of motion and sensation. They become three great divisions, the opthalmic which extends to the region about the eyes, forehead and nose; the superior maxillary, which is distributed to the upper teeth and a wide region of the face; the inferior maxillary, which is distributed to the lower teeth and the region about the lower jaw. This nerve is often the seat of much pain known as headache, toothache and neuralgia of the face or tic douloureux.

The sixth pair supply the external recti muscles of the eye.

The seventh pair or facial are distributed to the muscles of the face. They are motor nerves exclusively.

The eighth pair of cranial nerves, the auditory, are closely associated with the facial and were formerly regarded as a part of the seventh pair. They are distributed to the external ear.

The ninth pair are distributed to the pharynx and the back part of the tongue.

The tenth pair, the pneumogastric, is widely distributed reaching the pharynx, larynx, heart, lungs, œsophagus and stomach. From its wandering course it is often called the vagus nerve.

The eleventh pair receive their name, the spinal accessory, from their singular origin and course.

The twelfth pair of cranial nerves is distributed to the muscles of the tongue. The nerves of special sense not only originate in the

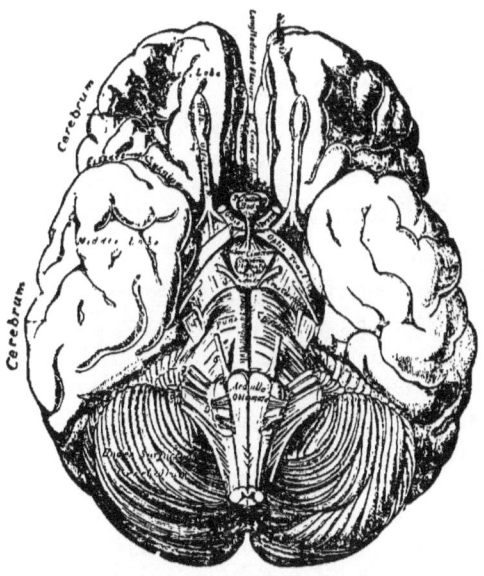

The base of the brain, showing the Cerebrum, Cerebellum, Pons Varolii, Medulla and the origin of nine pairs of the Cranial Nerves.

1, olfactory; 2, optic; 3, motor oculi; 4, patheticus; 5, trifacial; 6, oculi abducens; 7, facial; 8, auditory; 9, glosso-pharyngeal.

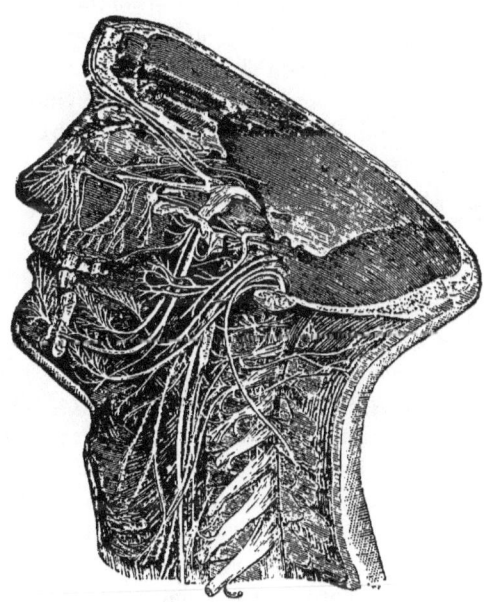

The cranial nerves on the left side.

brain but also terminate in a neighboring portion of the head except the nerves of touch, which pass to every portion of the external surface of the body.

II.—THE NERVES AND SPINAL CORD.

The nerves form a network of the entire body. They convey impressions to the brain and control movements in conformity to the will. This subject is one of unusual interest. There are two kinds of nerve structure, the gray, in which impressions originate and the white, which transmits the impression.

The nerve substance originates and conveys impressions to control the action of the various organs. There are two systems; viz: the cerebro-spinal and the sympathetic. The cerebro-spinal system is made up of the brain, the spinal cord and their branches. The cerebro-spinal system presides over the functions of animal life and the intellectual processes.

The sympathetic system presides chiefly over the work of nutrition and growth. It is indirectly connected with the brain and spinal cord and their functions are not so absolutely separate as was once supposed. The sympathetic system is known to be connected with the cerebro-spinal system by means of interlacing branches which are the channels of communication. The sympathetic system consists of a series of ganglia on either side and in front of the spinal column connected together by means of nerve fibers.

The Spinal Cord.—This is the great line of communication between the brain and other portions of the body. It occupies the canal formed by the vertebræ and is surrounded by fluid to prevent its injury. On its passage from the brain it gives off branches on each side forming thirty pairs of nerves.

The branches which go to the upper and lower extremities are necessarily large. The spinal cord in structure resembles the brain. The internal portion of the cord contains the gray substance which is surrounded by white fibers that pass in longitudinal, transverse and oblique directions. These membranes envelop the cord; the outer is the dura mater, the middle the arachnoid, and the inner the pia mater, a continuation of the enveloping membranes of the brain. The front portion of the cord transmits impressions from the brain to the muscles.

The gray substance carries sensations from without to the brain. The back portion of the cord controls the co-ordination of muscular movements. The spinal cord also produces reflex or unconscious

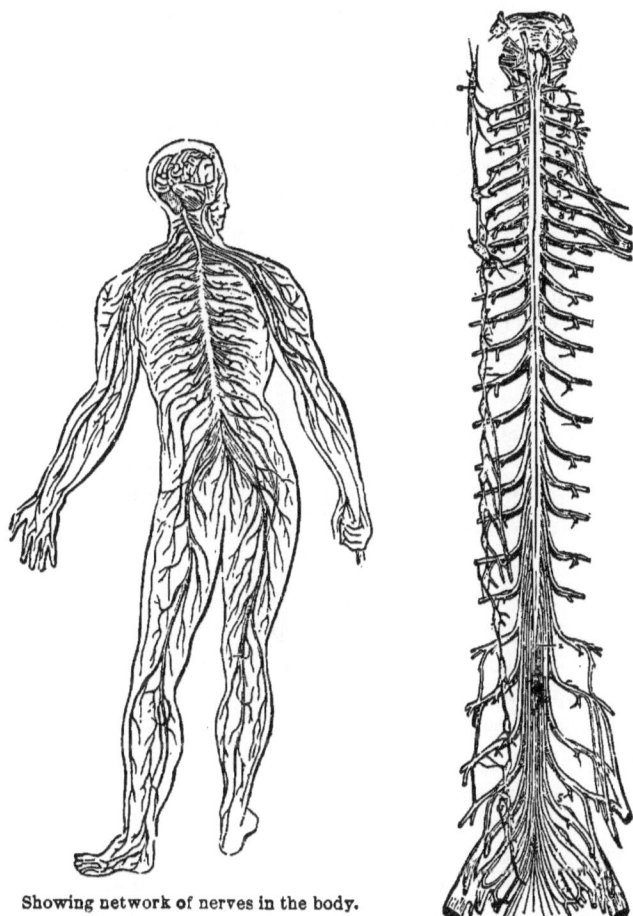

Showing network of nerves in the body.

SPINAL CORD.
Showing also on the left side the sympathetic ganglionic masses.

movements. Reflex movements are such as are produced independent of the will. The acts which we do in sleep are reflex.

As a branch passes out from the cord it contains fibers from the anterior and posterior columns of the spinal cord, so that these spinal branches are mixed nerves, or nerves of motion and sensation; and however much these nerves are divided and subdivided they are always mixed, containing the two sets of motor and sensitive fibers. The nerve force is peculiar. It passes as rapidly along a nerve as electricity does a wire. It is owing to the action of the nerve force that muscular movements are skillfully performed.

III.—HYDROCEPHALUS, OR DROPSY OF THE BRAIN.

This is a disease characterized by an excessive amount of fluid in the spaces and tissues of the brain. It is in many cases a congenital affection and exists at birth.

The first thing noticed is the excessive size of the child's head, it being out of proportion to the rest of the body. Children born with hydrocephalus usually die within a year but a few cases of recovery have been reported.

CAUSES.

When this disease comes on after birth the exciting causes to be considered are fevers, falls, blows upon the head, tumors of the brain, diseases of the heart and lungs, Bright's disease of the kidneys, unfavorable surroundings and disturbances of the nervous system.

SYMPTOMS.

In congenital cases the digestion is poor and much disturbed, the face has an old, wrinkled look, the intellect is impaired, standing upon the feet or walking is delayed and the weight of the head seems too great for the strength of the body.

When the disease comes on suddenly the symptoms at first are headache, intolerance of noise and light, delirium, restlessness followed by stupor and coma. Or the disease may approach with nausea, vomiting, fever, twitchings and finally convulsions. The pupils of the eyes may be of unequal size, the pulse irregular and the bowels constipated. The symptoms increase in severity till a state of complete stupor is reached and recovery cannot be predicted.

TREATMENT.

Only mild cases, when the symptoms are arrested previous to convulsions, recover. Congenital cases need pure air, nutritious food, suitable tonics and aids to digestion. Acute cases are to be treated as the symptoms require with brain sedatives, antispasmodics and perhaps stimulants.

IV.—MENINGITIS OR INFLAMMATION OF THE BRAIN.

This disease was formerly known as brain fever. There are several varieties. Simple meningitis is an inflammation of the pia mater, or outer covering of the brain.

Tubercular meningitis is another and more serious form of inflammation of the brain. Its beginnings are insidious, its progress chronic, and its termination usually fatal. The diagnosis of the second form during life is uncertain and difficult, for the symptoms are often mistaken for malarial fever or worms. This form of meningitis is more likely to occur where there is a marked history of tubercular consumption in the family. Tubercular disease attacks not only the lungs, but sometimes the brain and bowels.

Cerebro-spinal meningitis is an acute inflammation of the brain of intense character. It involves the base of the brain and extends into the spinal cord, and hence its name. It attacks young persons, especially between the ages of fourteen and twenty-five. It occurs sometimes as an epidemic, and on account of the peculiar character of the fever which accompanies it, it was formerly called spotted fever.

CAUSES.

The causes of inflammation of the brain are quite varied, as blows upon the head and falls of so serious a nature as to injure the tissues of the brain. It is sometimes the result of prolonged exposure to the excessive heat of the sun's rays, and begins as a congestion, followed by fever and other symptoms.

The excessive use of alcoholic stimulants causes a condition of congestion, and if long continued may result in meningitis.

In childhood it often follows and terminates in other serious diseases, as cholera infantum, scarlet fever, or pneumonia; also other acute affections of the adult, as erysipelas, rheumatism, Bright's disease, and typhoid fever. It may also result from chronic disease of the ear, and in such cases the destruction of tissue due to the continued flow of pus at length reaches the brain and sets up inflammation.

SYMPTOMS.

The more common symptoms are severe headache, vomiting, restlessness or stupor, delirium and convulsions. The face is pale, the features are sunken, the pupils of the eyes may be dilated or contracted, the urine is scanty, and the bowels constipated. The pain in the head is often acute, causing the patient to cry out or scream when a change of position is attempted. Light and noise increase the suffering. There is great restlessness, often inability to sleep, the skin is hot and dry, twitchings and convulsions are prominent, and in fatal cases coma precedes death.

In tubercular meningitis the early symptoms approach gradually, the patient is languid and feverish; vomiting may occur, and for this disturbance no cause appears. The patient loses flesh and strength, grows pale, and seems disinclined to make exertion of any kind. The sleep is disturbed, the child often starting or moaning, grinding the teeth and rolling the head from side to side. The thermometer shows a continued rise of temperature. In brain troubles the respiration is slow, the pulse is slow and intermittent when the temperature is high; this is an important symptom.

TREATMENT.

A disease so grave demands professional skill and no line of treatment could be safely followed by the household. Meningitis is always serious and often fatal and requires careful attention. In the acute forms with much fever cold applications to the head are indicated, either cold water or ice. The bowels should be kept open by gentle physic. Tincture of aconite is a valuable remedy to relieve congestion of the brain. To produce rest chloral is preferable to opium. Bromide of potash and other brain sedatives are beneficial.

Gelsemium and ergot are remedies which in skillful hands may be successfully used. The diet should be nourishing and consist of milk, beef tea and other liquid food. If stimulants are indicated the aromatic spirits of ammonia in teaspoonful doses well diluted for an adult or brandy may be used. The patient ought not to be disturbed by noise and excitements. The nurse should move about carefully and exclude most of the light from the room. Medicines given in the early stages may avert the fatal consequences of this disease. Preventive remedies such as proper diet, ventilation and keeping delicate children away from school until a suitable age will do much toward building up the constitution where there is danger to be feared from the development of tubercular disease.

V.—NEURALGIA.

Neuralgia is pain of a nerve, often due to an overtaxed or impoverished condition of the nervous system. It is in such cases the cry of a hungry nerve for nourishment. Neuralgia is an exceedingly common affection. It exists apart from fever and inflammation, and without any apparent cause. Pain is the most prominent and often the only symptom present. The pain is sharp and cutting, of a movable character, often obstinate and more severe at some times than others. While the skin may be sensitive to the touch, firm pressure usually relieves the pain, and distinguishes neuralgia from any ordinary inflammation. Motion of the affected parts increases the pain.

Some persons are much more subject to neuralgia than others, especially those of a nervous temperament, as frail women, and those who inherit a tendency to nervous troubles.

The duration of an attack of neuralgia is indefinite. It may last only a few hours, or it may continue for days and weeks and the termination is often gradual. There are many different varieties of neuralgia, and the locality of the affection furnishes the particular name which designates it.

Neuralgia of the head is called migraine, and is usually confined to one side of the head. Other names which may be applied are nervous headache, hemicrania, and neuralgic headache.

Neuralgia of the face is called tic-douloureux. The pain is usually very severe, and is increased by exposure to cold air, wind and dampness.

Neuralgia of the chest is called intercostal; that about the heart, angina pectoris; that of the stomach, gastralgia; of the back and loins, lumbago; of the ovaries, ovarian; of the thighs, sciatica; and that of the skin accompanied by eruptions, herpes zoster or shingles. These form a class of common affections frequent in occurrence and often troublesome.

CAUSES.

Among the predisposing causes are heredity and certain periods of life. Women are much more frequently the victims of neuralgic pain than men as might be expected from their liability to uterine diseases. Certain other diseases as rheumatism, gout, anæmia, syphilis and malaria have much to do with the development of neuralgic troubles. Among exciting causes the following are sufficiently prominent to mention: atmospheric changes as heat, cold and dampness, bad teeth, broken bones, the pressure of tumors and other growths, injuries, irritation or pressure upon a nerve, the poison of any miasm acting upon the nervous system, the presence of worms, in fact whatever overtaxes or impoverishes the nervous system.

It is especially noticeable that neuralgia is common in cold and damp weather, in damp locations or as the result of exposure to storms.

TREATMENT.

The successful treatment will depend much upon the cause and hence no special line can be proposed. Local causes of irritation should be remedied and removed. Decayed teeth, errors in refraction and uterine troubles ought to receive appropriate attention.

When dependent upon anæmia, malaria, rheumatism, gout or syphilis these diseases must receive attention adapted to each case. In the great majority of cases some fault of nutrition exists and for these cases nerve tonics such as phosphates are excellent. Overwork and excessive nerve strain should be avoided and their past effects corrected. Change of climate, rest from wearying occupations and an improved diet will help many cases. Indigestible foods, hot bread, pastry and cakes aggravate digestive troubles and should be avoided. The habits if bad should be corrected as late hours, late suppers or the use of tobacco and alcohol.

A proper amount of sleep should be secured. Baths, if possible salt water baths, and friction of the skin with a rough towel or flesh brush are especially serviceable for those who experience inconvenience from atmospheric changes. Suitable clothing, preferably woolen, should be worn next the skin at all seasons. In summer it may be of very light weight.

Electricity may sometimes be used to advantage. Local applications of heat and of stimulating liniments may afford considerable temporary relief; counter irritants, as mustard, turpentine, or perhaps chloroform stand highest in the list of local remedies. Menthol liniment will often relieve headache and neuralgia of the face. The following mixture makes a liniment of considerable efficiency:

℞ Oil of mustard   one dram
   Camphor liniment   three and a half ounces
   Chloroform   four drams

Mix, and apply on a piece of flannel or muslin.

The most efficient internal remedies are the phosphate of iron, quinine, arsenic and strychnine, combined in a pill or tablet form. (See Anæmia.)

VI.—HEADACHE.

Headache claims many sufferers; it is not only of frequent occurrence, but of great variety. The brain is a delicate and complex structure. It is no wonder that in the severe struggle of modern life this great group of nerve centers is liable to suffer from such opposite conditions as congestion and exhaustion or anæmia. The nervous system is liable to be overtaxed by the frequent demands made upon it without sufficient opportunity for rest and recuperation.

The brain is subject to constant burden and overwork. There can be no thought and no emotion which does not reach and often thrill it. There can be no anxious care which does not add to its burden. Every part of the human body communicates directly with the brain, and hence our various ills all tend to depress and exhaust it. Any functional or organic disease of the various organs is likely to act as a debilitating force upon the brain.

CAUSES.

Digestive troubles and all affections of the stomach, liver, womb, or ovaries are frequent causes of headache. Defective vision, causing eye strain, or malarial poison circulating through the system produce headache of a persistent type. Any excessive indulgence at the table, the use of alcoholic drinks, or narcotic medicines are liable to cause headaches.

Gratification of the sensual passions tends to consume the vital forces and debilitates the nervous system, and may be a frequent cause of this affection. The two most prominent factors in headaches appear to be excitement, causing congestion of the brain, and exhaustion, causing anæmia. Thus we have two opposite conditions producing the same symptoms.

In congestive headache the blood vessels of the brain are dilated and distended, the face is often flushed, the eyes red or bloodshot and the arteries full and throbbing. Congestive headache may be due to an enlarged heart or to its excessive action so that the tissues of the brain receive too much blood. Or there may be some obstruction which prevents the rapid return of the venous blood. Excessive or prolonged mental work may attract sufficient blood to the brain to cause congestion and a resulting headache. In fevers the headache is of the congestive variety. The heat of the sun sometimes causes an intense congestive headache.

Anæmia causes a headache due to an impoverished and watery condition of the blood, and the brain suffers for want of nourishment. The sufferer from this form of headache is weak, faints easily, has cold feet and poor circulation. There is a marked lack of vitality, inability to sleep, irritability and nervousness. This is the headache of exhaustion and nervous prostration, and is very similar to neuralgia, the hungry nerves uttering their constant protest against starvation.

Headache may result from many other causes, as poorly ventilated rooms, the inhalation of carbonic acid gas from burning charcoal, overstudy, colds, catarrh, gout, rheumatism, fevers, syphilis, or whatever affects, either temporarily or permanently, the delicate tissues of the brain. The duration of a headache may be a few minutes or several days, or even months.

TREATMENT.

Much skill is often required in managing this affection which at first appears so innocent. If the cause is known the treatment is usually simple. Cold applications to the head often relieve a congestive headache. Wet a towel in equal parts of strong vinegar and water and tie about the head. It will help the result to soak the feet in hot mustard water. If constipation exists or biliousness is suspected open the bowels freely. Fifteen grains of the bromide of lithium or sodium, or a five grain tablet of acetanelid or a dessert spoonful of the effervescing hydrobromate of caffeine are all efficient remedies.

For the headache of exhaustion and overwork nerve foods or tonics are indicated. In headache of this variety the phosphates are valuable. Tablets of the phosphate of iron, quinine and strychnia may be used. Rest, change of climate and a nourishing diet are often quite as curative as medicines.

Headache is a symptom of many other diseases, as malaria, hysteria, constipation, uterine disturbances, fevers, and diseases of the kidneys. Menthol applied externally is beneficial in some forms of headache.

For hysterical headache use one teaspoonful of the ammoniated tincture of valerian mixed with a wine glass of water.

The following may be used for anæmic headache:

℞ Reduced iron   ten grains
   Arsenious acid   one-half grain
   Podophyllin   one grain
   Ext. gentian   twenty grains

Mix, and make into twenty pills. Dose, one three times a day after meals.

For nervous headache the following will afford temporary relief:

℞ Aromatic spts. of ammonia   one ounce
   Spts. of chloroform   one dram
   Water q.s. to make   two ounces

Mix. Dose, a teaspoonful in water.

VII.—VERTIGO OR DIZZINESS.

Vertigo is a symptom of various conditions rather than a disease in itself. It is caused by a disordered circulation of the brain, or a congestion of that organ. A sedentary occupation, with little exercise and a hearty, unrestrained appetite is liable to bring it on. A disordered condition of the digestive organs, especially the stomach and liver, are among the more prominent causes. The arrest of digestion, chronic dyspepsia, constipation, intellectual or physical fatigue, fevers, inflammation, blood poisoning, malaria, exhausting hemorrhages, derangement of the menstrual functions, exposure to the heat of the sun, or similar causes, may favor attacks of vertigo. The irritation resulting from disease of the ear, or from foreign bodies in the ear, or organic disease of the brain, may result in vertigo. Certain drugs, as alcohol, tobacco, belladonna and others, may act as causes. The most frequent cause, however, is disordered digestion.

An attack of vertigo may be momentary, or it may last an indefinite period. The degree and duration will be likely to depend upon the cause. Old people are more subject to attacks of vertigo than any other class.

TREATMENT.

When vertigo is associated with flushed countenance and distention of the veins and arteries of the temple it is suggestive of apoplexy, and should receive prompt attention. When vertigo is associated with the opposite condition, as pallor and anæmia, it is usually due to weakness, indigestion and disorder of the uterine functions, and requires a line of treatment to enrich the blood and improve the general condition. The treatment demands a diligent search for the cause.

In all cases the diet should be regulated and the course of life made to conform to hygienic laws. If animal food has been used to excess let a milk and vegetable diet be substituted. When due to overwork, rest and change of air, as a summer at the seaside or a trip across the ocean, will be found preferable to medicine. Constipation should be relieved, the use of tobacco regulated or abandoned. Defective vision should receive attention. Diseases of the ear should be looked after and intelligently treated. When vertigo is caused by disease of the inner ear it is persistent and difficult to reach. When signs of cerebral congestion exist the following will be found efficient:

℞	Extract ergot, fl.	one ounce
	Tr. digitalis	two drams
	Bromide of potash	one ounce
	Syr. orange peel	two ounces
	Water to make	eight ounces

Mix. The dose of this is one dessertspoonful every four hours.

If anæmia exist the remedies recommended for that affection or for headache due to anæmia are reliable.

VIII.—INSOMNIA.

Inability to sleep is often a serious trouble to the brain worker. It is impossible to continue mental or physical exertion without a proper amount of sleep and not incur the danger of nervous exhaustion. In fact it is a prominent symptom of brain exhaustion.

CAUSES.

It is often the symptom of some affection, or it may be due to temporary emotions. Its chief cause is congestion of the tissues of the brain, a condition which is invited by overwork, great anxiety, depressing emotion, or excessive activity of the tissues of the brain. The patient is often nervous, sometimes hysterical, lies awake a long time after retiring, all the activities of the day pass in review, the brain is active, thought succeeds thought, plan succeeds plan, the head is hot, the heart beats heavily, and the reclining position seems less favorable to sleep than the upright posture. Some people are awake very early in the morning, at two or three o'clock, and are unable to get to sleep again. Among the causes may be mentioned chronic heart disease. Pregnancy often causes insomnia. It may be the indication of approaching insanity. The insane are usually poor sleepers.

TREATMENT.

Leave off mental work some time before retiring and take a walk out of doors. The head may be bathed with cold water and cooling lotions. Country air is good. Take a vacation, or sea voyage, especially in a sailing vessel. Hot foot baths or sponge baths are beneficial; avoid late suppers, and sleep in a cold room with the window open. Quiet the nervous system by good habits, regulate the daily life, attend to the digestion and relieve constipation.

Avoid spirits, as they only lead from bad to worse. Bromide of potash may be used with less danger than opium, but it affords no nourishment to the exhausted brain. Sulfonal in powder of five grains may afford relief. Chloral may be used sometimes with benefit to calm the excited brain and produce much needed sleep, but it is not safe to resort to such a remedy except as it is recommended by the medical adviser.

When sleeplessness is due to organic disease it must receive the attention of the doctor. The warm bath before retiring is an excellent remedy. The bath should be warm, 95 degrees or more, and continued from twenty minutes to half an hour. This may be followed, if necessary, with cold applications to the head.

IX.—INSANITY.

Insanity appears to be due to a disordered condition of some of the nerve centers of the brain, which is sufficient to produce derangement of the thoughts, feelings, or actions, or all combined. When the functions of the brain are so disordered as to render the patient incapable of fulfilling the ordinary relations of life, his condition is known as insanity.

While it is difficult to give a satisfactory definition of the term insanity, yet, according to modern investigation and teaching, it is a condition resulting from a disturbance or disease in some portion of the brain. Views respecting the character of this disease have undergone no little change during the past twenty years.

The history of insanity, if not as old as the race, runs back to a very remote period. It is a well recognized and unpleasant fact that the number of insane persons is steadily on the increase; yet it must be borne in mind in accepting this statement that the recognition of insanity has broadened very much, so as to embrace a large number not formerly included. The medical skill of today renders this disease more readily detected than formerly. It is not strange, too, that insanity increases when we consider the increasing demands of our exacting civilization, and the only cause for wonder is that so few brains are overwhelmed by the intensity and perplexity of modern life.

CAUSES.

These are both predisposing and exciting. Among the predisposing, the hereditary tendency to insanity stands first, and close to this stands the intermarriage of those who are so closely related as to be unable to produce a vigorous and healthy progeny. Such marriages result in deterioration of offspring although the reasons for such degeneracy cannot be easily explained. Other predisposing causes are long continued ill health, which finally results in a hopeless condition of melancholy; an overcrowded population, rendering the struggle for life, on the part of the poorer classes, desperate and severe.

The exciting causes are intemperance, overwork, mental anxiety and worry, disappointment, especially in love, political or religious excitement, prolonged domestic or business troubles, poverty, excesses which overtax the strength and debilitate the body, and especially the brain.

SYMPTOMS.

The symptoms of insanity are numerous and varied. They are usually classified under the three heads of illusions, delusion and hallucination. The more noticeable and common symptoms are a change of character, as a lowered moral tone, increased irritability, a loss of stability, a loss of memory, and a loss of interest in affairs.

There may be a loss of self-control, a manifestation of stupor or violence, and usually a disposition to be suspicious, cunning, and in nearly all cases sleeplessness. The usual classification of the different forms of insanity is mania, melancholia and dementia, and under one or the other of these heads every form of insanity may be placed.

TREATMENT.

The treatment of insanity requires the control and restraint of the patient for his own protection and for the protection of others. These are especially prominent requirements in that form of insanity known as acute mania. Attention must be given to the bodily functions in order to secure their healthful action. The tendency to constipation and wakefulness so often characteristic of the insane should be remedied. Sufficient nourishment is essential, and it is sometimes necessary to resort to artificial methods of feeding in order to fulfill this requirement. The treatment for insane cases can only be outlined in a general way, for each case needs to be studied and have a treatment especially appropriate for its own peculiarities.

Some cases do better at home, surrounded by friends, where freedom from restraint and care are secured; other cases do better in an asylum, away from friends and under the influence and control of strangers. Much improvement has been made in the treatment of the insane in recent years. Quite as much dependence is now made upon such remedial agents as rest, nutritious diet, baths, fresh air and agreeable occupation, as upon medicines.

When medicines are required they must be so chosen as to meet the individual requirements of the case in hand. Such medicines as improve the appetite and digestion are often needed. Medicines to relieve constipation, aid sleep and improve the general condition may be required. The sources of irritation should be ascertained and removed. Drugs to produce sleep should be chosen with care and used with good judgment. Rest and travel are often important aids to recovery.

X.—APOPLEXY.

Apoplexy is the result of pressure upon the brain due either to congestion or hemorrhage within the skull. If due to hemorrhage, there is the rupture of a blood vessel, and pressure upon the brain is caused by a clot of blood.

An attack of apoplexy is usually sudden, and for this reason it is sometimes called a stroke. It is unusual in children and young persons, but after sixty years of age it is quite a common cause of death.

SYMPTOMS.

Previous to an attack of apoplexy there may be some premonitory symptoms, as headache, vertigo, drowsiness, confusion of the mind, loss of memory for words, causing their wrong use, a changed disposition, weakening of one side of the body, and other similar warnings. In other cases the attack comes on suddenly, the patient falling insensible without warning. The facial muscles and tongue are drawn to one side, and the stupor is sudden, with snoring respiration. The pulse is slow, the face flushed, and the unconsciousness profound. Apoplexy is associated with more or less paralysis of a leg, arm, or of one side of the body. Partial or complete recovery may take place, but the mental force is ordinarily more or less permanently impaired.

CAUSES.

The cause of this disease is a degenerate condition of the blood vessels of the brain, which permits their rupture when the force of extra exertion or pressure is brought to bear upon them. Predisposing causes are high living, mental excitement, lymphatic temperament, age, and the use of alcoholic stimulants. Whatever determines an unusual quantity of blood to the brain and retards its return may help to cause the rupture of a blood vessel and result in a stroke of apoplexy.

TREATMENT.

When apoplexy is threatened, but has not occurred, means should be taken to relieve the brain from excessive blood pressure. Medicines which relieve congestion by contracting the blood vessels are beneficial. Mustard draughts may be applied to the feet, and cold applications, as vinegar and water, or ice, to the head. Rest should be maintained in a cool room, the bowels opened freely, and the head well elevated; and quiet is essential. Do not give solid food, but milk and beef tea are appropriate.

The aromatic spirits of ammonia, if stimulants are needed, may be given in teaspoonful doses. When it is known that hemorrhage has occurred it is usual to give a dose of physic. Aconite in one drop doses of the tincture every hour or two is beneficial.

After a few weeks, massage and electricity are appropriate to overcome the wasting of the paralyzed muscles and to aid in their restoration. Many other remedies could be suggested, but remedies are of little avail in this disease, unless adapted to the individual case in hand. A young and vigorous patient is more likely to recover than one who is aged and feeble.

Bleeding was formerly much resorted to in the treatment of apoplexy, but recent medical practice favors it only in rare cases and when the condition of plethora is well marked. In a few cases it may be advantageous. It is safe to administer medicines to act upon the bowels freely in every case.

XI.—VARIOUS OTHER DISEASES OF THE BRAIN.

Abscess of the Brain.—An inflammation sometimes takes place in the brain followed by a localized collection of pus. The cause may be stated as contusion and other injury, or caries of the cranial bones. The abscess may be as small as an almond or pea, or it may be much larger. The abscess is usually encysted or enclosed in a membrane. The symptoms are similar to those of brain disease in general, and the diagnosis cannot be made by ordinary individuals. These cases usually terminate fatally, but surgical interference has brought some recent cases to a successful issue.

Tumors of the Brain.—These growths within the brain are rare and can be dismissed with few words. Tumors within the brain affect it unduly on account of pressure. Cancer within the skull terminates fatally. The diagnosis is uncertain and the treatment unpromising. The symptoms resemble meningitis, apoplexy, and pressure. See general articles on tumors.

Aphasia.—This is inability to use language or express ideas. It is one of the common results of apoplexy.

Amnesia.—Is loss of memory, either real or apparent, temporary or partial. A familiar word or fact sometimes escapes a speaker which, for the time being, he is utterly unable to recall. Sometimes after severe acute diseases the memory for a time is left a blank. In some cases there is ability to recall the remote events of childhood, but no ability to recall the events of the present or immediate past. This may be due to the deterioration of the brain in old age, or to softening of the brain, and is known as amnesia.

Numbness and Prickling.—These may be due to pressure upon some large nerve. Numbness occurs in many nervous affections, in poisoning, in lesions of the brain, or of the spinal cord.

Hemiplegia.—This is a form of paralysis involving one side, or half of the body. It may result from embolism or from apoplexy. Embolism is the plugging of an artery by a clot. It causes arrest of nutrition, followed by softening of the brain.

Paraplegia.—This is a paralysis of the lower half of the body, and results from disability of the spine. It is due to inflammation, hemorrhage, or pressure from some cause, as syphilitic tumors. It comes on suddenly, or gradually, and it may be complete or partial. It may be due to disease of the membranes of the spinal cord, or to pressure from dislocation of a vertebra, or from a tumor or growth which cuts off connection with the nerve of the lower extremities.

Locomotor Ataxia.—This is a disease of the spinal cord. It is due to organic changes which take place in the posterior portion of the cord, causing atrophy and degeneration. These changes take place gradually, the disease reaching over several years. A hardening process takes place which affects the circulation, the nutrition and the muscular movements. The patient is unable to stand or walk in the dark or with the eyes shut. The locomotion is chiefly affected and is peculiar. In the early stages there are deep seated pains about the thighs, legs and back, which are mistaken for rheumatism. The disease may exist fifteen or twenty years. It is thought to result from dissipation and abuse of the sexual organs. It is sometimes the result of syphilitic disease.. The treatment in such hopeless cases is unsatisfactory, the preparations of gold and electricity perhaps doing as much good as anything.

Facial Paralysis.—This may be due to pressure upon the great nerves which supply the face. The features are distorted and drawn either toward the right or left, usually only one side being affected. It is the contraction of the muscles on the unaffected side which causes the distortion. The treatment of these cases is not as encouraging as of many other affections. Electricity will benefit some cases, and perhaps cure some of those of more simple degree. Phosphorus and strychnia are powerful remedies to nourish and stimulate disabled nerves, but their use should be left in the hands of the medical practitioner. Other forms of paralysis are known to physicians such as writer's cramp, wasting and shaking palsy, different forms of paralysis of the aged, infantile paralysis, etc.

Congenital Defects.—Congenital defects of the brain are of considerable interest to the physician, and such defects together with other deformities may be appropriately noticed here. Congenital defects exist at birth, and sometimes are of such a serious character as to limit the duration of life to a few hours, days, months, or years. Hydrocephalus may exist at birth, and indicates usually a brief existence. Other defects of the brain may exist, or there is in rare instances an imperfect development of the brain, or an absence of the brain itself. When this latter condition exists, independent existence cannot be established, and as soon as the link connecting the circulation of mother and child is severed death ensues. Respiration cannot be established nor can the heart beat be excited without the controlling energy and force of the great nerve centers. Other congenital deformities may be a failure of the spine to close at some portion, causing a tumor at that point (spina bifida). Congenital defects, such as hair lip and cleft palate are of more frequent occurrence. Congenital defects of the heart sometimes exist, so that life is continued but a brief period. Such defects are sometimes confined to the organs of generation, and many of these can be remedied by the surgeon, while others are too serious to remedy. This, however, is to be remembered by the prospective mother, that such defects are occasional, and belong to the exception rather than the rule. No one should allow life to be clouded by fear of such defects or deformities, and brooding over them may be the chief factor in their production.

CHAPTER XIII.

THE EYE, ITS APPENDAGES AND DISEASES.

I.—Description of the Eye: 1, The Orbits; 2, The Optic Nerves; 3, The Sclerotic; 4, The Choroid; 5, The Iris; 6, The Ciliary Muscle or Ligament; 7, The Ciliary Process; 8, The Retina; 9, The Interior of the Eye; 10, The Appendages of the Eye.

II.—Examination of the Eyes; Errors of Refraction: 1, Myopia or Near Sight; 2, Hypermetropia or Far Sight; 3, Presbyopia or Old Sight; 4, Astigmatism.

III.—The Use of Glasses, and Directions for Testing the Eyesight.

IV.—Care of the Eyes.

V.—Diseases of the Eye; 1, Ulcers; 2, Paralysis; 3, Twitching of the Lids; 4, Inflammation of the Eye; 5, Stye; 6, Blepharitis; 7, Wounds of the Eyelids; 8, Conjunctivitis or Ophthalmia; 9, Purulent Ophthalmia; 10, Granular Ophthalmia or Granular Lids.

VI.—Foreign Bodies in the Eye.

VII.—Inflammations of the Cornea (Corneitis): 1, Ulcers of the Cornea; 2, Corneal Opacities; 3, Staphyloma.

VIII.—Inflammation of the Iris or Iritis.

IX.—Inflammation of the Choroid.

X.—Sympathetic Inflammation.

XI.—Glaucoma.

XII.—Inflammation of the Retina.

XIII.—Inflammation of the Optic Nerve.

XIV.—Cataract.

XV.—Cross Eye, Squint or Strabismus.

XVI.—Various Other Affections: 1, Growths; 2, Inflammation of the Tear Duct; 3, Abscesses of the Lachrymal Sack.

I.—DESCRIPTION OF THE EYE.

THE apparatus for vision is both ingenious and complex. The eye is a beautiful and wonderful organ. This description of it includes not only the apparatus for seeing, but also the appendages of the eye.

In simple language, each eyeball forms a hollow sphere, composed of three layers, or tunics. The inside layer is blackened over by deposits of pigment, so that pictures are formed upon its surface. The interior of the eyeball contains fluid material and a double convex lens, which lies behind the two chambers of the eye and converges the rays of light, so that a distinct image is formed upon the retina, which is conveyed to the brain by the optic nerve.

The light passes from without in order, through the cornea, the aqueous humor, the chrystalline lens, the vitreous humor, and is focused upon the back part of the eye, where the images or outlines of objects are formed. This outline or impression is carried to the brain by the optic nerve, and a sensation is awakened which we call vision.

There are some things pertaining to this process which are difficult to explain to the ordinary reader.

The amount of light admitted to the eyes is regulated by the iris. The iris is so sensitive that it contracts the pupil when the light is too bright, and enlarges it when the light is too dim to produce perfect vision. In this way the rays are diminished or increased, as the requirements of perfect vision demand. A muscular arrangement also increases or diminishes the convexity of the lens so that objects can be seen far away as well as near at hand. Muscles are attached to the eyeballs which rotate them sufficiently to enlarge the field of vision and permit a wide survey at the same instant.

The two eyes also act in such harmony that the images formed upon each retina, though slightly different, are blended into one symmetrical whole. This is, in brief, a description of the apparatus for vision. It is very similar to the method employed in taking pictures with the camera obscura, which was no doubt suggested by a study of the human eye.

The Orbits.—The orbits are the bony cavities which give a secure abode for the eyeballs. They are shaped like pyramids, with the base in front and the apex extending backward toward the brain. Through an opening, called the optic foramen, at the apex, the optic nerve enters, accompanied by blood vessels, both essential to the functions of the eye. The orbits are lined with periosteum, and contain considerable connective tissue and fat, which forms an easy bed for the eye to rest upon, and favors its natural movements.

The bony structures, so prominent about the eyes, serve to protect these important organs from harm.

The Optic Nerve.—The optic nerves compose the second pair of cranial nerves; they have nothing to do with motion or sensation. They are nerves of special sense. The optic nerve, accompanied by an artery, penetrates the back part of each eyeball, and is spread out upon the retina so as to make it very sensitive to impressions, and for this reason the retina is sometimes termed the sensitive coat or tunic of the eye. Division of the optic nerve causes immediate blindness.

The Sclerotic.—The sclerotic is the outside coat or tunic of the eye, and forms its structure; it is called the fibrous tunic. It receives its name on account of its density and hardness. It is the toughness of this tissue which enables the eyes to preserve the shape of a globe. The sclerotic makes up about five-sixths of the external surface of the eyeball. The remaining one-sixth is situated directly in front, and is called the cornea. This is a continuation of the sclerotic, but for the purpose of vision is transparent. It is sometimes called the window of the eye, because it admits the rays of light. It sits upon the globe somewhat like the crystal of a watch, being the segment of a smaller sphere.

Around the margin of the cornea the sclerotic is seen as a white, glistening surface, which is known as the white of the eye. The cornea is composed of five distinct layers.

The Choroid.—Directly within the sclerotic coat is the choroid. This is a thin, delicate membrane, but so liberally supplied with blood vessels that it is sometimes called the vascular tunic. It has four separate layers. The choroid extends over the whole back part of the eyeball and reaches as far forward as the cornea. It terminates in the ciliary ligament, the ciliary processes and the iris.

The Iris.—It is a continuation of the choroid, and is a circular, muscular curtain, which hangs vertically behind the cornea, and in front of the crystalline lens.

It has an opening in the center called the pupil. The iris is differently colored in different persons by pigments, which accounts for the great variety of color and beauty of the human eye; some eyes appearing to be very light, and others blue, brown, hazel or black. The pupil is simply an opening in the center of the eye, which varies in size with the contraction or dilation of the iris. It appears to be black, because when standing in front of a person and looking into the eye the rays of light are intercepted, and you look into a dark chamber.

The Ciliary Muscles or Ligaments.—These are a continuation of the choroid, and cause the contraction and dilation of the iris, and hence are the prominent factors in accommodation.

The Ciliary Processes.—They are a continuation also of the choroid, and are composed of a circle of folds behind the iris, attached to the ciliary muscle and surrounding the margin of the lens.

The Retina.—Within the choroid is the retina; it forms the third or inner tunic of the eyeball, and from the fact that the optic nerve is spread out over this membrane it is sometimes called the sensitive tunic. It is a thin membrane, composed of three layers and very liberally supplied by nerves. It lines the interior of the globe from the optic nerve as far forward as the ciliary ligaments.

The whole surface of the retina is blackened over by deposits of pigment and, with the exception of a point where the optic nerve passes through it, it possesses the power of receiving visual impressions. This point is called the blind spot. The terminal fibers of the optic nerve are gathered together in bundles upon the retina, and from their resemblance are known as the layer of rods and cones.

The parts above described, viz.: the sclerotic, choroid and retina form the three tunics or coverings of the eyeball, also known as the fibrous, the vascular and the sensitive tunics.

The Interior of the Eye.—In the interior of the eye are the aqueous humor, the crystalline lens, and the vitreous humor; these are known as the refracting media or humors of the eye.

The aqueous humor is a clear, saline fluid and fills that portion of the eye between the cornea and crystalline lens known as the anterior and posterior chambers. The vitreous humor fills all the cavity of the globe back of the lens. It is perfectly transparent and about the consistency of thin jelly. It occupies four-fifths of the space in the eyeball.

The crystalline lens is situated behind the pupil, or opening in the iris. It is a transparent body, biconvex, or convex on both sides. It is enclosed in a capsule, and is held in place by the suspensory ligament. This lens is about a quarter of an inch in diameter. It separates the aqueous from the vitreous humor. The lens, acted upon by its muscular surroundings, has the power of increasing or diminishing its convexity, in order that a vision may be obtained of near or remote objects. The power imparted to the eye by the ciliary ligament, which dilates and contracts the iris, and by the suspensory ligament which increases or diminishes the convexity of the lens, is known as accommodation. By means of this faculty we can see objects far away as well as near at hand, for the rays of light are brought to a focus upon the retina whether we are reading a book or looking at some far away object. Some deficiency in the power of accommodation is a common fault of many eyes.

The motion of the eyeballs is due to six muscles, four recti and two oblique. The muscles of both eyes usually act in harmony. When the muscles do not act in harmony, owing to a loss of power, the result is a condition known as strabismus or squint. These muscles have their origin in the tissues about the apex of the orbits, and are inserted into the sclerotic a short distance back of the cornea. The oblique muscles run through a ring which acts as a pully, and increases the leverage. These muscles combine to give a wide range of motion to the eye.

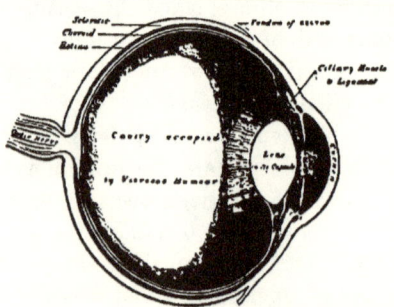

Section of the eyeball showing its internal structure and the entrance of optic nerve.

The various appendages of the eye are worthy of notice in this connection. The eyebrows are prominent ridges of skin on the upper borders of the orbits. They support a growth of short hairs, and are connected with certain muscles which somewhat control the amount of light admitted to the eye. The eyebrows are often marks of beauty.

The eyelids are two thin folds which open and close to protect the eye from injury. The upper lid is larger and more movable than the lower. The skin of the eyelids is thin, and beneath it there is some connective tissue, muscular fibers, cartilage, vessels, nerves and glands, lined up on the inside with a thin mucous membrane known as the conjunctiva. This not only lines the eyelids, but is reflected over the front portion of the sclerotic and cornea. That portion which covers the cornea is extremely delicate and does not appear to contain any blood vessels. Along the margin of each lid is a row of fine hairs, the eyelashes. The eyelids when open form an elliptical space, and the angles formed by the junction of the upper and lower lids are called the outer and inner canthus respectively. The inner canthus contains a small, triangular space, and on the margin of each lid is a little elevation with an orifice which is the commencement of the tear duct. Between the cartilage of the lids and the conjunctiva a row of glands is situated which may be seen by everting the eyelid, the Meibomian glands. There are between twenty and thirty in each lid. They open by means of little tubes on the borders of the lids. They secrete an oily fluid, which prevents the eyelids from sticking together. The eyelids are moved by means of delicate muscles which open and close the lids involuntarily, as in winking.

This act washes over the surface of the cornea, removes particles of dust, and also prevents the cornea from getting dry. The eyelids are abundantly supplied with delicate nerve branches and blood vessels.

In the inner canthus of the eye is a small, reddish, triangular elevation, containing a cluster of follicles, covered with mucous membrane. These follicles secrete a fluid substance which collects in the inner corner of the eye. The lachrymal or tear gland is about the size and shape of an almond, and is situated in a depression above the outer canthus or angle. Seven or more little ducts, opening at the reflection of the conjunctiva upon the sclerotic, connect this gland to the surface of the eye and convey the tears which it secretes. Unless the secretion is excessive this fluid is carried away in little canals into the cavity of the nose. But in excessive grief there is an overflow of these tears upon the face, as seen in the act of crying. Sometimes there is an obstruction of the canal which conveys away the tears, and then there is the condition known as watery or weeping eye. In old age the eye loses a great measure of its luster; the cornea and lens become flattened, rendering glasses a necessity for distinct vision. Near the outer margin of the cornea a grayish circle forms, called the "arcus senilis," and is the result of degenerative changes. Other similar changes take place to render the eye dim and vision less satisfactory in old age.

II.—EXAMINATION OF THE EYES. ERRORS OF REFRACTION.

The eye is one of the most delicately constructed organs of the human body, and while it is advisable to learn as much as possible about its different diseases, it is earnestly recommended that only skilled persons attempt to treat any except the most slight affections of this organ. Even to examine the eye thoroughly requires a large amount of practice and considerable skill.

For the examination of the interior of the eye the ophthalmoscope is everywhere extensively used. It is a concave mirror with an opening in the center. By means of this instrument light can be thrown into the back portion of the eye, and the optic nerve, the blood vessels and the retina become visible. The pupil of the eye is usually dilated with a solution of atropia before the examination is attempted.

The ophthalmoscope is an instrument of great importance, also for the diagnosis of certain diseases of remote organs, which first cause a disturbance in the delicate tissues of the eye. A skillful examination of the eye enables the examiner to detect the existence of Bright's disease and other important affections.

The appendages of the eye are readily examined and a diagnosis of conjunctivitis and other similar affections is easily made. The upper lid can be everted by lifting and turning it over the end of a probe or pencil. This is often essential in searching for some foreign body beneath the eyelid.

Myopia.—(Near Sight).—This is a congenital affection. It is that condition in which the rays of light entering the eye are brought to a focus in front of the retina. The patient can see only near objects distinctly, because the rays are brought to a focus too much in front of the retina for remote objects.

Hypermetropia.—(Far Sight).—This is the opposite of the condition just mentioned. The rays of light do not converge enough to come to a focus upon the retina. The ciliary muscle cannot increase the convexity of the lens sufficiently to see near objects distinctly. Hence the rays of light come to a focus behind the retina and vision

Lines to test the existence of astigmatism.

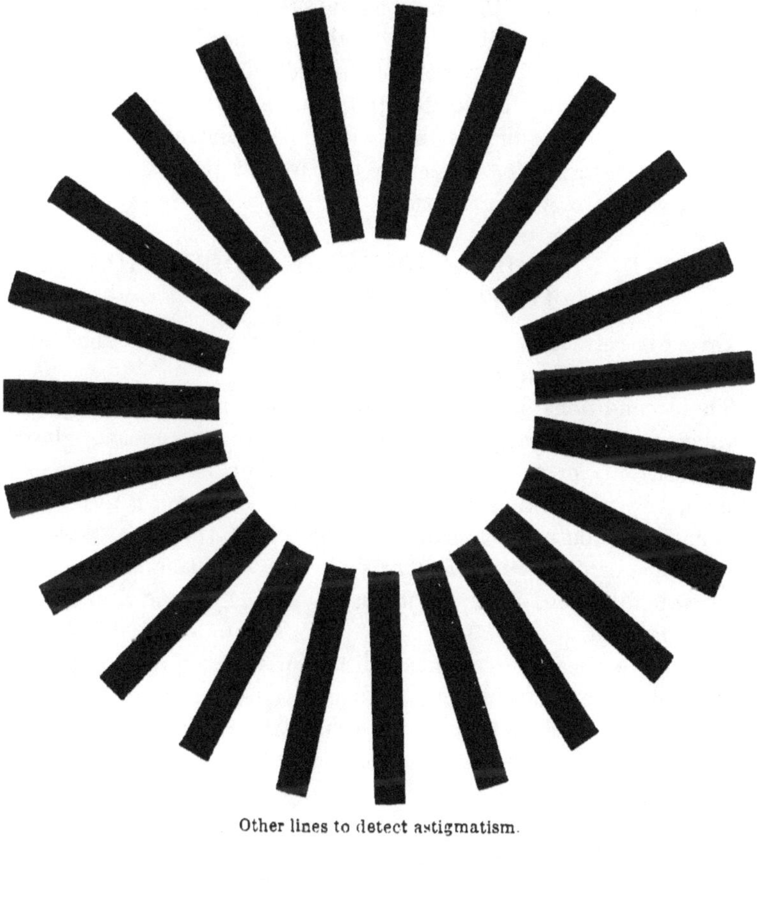

Other lines to detect astigmatism.

is indistinct. The attempt to see near objects wearies the muscles, produces headache and perhaps pain in the eyes, or eye-strain. Remote objects may be seen by the hypermetropic eye distinctly without strain, pain or weariness.

Presbyopia.—(**Old Sight**).—In this condition the patient does not see well, because the cornea is flattened and the lens does not respond to the action of the ciliary muscle sufficiently to increase its convexity. The vision is poor for near objects.

Astigmatism.—In this condition the cornea is not spherical, being warped, so to speak, and some rays of light entering the eye come to a focus sooner than others. This causes indistinct vision.

Examinations show that persons suffering from astigmatism can see horizontal lines more perfectly than perpendicular lines. The lines here represented may be used to detect this affection. Lines are also arranged in a circle radiating from a center about the size of a clock face. Some of the lines will appear blurred or indistinct if the eyes are astigmatic. Specially prepared or prismatic glasses are necessary to correct astigmatism.

III.—THE USE OF GLASSES AND DIRECTIONS FOR TESTING THE EYESIGHT.

Errors in refraction, as they are termed, are all nicely remedied by glasses suitably constructed and fitted.

These conditions can be made out by test cards or trial glasses. Myopia or near sightedness requires the use of concave glasses. Hypermetropia or far sight and presbyopia or old sight can also be remedied by well fitting glasses. Weakness of vision is usually due to some debilitating sickness, or overwork of the eyes, especially where some error of refraction exists. Loss of vision is usually due to organic disease of some of the tissues of the eye, and cannot be so easily remedied.

To use the eyes in a weak condition may result in changing an acute trouble to a chronic one, rendering a temporary affection permanent. It is often advisable to wear glasses during a temporary weakness of the eyes to prevent permanent injury, especially if complete rest is inexpedient and cannot be enjoined.

Imperfect and defective vision is largely the result of civilization. Close attention to books in schools is a prominent cause of the widespread and increasing affection known as myopia.

Hold this page, fourteen inches away from the eyes in a good light and select the smallest type that can be distinctly read with ease. The figures at the right show the focus and the number of glasses needed:

No. 1.
For age and want save while you may, no morning sun lasts all the day.   **55-60**

No. 2.
Work to-day for you know not how much you may be hindered to-morrow.   **50-55**

No. 3.
If you would have a faithful servant, and one that you like, serve yourself.   **40-48**

No. 4.
Experience keeps a dear school, but fools will learn in no other   **36-40**

No. 5.
Industry needs not wish, and he that lives upon hope will die fasting.   **30-36**

No. 6.
Want of care does us more damage than want of knowledge.   **24-30**

No. 7.
If you would know the value of money, try to borrow some.   **20-24**

No. 8.
What maintains one vice would bring up two children.   **18-20**

B
DE
BT

B E F

E T L F

P Z E D B

O L T Z B D

A C E O L N P

The power of vision is determined by means of cards containing letters of various sizes, which the normal eye can distinguish at a certain distance away.

A normal eye ought to distinguish the large letter B at a distance of fifty (50) feet; the next in size, D and E, at a distance of thirty (30) feet; the next in size, B and T, at a distance of twenty (20) feet; and the next in size, B, E and F, at a distance of fifteen (15) feet. The remaining letters in the four last lines should all be distinguished at a distance of thirteen (13) feet. Only one eye should be tested at a time; the other eye may be closed by the fingers.

Another practical method is the following:

Snellen's test type, to be seen distinctly at a distance of twenty feet.

If these letters can be distinctly seen at a distance of twenty feet there is but little, if any, defect of vision. If the patient is unable to see these letters distinctly at the distance mentioned he may be near sighted and need glasses.

Jaeger's Test Types —The method of testing the eyes by means of sentences printed in different sized type is practical. If the size of No. 1 cannot be read at any distance there is some fault of vision. If it is easily read at a distance of eight inches the vision is normal; if it can be easily read at a less distance than six inches the patient is probably near sighted; if it can only be read by holding it away more than eight inches the patient is far sighted.

IV.—CARE OF THE EYES.

The care of the eyes is exceedingly important, especially in the case of children.

Reading and fine work require plenty of light. It is better for the rays of light to fall over the left or right shoulder than to come from in front of the eyes.

The eyes are often strained or weakened by attempting to read in the twilight, or when the source of light is too far away. The eye is injured by reading upon moving trains, which, by their unsteadiness of motion, constantly change the focus and render reading difficult and tiresome. Books printed in very small type, or badly blurred, so as to be indistinct, should be avoided. Reading in bed is not a good habit. The position is unsuitable, the light unfavorable, and the eye is subjected to unusual strain, besides the danger of falling asleep and setting the house on fire.

Riding against the wind is sometimes injurious, and may cause congestion of the tissues about the eye. A foul atmosphere, or one filled with smoke, vapor, dust, or gas, is bad for the eyes. The vapor of acid is also injurious. The glare of the sunlight, especially upon the seashore, or from the pavements of the city, is trying, and the eyes should be protected from excessive light by a broad brim hat or appropriate glasses. The light reflected from fields of snow and ice is also trying, and requires their protection.

The eyes should receive especial care after certain diseases, as measles, scarlet fever and small pox.

The eyes are often weak during pregnancy, and for a long time after confinement. When the eyes are weak as the result of some especial tax upon the nervous system, or some disease, their use should be regulated and reading and study prohibited for a suitable period.

The eyes should be kept clean. It is safe to bathe them in warm or cold water, and for severe pain in the eye hot water may be applied for a few minutes every hour. The continuous use of moist heat, as produced by a poultice, is dangerous, and ought not to be employed, except advisedly, since it is liable to soften the delicate tissues and do great harm, or even destroy the sight. For eyes that are easily inflamed, an application of water, containing a little common salt, is said to be beneficial. A teaspoonful of salt to a quart of water is sufficient, and may be applied once or twice a day.

The habits exert their influence upon the eyes as well as upon the other tissues of the body. Incessant smokers and drinkers are liable to have diseases of the retina and optic nerve. Excessive sexual indulgence is liable to have a debilitating influence upon the eyes. Insufficient food, overwork, or whatever produces a profound impression upon the system, is liable to have a corresponding effect upon the eyes, for they are very sensitive to our habits, and sympathize with any constitutional impairment. General attention to the health, as exercise, bathing, nutritious food and correct habits, find corresponding approval and response in the eyes.

Life in the country strengthens the eyes and trains them for far vision, while life in the city favors myopia. Constantly looking at near objects favors near sight, while looking far out and away, over field and landscape, helps to perfect the eye and adapt it to a wide range of vision. When performing work which is difficult and exacting, frequently look away for a second, as this relieves and rests the eyes.

V.—DISEASES OF THE EYE.

Diseases of the eye and its appendages form a numerous class. Some of them, owing to difficulty of treatment or to their rarity, will be only briefly noticed.

Ulcers.—Ulcers occur upon the eyelids, sometimes as the result of syphilis. These are to be treated as similar ulcers elsewhere.

Paralysis.—Paralysis of the nerves which control the eyelids may occur. There is inability to close the lids. The lower lid falls away, the eye fills with tears and overflows owing to the displacement of the tear duct.

The treatment for this affection is the administration of strychnia, one-sixtieth of a grain three times a day, also the external application of electricity.

Twitching of the Lid.—This may be due to some affection of the cornea, or it may result from some nervous state or indigestion. The treatment requires attention to the general health, and the correction of any errors of refraction by glasses.

Inflammation of the Eyelids.—This may result after measles, scarlet fever, erysipelas, or from injuries or severe neighboring inflammations. This condition demands attention to the general health, cooling and soothing lotions.

Stye.—This generally occurs in persons of delicate health. It consists of a small red and painful swelling due to the closure and inflammation of the outlet of one of the glands. When pus has formed the stye should be pricked or opened and this will afford no little relief. When a succession of styes occurs, they indicate that the general health should receive attention, and suitable tonics should be administered.

Blepharitis.—This disease of the lids is characterized by the formation of dry crusts or scales along their margin about the eyelashes. If these crusts are forcibly removed they leave an ulcerated and bleeding surface about the hairs, and sometimes the lids become thickened along the margins. This disease occurs often among unthrifty children, and is very chronic in its course, sometimes resisting all remedies. It is sometimes caused by eye strain due to errors in refraction, and yields to the adjustment of glasses. A lotion containing four or five grains of alum to an ounce of water may be used three or four times daily. The crusts should all be removed, and then apply an ointment containing one grain of the yellow oxide of mercury to one ounce of vaseline.

Wounds of the Eyelids.—These should be cleansed by an antiseptic solution and sewed up with fine silk. The stitches should be carefully removed after three or four days.

Injuries produced by blows cause a rupture of some of the small blood vessels in the soft tissues about the eye, and an extensive extravasation of blood, called ecchymosis or black eye. Time will cause the absorption of the blood, or the result may be hastened by the following lotion:

℞ Chloride of ammonia one dram
   Water one pint

Mix and apply on a piece of muslin.

Conjunctivitis or Ophthalmia.—There are a number of varieties of this affection, but in all the eyes are red and inflamed. There is pain of a smarting, itching character, and the eyelids are glued together by the discharges of the glands during sleep.

This affection is best treated by astringent lotions, and the more chronic the trouble the stronger they may be. Weak lotions are sufficient for mild acute cases. The following are harmless and often beneficial:

℞ Alum three grains
   Distilled water one ounce

Mix and use as eye wash.

℞ Sulphate of zinc one or two grains
   Distilled water one ounce

Mix and use as eye wash.

A little vaseline may be used on the margin of the lids each night to prevent them from being glued together. Many other remedies are used by the surgeon, but these here recommended are mild and can be used by any one without danger. Catarrhal ophthalmia is the most common variety, and is caused principally by taking cold. The disease often commences in one eye, extending soon to the other. It spreads from one person to another by using the same towel, and in other ways. The above lotions are suitable for this affliction. If there is much smarting a grain of cocaine may be added to either prescription for its relief.

Purulent Ophthalmia.—This occurs in new-born children, and is due to the inoculation of the eye with the acid secretions of the vagina. The worst form is where the secretions are gonorrheal. The disease appears a few days after birth. The eyelids are swollen; the conjunctiva is highly congested; the eyes cannot bear the light; they are opened with difficulty, and there is an abundant discharge of whitish or yellowish matter. This affection among new-born children is known as ophthalmia neonatorum. There is much danger of implication of the cornea, which is sometimes destroyed, and the sight is lost.

Treatment.—Wash out the eye every hour during the day with a strong alum lotion: Alum, ten grains; water, one ounce, and apply vaseline or some simple ointment to the lids.

The conjunctiva is sometimes inflamed by hot lime or metals spattering into the eyes.

Examine the eye thoroughly and remove all foreign particles. For slacking lime, wash the eye thoroughly in water to which a little vinegar has been added. Then place a drop or two of sweet oil between the lids.

Granular Ophthalmia.—This is a disease which often results from unfavorable hygienic surroundings, and the crowding together of individuals in workshops, schools, and in the army. It is characterized by the enlargement of the little follicles in the conjunctiva which covers the eyelids, these appearing as little concave elevations in a state of inflammation. They sometimes irritate and injure the cornea, so as to destroy a measure of its transparency. The treatment used by the oculist is the thorough removal of the granulations without destroying the surrounding tissue. This is accomplished by applying the mitigated nitrate of silver stick twice a week, and using the following astringent lotion:

℞ Sulphate of copper   two grains
    Water   one ounce

Mix and apply four or five times a day.

Many eyes have been permanently injured by incompetent treatment. Other affections may complicate the existing trouble and require the exhibition of extraordinary skill.

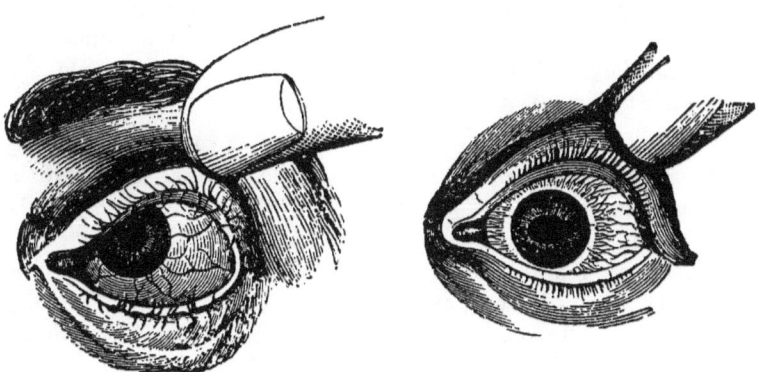

Conjunctivitis, showing congested blood vessels.

Iritis, showing change in shape of pupil.

VI.—FOREIGN BODIES IN THE EYE.

Particles of metal, cinders, the grit from emery wheels and other substances often strike the eye with such force as to become imbedded in the conjunctiva or cornea. They can be removed by a soft piece of cloth or by the surgeon with a spud or a pair of forceps

If the eye is much inflamed and intolerant of the light a little cocaine solution dropped into it a few minutes before attempting to remove the foreign body greatly facilitates the operation.

VII.—INFLAMMATIONS OF THE CORNEA (CORNEITIS).

Many diseases of the eye involve the cornea. They derive their importance from the fact that any impairment of the transparency of the cornea affects the vision unfavorably. There are several varieties of corneal inflammation. It is sometimes caused by injuries, as the lodging of foreign bodies upon or in the corneal tissue. There is pain, intolerance of light, an increase of tears, and a dull or hazy condition of the cornea, with congestion of the blood vessels surrounding the cornea. It is sometimes associated with inflammation of the iris.

Inflammation of the cornea may be suppurative. This is usually caused by some injury, as a blow from a twig, or some other substance. It also results from great debility, after severe sickness, as fevers, or it develops in those who have suffered for lack of food, or those who inherit scrofula or syphilis. Cases of such grave import should be submitted to a competent oculist.

Foreign bodies or other irritating causes should be removed. Constitutional remedies should be given, such as iodide of potash, and iron in pill form. The eye needs rest, protection from the light, and such other treatment as the symptoms indicate.

Ulcers of the Cornea.—These occur in great variety. They may be superficial, or involve all the layers of the cornea. They may be small or large, there may be one or several. They may injure the transparency of a single point or of the whole cornea.

Children are more subject to these affections than others. They occur after acute diseases, as measles and scarlet fever. They may result from a debilitated condition of the system, or from some defect in the nutrition of the eye.

The symptoms of corneal ulcer are smarting pain, intolerance of light, increased flow of tears, and the feeling as if there was something in the eye. The treatment varies with the condition of the patient and the character of the ulceration. The general health must be looked after, and the eye needs to be somewhat protected from the light. A lotion containing two grains of atropia to an ounce of water is much employed. Of this two or three drops are used in the eye quite frequently. A sloughing ulcer sometimes extends rapidly, and if not arrested perforation of the cornea takes place, followed by prolapse of the iris and loss of sight. To prevent this unfortunate occurrence surgeons resort to one of the following operations: The puncturing or tapping the cornea with a needle and allowing some of the fluid to escape. This relieves the pressure on the cornea from behind. Or, to iridectomy, which is the name given to the removal of a portion of the iris.

Corneal Opacities are either the result of injuries, inflammation or ulceration. The cornea is found, after healing, to have lost more or less of its transparency, and to have become hazy or cloudy. This condition may be present in varying degrees from a slight cloudiness to a dense white opacity, involving the entire cornea. Slight corneal opacities may improve or nearly disappear, as in the case of children, and their removal may be aided by applications which favor absorption.

Staphyloma.—This is the name given to a bulging of the cornea, from its fancied resemblance to a grape. It causes great disfigurement of the eye and is itself caused by ulceration of the cornea and prolapse of the iris. When the whole cornea bulges forward the disease is said to be total; if only some portion of it, it is said to be partial. The treatment of this affection when total is the removal of the eye, to prevent the sound eye from becoming diseased also.

VIII.—INFLAMMATION OF THE IRIS OR IRITIS.

There are three varieties of iritis: simple, rheumatic and syphilitic. There are several causes which may produce it, as an extension of irritation from foreign bodies in the conjunctiva or cornea, friction due to granulations upon the lids, injuries from accidents or operations, debility after disease, rheumatism, gout and syphilis.

SYMPTOMS.

These are a changed color of the iris, more or less severe pain, contraction of the pupil, a redness around the border of the cornea, dimness of vision, and intolerance of light. A simple attack may last from one to two weeks, or even longer. There is danger of adhesions forming between the iris and crystalline lens.

Rheumatic iritis occurs in those persons who are subject to gout or rheumatism. It tends to reappear again and again in the same individual, and from this fact it is termed recurrent iritis. It is sometimes accompanied by very severe pain in the eyeball. Its most distinguishing characteristic is its tendency to recur without any apparent cause, which is prevented by the operation of iridectomy.

The most common variety of iritis is the syphilitic.

TREATMENT.

The treatment should be directed to the removal of the cause, if it can be ascertained. This may be some foreign body which excites the inflammation, or irritation produced by granulation on the lids or inverted eyelashes. The pupil should be kept dilated by a solution of atropia, one or two grains to an ounce of water, as this prevents the iris from adhering to the lens.

Syphilitic iritis should, in addition, have constitutional treatment appropriate to that disease. Tonics may be necessary in debilitated conditions. Anodynes may be required to allay pain. The eyes may be protected, if necessary, by a suitable shade.

Many other successful remedies may be used for the benefit of individual cases. To mention them would be superfluous, as iritis cannot be treated properly by the unprofessional. Iridectomy is often necessary, and this delicate operation can only be performed by a skillful oculist.

IX.—INFLAMMATION OF THE CHOROID.

This is often associated with inflammation of the iris. It is unnecessary to describe this disease as its diagnosis can only be positively made by examination with the ophthalmoscope. It is quite commonly caused by syphilis. The treatment is very similar to that of iritis. Injuries of the choroid are treated the same as injuries of the sclerotic.

X.—SYMPATHETIC INFLAMMATION.

This is a peculiar inflammation coming on in the sound eye in consequence of the injury of the other. After injury of one eye, or the lodging of a foreign body within the globe, the other eye may become irritable or painful, and inflammation the same as has existed in the injured eye succeeds. Much damage or even loss of the uninjured eye is likely to result from sympathetic ophthalmia.

The way to prevent such an unfortunate result is by the timely removal of the injured eye. If the disease has become fully established it is doubtful if the removal of the injured eye will stop the progress of the inflammation. This condition requires the advice of a competent oculist.

XI.—GLAUCOMA.

Glaucoma is a disease of the eye due to an increase of the tension of the globe. The cause is not known. It is supposed to be due either to an excessive accumulation of the fluids within the eye, or else to some defect in their absorption and removal. The symptoms are not well marked, and the disease is quite insidious. The power of vision is gradually diminished; also the power of accommodation is lessened, the pupil is dilated and the lens cloudy. Hemorrhages may occur from the blood vessels of the retina, and there may be acute pain in the eyeball. The eyeball at length becomes very hard, the cornea loses its transparency, the humors of the eye become discolored and the lens opaque. The disease ends in blindness. The acute condition is liable to become chronic. It does not come on usually before fifty years of age. This disease is not benefited by medicines, and requires the operation of iridectomy, which should be done early.

XII.—INFLAMMATION OF THE RETINA.

Inflammation of the retina is generally the result of some constitutional disease, as syphilis, or Bright's disease of the kidneys. It may, however, occur from the plugging up of the blood vessels, or from hemorrhage, or from inflammation of the brain. The vision is impaired. Other symptoms are pain, dread of the light and colored vision.

The disease is diagnosed by means of the ophthalmoscope. There is sometimes a congested condition of the blood vessels of the retina, caused by eye strain, or by working over a hot fire, and constantly looking at a bright light. This condition is remedied by rest and by protecting the eyes from too much light by a shade or some other device.

Hemorrhage sometimes occurs from the vessels of the retina, a vessel becoming ruptured. The blood clot is absorbed in time, but rarely so but what traces of the injury remains.

XIII.—INFLAMMATION OF THE OPTIC NERVE.

The optic nerve is subject to inflammation or atrophy and paralysis from pressure of tumor or other diseases of the brain. The nature of these affections becomes known only by examination of the eye with the ophthalmoscope. The vision is impaired, and partial or complete loss of sight may be the result. Some cases are benefited by the judicious use of phosphorus, iron and strychnia, also galvanic electricity. It seems to be established that the excessive use of tobacco may cause atrophy of the optic nerve. The abandonment of the narcotic in such a case is followed by improvement.

XIV.—CATARACT.

This is a common affection, usually occurring after fifty years of age. It is an opacity of the crystalline lens and caused by failure of its nutrition. The disease approaches gradually. It may result from changes due to age, or from constitutional diseases, or from inflammation in the parts which surround the lens and from which it draws nutrition. It also results from injury. When the lens becomes opaque the rays of light cannot pass through it to the retina, and vision is cut off.

There are two varieties of cataract, hard and soft. The only symptom of the disease is a milky appearance in the center of the eye and the gradual loss of vision. There is absence of pain.

TREATMENT.

When the opacity of the lens is in the center and not complete, vision may be improved by enlarging the opening in the iris. This is accomplished by the operation of iridectomy, or the removal of a portion of the iris. When the whole lens has lost its transparency its removal should be undertaken. The operation is a delicate one. A cataract knife is passed through the upper half of the cornea near

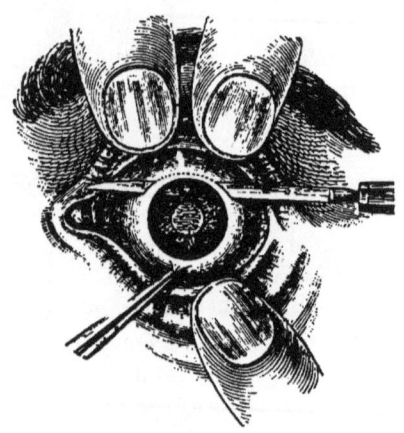

Cataract operation

its junction with the sclerotic. A portion of the aqueous humor escapes through the wound. Next a cystotome is introduced and the capsule of the lens is lacerated. This allows the lens to escape forward, and by skillful manipulation it advances through the cut made by the knife in the cornea. The eye is then bandaged, and after recovery a convex lens in front of the eye restores its vision if the operation has been successful and the eye is otherwise sound.

XV.—CROSS EYE, SQUINT OR STRABISMUS.

This is a common defect, and is caused by inequality in the strength of the muscles, which control the movements of the eye.

The two varieties of cross eye most frequently seen are convergent and divergent. In convergent squint the eye turns inward toward the nose, in divergent squint it turns outward. It is sometimes difficult to tell which eye is at fault, but various methods in use avail for this purpose.

TREATMENT.

Unless the degree of squint be slight, it can only be remedied by an operation. The muscle which contracts with the most strength, pulling the eye too far out or in, is divided at its tendinous insertion into the sclerotic. Before this can be done a little cut is made through the conjunctiva just in front of the muscle, a blunt hook is passed into this opening, the muscle is brought into view and wholly or partly divided with a pair of curved scissors close to the sclerotic.

It is often necessary to fit glasses to correct the vision, complete the success of the operation and prevent the recurrence of the trouble. It is sometimes necessary to repeat the operation or to perform it upon both eyes in bad cases.

XVI.—VARIOUS OTHER AFFECTIONS.

Growths—Tumors, growths and cancers within or about the eyeball are not of frequent occurrence, but they usually require the removal of the eyeball sooner or later, and hence should be submitted to the care of an experienced hand. It would be impossible to describe all these rare affections fully enough to be of service to non-professional readers.

Suppuration sometimes occurs within the eyeball, and rapid failure of vision results, accompanied by severe pain. The sight is generally lost, whether the pus is evacuated through an opening made or left to rupture its way out.

Inflammation of the Tear Duct.—This may be caused by injury or burns and tears overflow upon the cheek owing to the obstruction of the canal. The obstruction is removed by slitting the canal with a narrow knife.

Abscesses of the Lachrymal Sac.—The lachrymal sac, situated under the inner corner of the eye beside the nose, is sometimes the seat of an abscess due to inflammatory action. The pus should be evacuated by an opening into it, or by slitting the canal and allowing it to escape.

If the abscess takes its own course and ruptures through the skin a fistulous opening is liable to be established.

CHAPTER XIV.

THE EAR AND ITS DISEASES.

I.—Description of the Ear: 1, The External Ear; 2, The Auditory Canal; 3, The Middle Ear or Tympanum; 4, The Eustachian Tube and the Ossicles; 5, The Internal Ear or Labyrinth. II.—Diseases of the Ear: 1, Deafness; 2, Impacted Wax or Cerumen; 3, Foreign Bodies in the Ear; 4, Inflammation of the Ear; 5, Polypi. III.—Diseases of the Middle Ear: 1, Rupture of the Drum; 2, Acute and Chronic Catarrh of the Middle Ear or Otitis Media; 3, Inflation of the Middle Ear; 4, Congenital Defects of the Ear. IV.—Mastoid Disease.

I.—DESCRIPTION OF THE EAR.

THE ear exists for the purpose of collecting and conveying the impressions of sound to the brain. The process is quite intricate.

The External Ear.—The external ear assists in collecting the waves of sound and these are conveyed through the external canal and reach the drum, which is thrown into vibration.

By an arrangement of three connecting bones these vibrations are conveyed to the fluid in the labyrinth of the internal ear, and to the auditory nerve which transmits the impression to the brain, where these vibrations are perceived as sounds.

The anatomy of the ear is generally divided into the external, the middle ear or tympanum and the internal ear.

The external ear consists of that portion of the face known simply as the ear and the auditory canal. In man the muscles of the ear are rudimentary and permit of only very slight motion. The external ear consists of a layer of cartilage, which enables it to preserve its form, and various blood vessels and nerves which supply its nutrition.

The Auditory Canal.—This extends from the external opening to the drum. It is nearly circular, about an inch long and somewhat crooked. This canal is lined with a thin skin containing sebaceous glands and a special set of glands, which secrete wax and prevent insects from entering the ear.

The Middle Ear or Tympanum.—This consists of the drum, called the membrana tympani, and the cavity behind it, also the mastoid cells behind the ear and the Eustachian tube. The drum lies at the bottom of the auditory canal and separates it from the cavity behind it. It is a thin inelastic transparent membrane composed of three layers. The cavity behind the drum is called the cavity of the tympanum, and it is lined by mucous membrane which is a continuation of the lining of the pharynx and Eustachian tube.

The Eustachian Tube and the Ossicles.—The Eustachian tube is about one and one-half inches in length, and extends from the throat to the cavity of the tympanum. It contains and conveys air which aids the process of hearing. There are three small bones, called the ossicles of the tympanum, stretched across the cavity of the tympanum. They connect the drum with the labyrinth, and serve to convey vibrations of sound from the drum across the cavity of the tympanum to the internal ear. They are joined to each other and to the walls of the tympanum by ligaments. Their names are the malleus (hammer), the incus (anvil), and the stapes (stirrup).

The Internal Ear or Labyrinth.—This is the portion of the ear most essential to hearing, and to it the nerves of hearing, the auditory, are distributed. It is called the labyrinth on account of its winding, irregular shape. Its parts are the vestibule, semicircular canal and the cochlea. These parts are bony cavities lined with a thin membrane which secretes and contains fluid. Upon the walls of this membrane the nerves of hearing are distributed or spread out. These parts are so complex and so difficult to describe plainly and briefly that those who desire to pursue this subject are referred to special works upon the ear.

II.—DISEASES OF THE EAR.

Deafness.—Persons having normal hearing ought to hear a watch tick twenty inches away. Deafness may be due to several causes, as obstruction from the secretion of hardened wax or other foreign body, and disease of the middle or internal ear.

Deafness occurs, though rarely, as the result of such acute diseases as scarlet fever and cerebro-spinal meningitis. The acuteness of the hearing is tested by several methods, as the tick of a watch, the human voice, and the tuning fork. The voice test is considered as the most practical one for estimating the hearing power.

The hearing is often affected by the general health or by previous illness.

Deafness for various purposes is sometimes feigned. The clink of a coin dropped behind the pretender usually discloses the deception.

Examination of the auditory canal is conducted by means of reflected light from a mirror, as in the examination of the eye. The mirror gathers the rays of light and reflects them into the ear.

Impacted Wax or Cerumen.—This occurs frequently, and is due to an increased secretion of the glands, and is similar to a catarrhal condition of the mucous glands. It is sometimes secondary to other diseases.

SYMPTOMS.

These are a sense of fullness, sudden loss of hearing, sometimes pain, vertigo and ringing in the ears (tinnitus), due to the pressure of the hard mass upon the nerves. The hardened wax, owing to the drying action of the air, may resemble a stone, or it may be soft, and about the consistency of syrup. The accumulation of this material is so gradual that deafness does not come on until the canal is completely obstructed, and this may occur suddenly from a jar that changes its position and closes up the canal.

Sometimes there is other deep seated disease of the middle or internal ear, so that the removal of the wax will not cure the deafness, but in many cases it is sufficient to remove it.

TREATMENT.

Use a soft rubber syringe and throw warm water into the canal to soften the mass. The addition to the water of a little glycerine and bicarbonate of soda renders it more efficient, or a few drops of the following may be dropped into the ear several times a day to soften the wax:

℞   Bicarbonate of soda   ten grains
    Glycerine   one-half ounce
    Water   one-half ounce

Mix. The above prescription may be added to the wash and used in the syringe in the proportion of one dram to an ounce of water.

Foreign Bodies in the Ear.—Foreign bodies, as insects, beans, beads, orange or lemon seeds, buttons and the like are often lodged accidentally in the ears, especially of children.

Insects may be dislodged by syringing out the ear with warm water, after which a little sweet oil may be dropped into the ear, or the warm water, before using, may have in it five or six drops of carbolic acid to the ounce of water. Beans, peas and other seeds after being lodged in the canal of the ear for some time swell and are quite difficult to remove. To do this requires a practiced hand, and it is not possible to give sufficient instruction here to enable every one to perform such delicate work.

Inflammation of the Ear.—This may be due to a cold or other obscure cause.

SYMPTOMS.

These are a state of fullness and severe pain. If pus forms under the periosteum the pain is very severe, as in a felon. The child cries and cannot sleep. Relief comes with an incision down to the bone, or the more tedious rupture of the gathering into the auditory canal. The process may be hastened by hot fomentations and poultices. The pus which is discharged into the auditory canal should not be allowed to remain and dry on to the membranes as is often the case. The canal should be cleansed out with warm astringent solutions, as warm water containing boracic acid or pulverized alum, three or four grains to each ounce of water, or one or two grains of sulphate of zinc may be used to each ounce of warm water.

TREATMENT.

After cleansing out the auditory canal as above directed wipe it dry with absorbent cotton wound about a pine stick or probe, then dust into the ear a little pulverized boracic acid powder or iodoform.

Powder blowers, made of glass or hard or soft rubber, are now made which are both cheap and efficient for blowing a little antiseptic powder into the ear and add much to the convenience and success of treating these diseases.

Other inflammations, as abscesses, may occur in the vicinity of the auditory canal. They are often painful in the extreme, and cause temporary deafness by closing the canal. If the abscess points so that the place of its future rupture can be determined, instead of waiting for this event to occur it should be opened with the sharp point of a surgeon's bistoury, and afterward use the same treatment as recommended above for cleansing and healing.

Polypi.—Polypi of the ear are exuberant granulations, the results of prolonged suppuration. They may occur in the auditory canal or in the cavity of the tympanum behind the ear drum. Wherever located their treatment is the same and must devise their destruction, either by the application of caustic, as chromic acid, or their removal by the wire snare. If the caustic is used it must be cautiously. To remove polypi by means of caustic or a snare is such a delicate operation that only a skilled surgeon would care to attempt it. There are a few other rare diseases of the auditory canal, as fungus growths, syphilitic ulcers and abnormal growths of bone (exostosis). The description and treatment, however, of such rare diseases is unnecessary here, as considerable professional skill is required to treat them successfully.

III.—DISEASES OF THE MIDDLE EAR.

Rupture of the Drum.—This may be caused by the concussion from an explosion near at hand, blows on the side of the head, a wave striking the side of the head in surf bathing, violent vomiting or coughing, sneezing or blowing the nose, thrusting a hairpin or ear scoop carelessly into the ear, or the unskillful use of instruments in the ear. The most frequent cause of rupture of the drum is the formation of pus in the middle ear. Rupture of the drum from injuries usually heals kindly, and without affecting the hearing. Rupture of the drum from concussion is more serious, and usually injury is done to other parts.

Acute and Chronic Catarrh of the Middle Ear, or Otitis Media.—This is the most common of all the affections of the ear. It is known as ear ache, from the severe pain which accompanies it.

The causes are numerous, as exposure to cold, or taking cold, especially in the head, scarlet fever, diphtheria, measles, pneumonia, small pox and syphilis. The nasal douche, once so much employed for nasal catarrh, has fallen into disuse, because it often permitted water to pass up the Eustachian tube, into the cavity of the tympanum, and was a cause of this affection.

SYMPTOMS.

These are ringing in the ears, a sense of fullness, impaired hearing, swelling, causing the ear drum to bulge forward, catarrh of the pharynx, fever, and sometimes delirium. The common and uniform symptom is ear ache, a peculiarly severe pain. It is sometimes difficult to tell what is the matter with a baby suffering from this affection. The child cries, and manifests symptoms of extreme pain. The following will usually settle the difficulty. Pressure against the ear causes the child to squirm and cry. Dropping warm water into the ear produces a temporary quiet.

TREATMENT.

Specialists speak of leeches placed in front of the ear as of foremost importance. Other remedies are warm water syringed into the ear for a few minutes at frequent intervals, steam, tobacco smoke, dry heat, as from the heart of a roasted onion, and laudanum or chloroform dropped into the ear. The following may be used:

℞	Laudanum	one dram
	Chloroform	one dram
	Sweet oil	one or two drams

Mix and drop one, two or three drops into the ear as needed, or a piece of cotton wet in the mixture may be placed in the ear. Physicians often find it necessary to control the pain by the administration of an opiate, or the hypodermic injection of morphia. In order to prevent the disease from becoming chronic, prompt and efficient treatment should be employed. Unless simple means avail for curing the discharge the case should be intrusted to a medical adviser.

Mild cases of this disease occur in persons who are in a run down, or scrofulous condition. In these cases the disease soon becomes chronic as the discharge continues in preference to healing. The chronic form of this affection is known as otitis media, otorrhœa, or running ear. There is no pain accompanying the chronic form of this affection. The discharge may be periodic, scanty, profuse, or purulent. Sometimes the whole canal is found to be full of dried pus. The drum head in some of the chronic cases is missing, having sloughed away. This stage of the disease is tedious, and requires patient treatment. It will be necessary to improve the patient's general condition and attend to his hygienic surroundings.

Tonics are to be prescribed and everything attended to which will contribute to the more successful cure of this tedious affection. Cases have been known to continue for a life time which ought to have been cured. In the treatment of otorrhœa, cleanliness is of great importance. The ear should be washed out daily with some simple astringent solution, and then dusted with some antiseptic powder, as iodoform or boracic acid. The treatment must be varied to suit the conditions of each case and persisted in till a cure results. Polypi sometimes have their origin in this chronic suppuration which causes defects in the bone and its covering that become the site of these growths.

Inflation of the Middle Ear.—This is beneficial in curing chronic affections, such as a running ear. The process is simple. It is known as Politzer's method. It consists of a rubber bulb and a tube with a hard rubber nozzle. The nozzle is placed in one nostril, the opposite nostril is pressed against the septum and closed, also the tissues are held close to the nozzle to prevent the entrance or exit of air. The patient holds water in his mouth and at a given signal is told to swallow, at the same time the bulb is compressed, this act inflates the Eustachian tube and the cavity of the middle ear. If the patient is an infant the inflation can be accomplished during the act of crying.

Congenital Defects of the Ear.—The real cause of these defects is somewhat obscure. Children are sometimes born deaf, and all cases of congenital deafness are also mute. All those cases where the hearing is lost during the first years of life, before language and sounds are acquired, are mute. These are usually hopeless cases which resist treatment.

IV.—MASTOID DISEASE.

The mastoid process lies directly behind the external ear. The bone is honeycombed or made up of a large number of little openings or cells, separated from each other by a thin tissue of bone.

When disease invades these cells the bone tissue breaks down or suppurates and the pus in seeking an outlet may advance to the brain. The cause of this disease is the extension of the inflammatory process from the middle ear. The treatment requires making an external opening into the diseased bone for the exit of pus. The opening must be kept open and the healing process extend from below to the surface. Suppuration of the middle ear is sometimes followed by paralysis of the seventh cranial nerve.

CHAPTER XV.

THE NOSE AND ITS DISEASES.

I.—Description of the Nose. II.—Acute Coryza, or Cold in the Head. III.—Ulcers in the Nasal Cavity. IV.—Other Minor Affections: 1, Warts; 2, Polypi; 3, Tumors, etc. V.—Hemorrhages from the Nose. VI.—Chronic Nasal Catarrh. VII.—Hay Fever, Rose Cold, or Summer Catarrh.

I.—DESCRIPTION OF THE NOSE.

THE nose is composed of bone, cartilage and other tissues, together with the internal openings or the nasal fossa.

The destruction of the cartilage and soft tissues gives to the skull a hideous appearance, as seen in a prepared skeleton.

The nostrils are the openings of the nose, and are separated in the center by a partition of cartilage called the septum.

The nose has a number of small muscles, situated just beneath the skin, which assist in the various expressions of the face.

The mucous membrane lining the nasal cavities has a pink color, and is called the Schneiderian, after a celebrated anatomist. This lining membrane is abundantly supplied with glands which secrete sufficient mucous to keep it in a moist condition, but when these glands are inflamed they may secrete an enormous quantity.

The nasal cavities are of irregular shape, and extend from the nostrils to the larynx or throat. Through these the air passes to the lungs in the act of respiration. Their entrance is guarded by moisture and hairs in order to prevent noxious substances and particles of dust from entering the lungs. Moist air does not irritate the lungs, but dry air or dust would be very difficult to breathe.

In passing through these long, irregular nasal cavities the air is moistened, strained, warmed, and especially fitted for respiration at all seasons of the year.

The terminal branches of the olfactory nerves are spread out over the mucous membrane. The nerves recognize odors and convey the impression of them to the brain.

The sense of smell is important; it helps us to make choice of suitable foods and warns us of many dangers that lurk in the atmosphere. The odor of food arouses the appetite, stimulates the glands of the mouth and stomach and thus not only strengthens the appetite but aids the process of digestion, while it contributes to the pleasure and happiness of our condition.

A healthy or normal state of this membrane is essential. When it is inflamed as in acute or chronic catarrh, not only is the sense of smell interfered with but the ability to enjoy the flavor of food is largely destroyed, while the natural process of breathing is obstructed.

In speech, too, some of the sounds are nasal, their correct use is pleasing and their absence disagreeable. We hear it sometimes wrongfully observed that a person talks through the nose when the nasal cavities are obstructed and the nasal sounds cannot be employed. The importance of the normal condition of the nasal cavities may be learned by listening to the attempts of a person to talk who has a cleft palate.

II.—ACUTE CORYZA, OR COLD IN THE HEAD.

This is of frequent occurrence for many persons are subject to a cold in the head from slight cause, such as sitting or sleeping in a draught of air, damping or wetting the feet, breathing dust or inhaling gases, or cooling off too quickly after getting heated.

SYMPTOMS.

The mucous membrane is at first congested or dry, there is a disposition to sneeze, there is a stuffed feeling about the nose owing to the swelling or congestion of the mucous membrane. In the more severe cases there is headache, weariness, fever, hot and chilly sensations, or perhaps severe frontal pain or neuralgia of the face. The dry stage is followed in about twenty-four hours with a profuse watery discharge from the eyes and nose and later on an abundant flow of mucous. The duration of the attack may be four or five days and the termination of it may result in the complete restoration of health or in a chronic catarrhal condition.

TREATMENT.

Those liable to colds should use especial care to guard against them. Living in too warm rooms or muffling the neck and face with extra coverings so as to favor perspiration invites rather than prevents attacks of this common affection.

Sponging the head, neck and shoulders each morning with cold water and then rubbing the skin thoroughly dry with a coarse towel is good to toughen the external surfaces and prevent colds.

When a cold is contracted a good sweat if taken early will sometimes break it up. Sweating is favored by the hot foot bath and hot drinks as lemonade or herb tea. Wrap in warm blankets and go to bed. Perspiration is favored by a five-grain Dover's powder. A person who uses such treatment to break up a cold should remain in the house several hours to prevent contracting a second cold which would most likely be more aggravated than if no remedies had been used. If there is some fever tincture of aconite in one drop doses may be taken hourly.

When the discharge from the nose is profuse a solution of borax, alum or chlorate of potash may be used, snuffing it up the nose and also gargling the throat with it. It should be milder for the nose than for the throat. A teaspoonful of common salt to a pint of warm water is a good remedy to snuff up the nose. Medicated solutions may be syringed into the nostrils or sprayed with an atomizer.

III.—ULCERS IN THE NASAL CAVITY.

The most common cause of intractable ulcers in the nose is syphilis. The ulcerative process may advance till it reaches the cartilage or bone, and dead bone may be discharged. The odor of decaying bone is almost intolerable. Scrofula may cause ulceration in the nasal cavities.

Foreign bodies in the nostrils, as a button, bean, kernel of corn, a pebble and such substances, will cause ulceration of the nose if allowed to remain in long enough. The treatment depends upon the cause of the ulceration, and must be adapted to each individual. (See syphilis and scrofula.)

When dead bone exists its speedy removal is desirable. Foreign bodies should be at once removed. Iodoform in powder or ointment is one of the best applications that can be made to an ulcer which is loath to heal. Aristol powder possesses similar efficiency and is preferable because it has a less disagreeable odor.

IV.—OTHER AFFECTIONS.

Growths in the nostrils are not uncommon; they consist of warts, polypi, cancers and other tumors.

Warts.—These should always be removed; this can be done by applying a small amount of chromic acid carefully. (See warts.)

Polypi obstruct the nose and affect the speech. They swell or become enlarged in damp weather and are otherwise disagreeable. They are soft, pear shaped, and usually hang by a small pedicle; they should be twisted off. Their removal is neither difficult nor very painful.

Tumors.—For treatment of cancer of the nose see general article on cancers. The treatment of a cancerous growth is similar wherever placed. Hemorrhage of the nose is of frequent occurrence and has received sufficient attention in the special article upon this subject which follows.

Surgical deformities of the nose cannot be treated in domestic practice, and are omitted intentionally.

V.—HEMORRHAGE FROM THE NOSE.

This occurs so often and is of such trifling importance in young persons who make blood rapidly as to occasion but little concern. It may occur from a fall or slight injury and usually requires no interference.

In persons who are too full blooded it is frequently beneficial, relieves headache and promotes the general well being and should not be checked unless it continues too long and is too abundant.

In the early stage of fevers when the veins are congested, the face flushed, the pulse rapid and bounding, a slight amount of nasal hemorrhage is rarely productive of evil.

When, however, it occurs in debilitated persons or is so severe as to threaten life it requires energetic measures.

TREATMENT.

Cold applied to the forehead and back of the neck will often check it. The feet may be placed in hot water; this tends to relieve congestion of the blood vessels of the head while at the same time ice or cold lotions may be applied to the head and neck. Equal parts of vinegar and water make a convenient and cooling domestic lotion to apply to the head. It is excellent to relieve some kinds of headache. Pinch the nose close together with the thumb and finger and hold the head forward while the patient breathes through the mouth; this is a method which will often succeed if continued till clots are formed to stop the hemorrhage. A solution of iron, (Monsel's solution) twenty drops in half a cupful of water, snuffed into the nostrils is a remedy of considerable efficiency. It may be used in an atomizer or as a nasal douche. In some instances, where life is threatened, plugging the nose in front and behind has been found to be an effective method. The operation requires considerable professional skill.

VI.—CHRONIC NASAL CATARRH.

This is chronic inflammation of the mucous membrane which lines the nose and the cavities connected with it. These mucous linings become congested and the little glands which secrete mucous are unduly stimulated, so that the secretion becomes abundant. As the inflammatory action progresses the secretion becomes thicker and more disagreeable. The nasal passages are more or less obstructed.

CAUSES.

Nasal catarrh is caused chiefly by damp climates, sudden changes of temperature, exposure to draughts of air, repeated wetting or damping the feet, unsuitable clothing, changes in clothing before the weather becomes settled, leaving a warm room in a state of perspiration and going into the cold air, wearing thin shoes so that the feet become cold and chilled, and many other improprieties due to carelessness or lack of the means of comfort.

SYMPTOMS.

The first symptom is a cold in the head. The nose feels stuffed by the swelling of the lining membrane, or perhaps by retained secretions, or both, so that the patient complains of being unable to breathe through the nose. There is frequent headache especially between the eyes. The mucous membrane is at first dry and irritated; there follows later a free discharge from the nose of thin mucous, and the handkerchief is a constant necessity. Soon the discharge becomes thicker and perhaps yellowish in color. Often a second cold is contracted before recovery has had time to take place, or there may be a succession of colds until recovery is retarded and a chronic catarrhal condition is established. The discharge becomes thick, greenish, and in time exceedingly disagreeable and offensive.

While an acute attack reaches its height in a few days at most and tends to recovery in the course of one or two weeks the chronic form is persistent, and though better at times it may last for years, gradually increasing in disagreeableness and severity.

It is not so troublesome in summer but winter and spring awaken the disease to its fullest vigor. The chronic form is difficult to cure and when cured is unwilling to remain so for any considerable length of time.

TREATMENT.

When the disease has become chronic it is necessary first of all to cleanse the nasal passages for these are often ulcerated and in an unhealthy condition. For cleansing a solution of common salt and water snuffed up the nose till it can be tasted in the throat may be used. As the mucous lining is sensitive the solution must not be too strong. A teaspoonful of salt to a pint of water is about right.

The following can be used in an atomizer or snuffed up from the hand. If strong enough to produce discomfort reduce with pure water.

℞ Sulphate of zinc   four grains
   Cocaine   three grains
   Carbolic acid   four grains
   Rose water   six ounces

Mix and use three or four times a day.

The following is highly recommended by excellent authority.

℞ Tannin   one dram
   Iodoform   ten grains

Mix and apply a small quantity of this powder by means of an insufflator to the parts after their thorough cleansing with salt and water solution.

The following is excellent. Its strength can be varied as required by the addition of more benzoinol.

℞ Menthol   one dram
   Cocaine   ten grains
   Aristol   twelve grains
   Benzoinol   four ounces

Mix and use in hand atomizer two or three times a day.

VII.—HAY FEVER, ROSE COLD, OR SUMMER CATARRH.

This is a catarrh which chiefly affects the mucous linings of the nose and air passages. It is likely to appear at about the same season each year.

It is noticed that hay fever is more common among persons of a nervous temperament.

Negroes are not troubled with it, neither does it occur among the natives of India.

CAUSES.

The two principal factors in the production of this disease are sensitive nerves and irritating substances floating in the atmosphere, as the pollen of certain plants and grasses, the pulverized dust in the streets and the dust of rooms.

Some persons are seized by an attack in consequence of passing a hay field, or riding behind a load of hay, or entering a barn containing hay in the lofts. The fact that patients are more comfortable in damp, cloudy weather, or after a rain, seems to prove that the odor of the hay does not cause the trouble.

The bloom of wheat, oats, rye, corn, barley, the rag weed and golden-rod excite the disease. The dust in furnace-heated houses and railroad cars, as well as many other irritating substances, may be regarded as helping to cause this disease.

SYMPTOMS.

It usually comes on with sneezing. If you look towards the light or sunshine an irresistible impulse to sneeze seizes you, but sneezing brings no relief. You continue to sneeze in spite of every effort to refrain; there is an increase of the secretions of the mucous tract, and the eyes and nose overflow.

You feel an itching in the throat which extends toward the ear, but you cannot reach it, and there is a stuffy, obstructed condition of the nose, which compels you to breathe through the mouth. Some persons suffer from an itching of the skin, especially about the nose, pain in the head, slight fever and loss of appetite, also a tickling sensation in the upper part of the windpipe. The mucous linings of the nose and throat are congested and swollen. There is cough and more or less catarrh. The patient feels extremely uncomfortable and unwillingly yields to a wretchedness which renders life burdensome.

The discomfort seems greatly out of proportion to the disease. It is persistent. You feel relieved perhaps for a time but your peace is brief. This condition may continue for days and even weeks. Each year the attack tends to greater severity and discomfort. The disease of itself is never fatal, simply annoying. Sometimes it extends downward to the lungs and develops an asthmatic condition.

TREATMENT.

The most certain treatment for those who can afford it is a change to regions where it does not exist. Sea voyages are beneficial and curative, but all catarrhal troubles are liable to recur.

The syrup of hydriodic acid is an efficient remedy. The dose is one teaspoonful in water before each meal. This syrup when fresh and suitable for use is colorless.

When the secretion of thin, watery mucous is very abundant the sulphate of atropia affords marked relief. A tablet containing $\frac{1}{100}$ of a grain once or twice a day is a suitable dose for an adult.

The inhalation of menthol affords some relief. It does not cure; it is simply palliative.

Tincture of iodine sufficiently reduced with water may be used as a spray for the nasal passages with a hand atomizer.

The following prescription is one of great value and affords much relief:

℞	Sulphate of zinc	six grains
	Carbolic acid	ten grains
	Cocaine	six grains
	Glycerine	two ounces
	Rose water	four ounces

Mix. Use in atomizer by throwing it up the nose freely and repeat with the return of sneezing or other symptoms.

CHAPTER XVI.

THE MOUTH AND ITS APPENDAGES.

I.—Description of the Mouth an Its Appendages: 1, the Mouth; 2, the Upper and Lower Jaw; 3, the Mucous Membrane; 4, the Lips; 5, the Cheeks; 6, the Glands; 7, the Tongue; 8, the Gums; 9, the Antrum; 10, the Palate; 11, the Teeth. II.—Diseases of the Mouth, Tongue and Vicinity: 1, Alveolar Abscess, or Gum Boil; 2, Catarrhal Stomatitis; 3, Canker, or Apthous Sore Mouth; 4, Gangrenous Stomatitis, or Cancrum Oris; 5, Toxic Stomatitis; 6, Other Minor or Rare Affections—*a*, Calculus of the Ducts; *b*, Salivary Fistula; *c*, Growths; *d*, Hare Lip; *e*, Hypertrophy of the Lips; 7, Diseases of the Tongue—*a*, Tongue Tie; *b*, Enlargement of the Tongue, or Hypertrophy; *c*, Inflammation of the Tongue, or Glossitis.

I.—DESCRIPTION OF THE MOUTH AND ITS APPENDAGES.

THE MOUTH.—The mouth is a roomy cavity adapted to various purposes, as the reception, mastication and preparation of food for the stomach, the origin and insertion of powerful muscles which open and close the jaws, muscles which control speech and some of the muscles of expression.

The mouth takes the place of the nostrils when they are obstructed and admits the air on its way to the lungs. It provides lodgement for the nerves of taste, and is supplied with a correspondingly large number of associate organs as the tongue, gums, teeth, lips, palate and glands.

The Upper and Lower Jaw.—The mouth is surrounded by a bony framework which protects it from injury, gives insertion to powerful muscles used in chewing the food, affords firm ridges for enclosing the roots of the teeth and protection for the arteries and nerves which are abundantly supplied to these and neighboring organs.

The Mucous Membrane.—The whole cavity of the mouth is covered over with a thick layer of mucous membrane which is much less sensitive than that about the eye or which lines the nose. Its beginning is seen along the border of the lips where the skin and mucous membrane unite. It extends throughout the whole alimentary canal. The lips are composed chiefly of muscles and muscular fibres, which control the expressions of the lower portion of the face. These, with the other muscles of the eye and face, are trained and developed by the contortionist to a remarkable degree.

The Lips.—The lips guard the entrance to the mouth. They are well supplied with delicate nerves of sensation and it is probably owing to this fact that they are the organs chosen to express affection. They also contribute their part to the complex process of articulation.

The Cheeks.—The cheeks cover over the sides of the mouth and contain muscles which help to open and close the lower jaw.

The Glands.—In front and below the lower half of the external ear lies a large salivary gland, the parotid, and this is the gland which is inflamed in mumps. Its secretions are poured out into the mouth through a duct two and one-half inches long (Steno's duct). This duct opens upon the inside of the cheek opposite the second molar teeth. The duct is about the size of a crow's quill. It sometimes becomes obstructed, which is the primary cause of a salivary fistula. The parotid gland is stimulated to action by the movement of the lower jaw in eating and pours out a large amount of fluid to moisten the food. The mucous membrane of the mouth is supplied with numerous other glands as the buccal, which also supply lubricating material. There are other large glands as the sub-maxillary, in front of the angle of the lower jaw; and the sub-lingual, under the forward portion of the tongue. These glands open by means of tubes or ducts under the tongue; they secrete a large amount of fluid to keep the mouth moist and to aid in the mastication of food.

The Tongue.—The tongue lies in a depression at the bottom of the oral cavity between the two sides of the lower jaw. Its free end extends forward and rests against the gums and teeth. With very slight exertion it can be protruded from the mouth or moved from side to side. It becomes thicker, wider and larger as it approaches the roots in the throat or back part of the mouth, where it is held in place by a number of muscles attached to the hyoid bone. The tongue is the organ of taste. It is supplied by a special nerve, the gustatory, the terminal ends of which are gathered up into little elevations, or papillæ, which can be seen as little red, pointed elevations upon its upper surface. On the back part of the tongue there are a number of these papillæ which are much larger than the rest, arranged in the shape of a harrow, with the point directed backward. The tongue is composed of muscular fibres which are liberally supplied with blood vessels and nerves. The muscular arrangement divides the tongue in the middle into two separate halves, with a fibrous septum in the center binding them together. The tongue assists in moving the food about in the mouth and rolling it up into a bolus to swallow. It is an important organ of speech.

The Gums.—The gums are ridges of firm tissue overlying a bent framework and the alveolar process which is covered in by them. The gums, with the alveolar process, surround the teeth and hold them in position, affording them a firm and permanent lodgement, so that the biting and chewing of hard substances is easily accomplished and does not loosen them.

The Antrum.—Within the bone on each side of the upper jaw is contained a large opening called the antrum. It extends from under the floor of the orbits to the roots of the molar teeth. This cavity is of interest because it is sometimes the seat of a painful abscess. It is nearly or quite penetrated by the roots of the molar teeth and the irritation of their fangs is probably the usual cause of the abscess which sometimes forms here. The natural outlet of this cavity or antrum is large enough to admit the end of a probe and terminates in the nasal passage.

The Palate.—The roof of the mouth is known as the hard palate until it reaches back to that portion which has no bone above it and at this point the soft palate begins. The soft palate terminates behind in a central, cone-shaped projection, with the apex pointing downward into the throat; this is called the uvula.

The uvula sometimes becomes elongated or hypertrophied and causes so much irritation that astringents have to be applied to it to shrink it up or the bottom portion of it has to be snipped off with a pair of scissors or some similar method.

The Teeth.—These are important and fully considered elsewhere because of their value in the reduction and preparation of food for the stomach.

II.—DISEASES OF THE MOUTH, TONGUE AND VICINITY.

The mouth and its appendages are subject to a great variety of diseases, from the slightest to those of the most serious consequence.

Alveolar Abscess or Gum Boil —This is a common affection, and often occurs even when the teeth are well cared for.

SYMPTOMS.

Soreness of a tooth to the touch, or on closing the jaw, is usually the first thing noticed. This sometimes continues for a day or so when pain is established, which continues in an increasing manner for four or five days, when it begins to decline. The face swells and at length pus is discharged through the gum at the point where the swelling was greatest. Repeated attacks are likely to occur.

TREATMENT.

The common practice of poulticing the face should be discouraged. It may ease pain but is likely to increase the damage to the surrounding tissues. Cold applications or menthol liniment may be used until a dentist can be consulted.

Catarrhal Stomatitis —When the mucous membrane lining the mouth is inflamed the affection is known as stomatitis. There are several varieties of this disease as catarrhal, aphthous, parasitic, ulcerous, gangrenous, toxic and mercurial. Catarrhal stomatitis is simply an inflamed condition of the oral cavity, which may be due to a great variety of causes, as too hot drinks, the abuse of tobacco or stimulants, acrid substances, irritating dust, gases, smoke and steam. It may be difficult to ascertain the cause. In the newly born a form of catarrhal sore mouth is common, and this is sometimes called thrush. It may be caused by nursing an exhausted breast, or perhaps by protracted crying.

Canker or Aphthous Sore Mouth.—Canker sore mouth prevails chiefly in warm weather. It occurs in pale, delicate children or those of a scrofulous condition, but sometimes in connection with neglected or decayed teeth. It appears within the mouth, either upon the inside of the cheek, upon the gums or tongue, as a small circular ulcer, having irregular edges and a whitish appearance. Often several of these ulcers unite and form a large irregular ulcerated surface, and in such cases the disease is confluent. Canker may occur in children of all ages or in adults.

SYMPTOMS.

The constitutional disturbances are often mild and consist in a coated tongue with indigestion. In severe cases there is occasionally some fever and loss of appetite. These little ulcers are exceedingly sensitive, disagreeable and painful, accompanied with a constant smarting or burning sensation. Eating, if possible, is painful. In a few days they lose their disagreeableness and heal kindly.

TREATMENT.

Very simple treatment avails, as a mild cathartic dose of castor oil or citrate of magnesia when the bowels are constipated. A solution of borax, alum or chlorate of potash may be used with benefit as a mouth wash. Other vegetable washes may be made of hydrastis, gold thread, witch-hazel or sage tea. The ulcers may be touched if painful with a solution of cocaine. Cold milk is soothing and makes an excellent article of diet in these cases. Tonics and digestive aids are often beneficial to these patients.

Gangrenous Stomatitis, or Cancrum Oris.—This is a disease of debilitated and underfed children. It is a rare and dangerous disease and by some regarded as contagious. It occurs most frequently in public institutions after measles, scarlatina, whooping cough, malaria and pneumonia. The disease spreads by ulceration and sloughing which sometimes causes hemorrhage. The chief characteristic of this disease is ulceration, beginning just inside the mouth and extending to the cheek, and accompanied by gangrene or death of the part. The real cause is not generally known.

SYMPTOMS.

Among the symptoms there may be rapid pulse, rapid swelling of the mouth and cheek, a foul odor and sometimes delirium.

TREATMENT.

Local applications should be made to arrest the progress of the disease and the most efficient are caustics, as muriatic acid or nitrate of silver. Only the unhealthy tissue should be destroyed and next the parts should be dressed with antiseptic and healing lotions, as carbolic acid solution. Nutritious food and supporting tonics are demanded.

Toxic Stomatitis —This is due to the action of caustic drugs taken intentionally or accidentally. It should be treated with emollient and soothing lotions as the following:

℞		
Cocaine	six grains
Carbolic acid	ten grains
Glycerine	one-half ounce
Syrup of acacia	one ounce
Fluid ext. hydrastis	one-half ounce
Rose water	one ounce

Mix and use as a mouth wash. Dilute with water if necessary. The diet should consist of milk, raw or slightly cooked eggs and albuminous foods.

Other Minor or Rare Affections. (*a.*) *Calculus of the Ducts.* —There are a few other rare affections of these parts which belong more to the domain of surgery than medicine. A calculus sometimes forms in one of the ducts leading from the glands under the tongue. It can be easily removed.

(*b.*) *Salivary Fistula.*—The duct of the parotid gland may become obstructed and a fistulous track open for the discharge of the saliva. This occurs sometimes upon the outside of the cheek instead of within the mouth. This trouble requires early attention and surgical interference.

(*c.*) *Growths.*—Tumors or cancerous growths about the mouth or tongue require prompt and energetic treatment, and hence should be submitted without delay to the experience and judgment of the skillful.

(d.) *Hare Lip.*—There is sometimes a congenital opening in the center of the upper lip; it may extend backward through the roof of the mouth or hard palate. This failure of nature or deformity can only be remedied by a surgical operation.

(e.) *Hypertrophy of the Lips.*—The glands of the lips are liable to enlarge in scrofulous children. This enlargement is sometimes so extensive as to suggest an idiotic appearance. Not only the glands but the surrounding tissues become hypertrophied or swollen.

Attention to the general health may suffice to remedy this unsightly thickening of the lips, but if not, it is advisable to remove a V-shaped piece of the redundant tissue, using sufficient caution to prevent future disfiguration.

Diseases of the Tongue. *(a.) Tongue Tie.*—This is caused by a thin band which binds down the tip of the tongue so that it cannot be extended. It interferes with nursing on the part of an infant and later on with speech. It is easily remedied by cutting through this thin band with a blunt pair of scissors.

When the tongue is wounded it tends to bleed very freely. Wounds of the tongue are dressed by drawing the separated portions together with stitches. They unite readily owing to an abundant vascular supply.

(b.) Enlargement of the Tongue, or Hypertrophy.—This is a rare and troublesome affection in which the tongue hangs outside the mouth. Medicines are of little or no avail. A portion of the tongue usually has to be removed and this operation yields a satisfactory result.

(c.) *Inflammation of the Tongue, or Glossitis.*—This is not a very frequent affection. It may be superficial or involve the whole substance of the tongue. The symptoms appear suddenly and increase rapidly. They are heat, swelling, stiffness of the tongue and impaired mobility. The tongue becomes dry and heavily coated and it may swell to an enormous size so as to fill the whole oral cavity. The symptoms are sometimes preceded by chills followed by fever, headache and pains in the neck. Sometimes the disease is so aggravated as to threaten suffocation. In such cases speech is difficult and eating is impossible. The glands, lingual and sub-maxillary, are also swollen and give pain. Sleep and respiration are disturbed and the expression is anxious. The pulse is quick and the temperature high.

CAUSES.

The causes are various. It may be due to some injury or it may result from decayed teeth or from debilitating diseases. It may originate from syphilis, the excessive use of mercury, and the use of toxic or poisonous substances. It prevailed in this country about the year 1845, under the name of black tongue, and appeared to be epidemic. Many cases were fatal within two or three days.

TREATMENT.

Warm washes of borax or alum, five grains to the ounce of water, or tannin dissolved in glycerine may be sufficient for the superficial variety; but when the entire tissues of the tongue are involved other remedies are required. The bowels should be moved freely. Tincture of aconite in one drop doses, associated or alternated hourly with tartar emetic in doses of one-fortieth of a grain will prove valuable treatment. If relief does not ensue it is customary to make deep incisions in the tongue. Free hemorrhage follows these incisions which relieve the inflammation. If the breath is fetid a mouth wash containing permanganate of potash, two or three grains to the ounce of water, should be used or a carbolic acid solution of proper strength.

A serious case of glossitis should be given into the hands of a competent physician, who will treat it as the symptoms demand.

CHAPTER XVII.

THE THROAT, LARYNX AND THEIR DISEASES.

I.—Description of the Throat and Larynx: 1, the Throat; 2, the Larynx. II.—Affections of the Throat: 1, Getting Choked; 2, Taking Cold. III.—Acute Sore Throat, or Laryngitis. IV.—Chronic Sore Throat, or Clergyman's Sore Throat. V.—Loss of Voice, or Aphonia. VI.—Quinsy Sore Throat, or Tonsilitis.

I.—DESCRIPTION OF THE THROAT AND LARYNX.

THE THROAT.—That portion of the oral cavity back of the mouth and behind the roots of the tongue is known as the throat. It is bounded in front by the uvula and base of the tongue, and behind by a lining of mucous membrane known as the walls of the pharynx. It extends downward to the opening into the trachea, called the larynx; and the opening into the œsophagus, sometimes called the gullet. The portions of the throat visible without a mirror are the tonsils and pharynx.

The Larynx.—The opening into the windpipe is called the larynx. It lies in front of the œsophagus.

The larynx has a cartilaginous structure which may be seen and felt in the front part of the neck. It is known as the Adam's apple. It moves up and down in the act of swallowing. Its upper extremity forms a cavity or box for the vocal cords, which are stretched across it. It is the organ of voice. On account of its rigid structure it remains open constantly, while the sides of the œsophagus fall together, except when food is passing into the stomach.

II.—AFFECTIONS OF THE THROAT.

Getting Choked.—If one talks or laughs while swallowing there is danger from bits of food or drink being drawn into the larynx, which will occasion energetic coughing for its removal. Sometimes a piece of meat or other food is drawn into the larynx which is large enough to completely obstruct it and prevent the entrance of air. This is the condition known as being choked, and unless relief is speedy death soon ensues. Fortunately this accident is so well guarded against by the epiglottis that it does not occur frequently.

Taking Cold.—Colds from exposure and changes of temperature are very liable to attack the throat, producing inflammation and soreness of the mucous membrane and tonsils. Not only are climatic changes liable to affect the throat unfavorably, but polluted air from close sleeping rooms, sewer gas and bad sanitary conditions in or about the house. Persons who live in hot and badly ventilated rooms are more subject to colds and throat diseases than those who give proper attention to their surroundings.

When going out from a warm room it is advisable to breathe only through the nose in order to warm and moisten the cold air before it reaches the lungs. From the liability of the mucous membrane of the nose to become congested and the nostrils to become obstructed, ample provision is made for the passage of air to the lungs by way of the mouth.

III.—ACUTE SORE THROAT, OR LARYNGITIS.

The term sore throat has reference to an inflammation of a greater or less degree of one or more of the structures or neighboring tissues of the throat. It may extend to the larynx or be confined to the tonsils, palate or the pharynx. Sore throat accompanies many diseases as scarlet fever, diphtheria, erysipelas and small pox. It is frequent in the last stages of consumption and in the early stages of syphilis. It may be caused by accident as when hot or corrosive fluids are swallowed. It is sometimes occasioned by the inhalation of poisonous gases or breathing air containing dust and other impurities. It may result from the excessive use of tobacco or alcoholic liquors. The most common cause of sore throat, however, is the sudden taking of a cold from exposure, especially when the body is overheated.

SYMPTOMS.

The symptoms are pain, irritation, redness, swelling, difficult breathing, pain in swallowing, hoarseness and cough. At first the throat may seem dry but afterwards there is an accumulation of tough mucous and sometimes there is complete loss of the voice. The symptoms may be slight and occasion but little attention or they may be so severe as to interfere with all labor, causing great distress and concern. The symptoms will depend upon the severity of the attack, the amount of tissue involved and the progress and extent of the inflammation.

TREATMENT.

For a mild case rest, protection from exposure and a spare diet are appropriate. In the early stages it is proper to soak the feet in hot mustard water. Take a bowl of hot drink, go to bed and wrap up warmly. A flannel wet in camphor liniment may be placed around the neck. If there is severe irritation and inflammation of the throat the following gargle will help to allay it and afford relief.

℞	Cocaine	ten grains
	Carbolic acid	twenty grains
	Chlorate of potash	two drams
	Glycerine	one ounce
	Rose water	three ounces

Mix. Gargle a teaspoonful every hour.

Tartar emetic given in doses of one-sixtieth of a grain every hour promotes the activity of the secreting glands, and is an excellent remedy in these cases.

IV.—CHRONIC SORE THROAT, OR CLERGYMAN'S SORE THROAT.

This disease may result from a succession of acute attacks which leave the throat in a debilitated and inflamed condition. It may last for years, involving usually both the pharynx and larynx. It is common to those persons who use the voice constantly, as clergymen, singers, teachers, actors, auctioneers and many others.

SYMPTOMS.

The blood vessels are congested and the throat is inflamed and more red than natural. There is irritation in the throat and a constant effort to relieve it by hawking. Sometimes there is very marked hoarseness when the larynx is involved. More or less catarrh attends this affection.

TREATMENT.

The treatment requires rest of the voice and the use of astringents to relieve the congestion. Gargles of alum, chlorate of potash and similar remedies are beneficial. A hand atomizer throws the finely divided spray with force and causes the remedies to reach the parts better than when gargled.

The general health must be looked after and the voice used cautiously. Local applications of the tincture of iodine and glycerine, equal parts, or a solution of nitrate of silver are often required to effect a cure.

V.—LOSS OF VOICE, OR APHONIA.

This may occur from one or several causes, as hysteria or other nervous disorders, from growths which press upon and paralyze the nerves, ulceration, and from laryngitis, either acute or chronic.

Before much successful treatment can be instituted it is necessary to ascertain the cause of the affection. Tonics are often necessary as quinine, iron and strychnia, thus:

℞	Quinine	thirty grains
	Reduced iron	twenty grains
	Strychnia	one-third of a grain

Mix. Make into twenty pills or tablets. Dose, one three times a day.

Electricity may be tried in paralysis of the vocal cords. The inhalation of medical sprays from a steam atomizer is a rational method of treatment. Solutions of alum or borax are suitable for such a use. Atropia given in doses of $\frac{1}{100}$ of a grain usually gives satisfactory results.

VI.—QUINSY SORE THROAT, OR TONSILITIS.

This is an acute and painful disease, characterized by a rapid inflammation of one or both of the tonsils, accompanied by restlessness, fever and much distress.

The cause of this disease is often thought to be a scrofulous condition of the system. Persons who have large tonsils are liable to have repeated attacks. After middle life liability to attacks of this disease diminishes. The poison of sewer gas and defective drainage or unwholesome surroundings are favorable to the development of tonsilitis.

SYMPTOMS.

These are headache, chilly sensations, followed by pain in the limbs, restlessness with fever and high temperature, sometimes reaching 104 degrees, rapid pulse, coated tongue, fetid breath, soreness in the tonsils and difficulty in swallowing, which may so increase as to render the act almost impossible. There is an increase of the secretions of the salivary glands, which are viscid and expectorated with difficulty. Sometimes the pain in attempting to swallow even fluids is very severe, extending into the ear, and the fluid may be forced back through the nose. Sometimes the tonsilar glands become so enlarged as to push clear across and fill the throat, or if both are inflamed they crowd against each other in the center. The symptoms are proportionate to the severity of the attack. Tonsilitis is common during epidemics of measles, scarlet fever and diphtheria, and often a membrane forms which renders the early diagnosis confusing. The disease may last from five to ten days.

Sometimes the swelling gradually subsides and full recovery ensues in a short time or the disease may advance to suppuration. When the latter takes place the symptoms are augmented in severity and the temperature and fever correspond to this septic condition. The patient is very restless, tossing and unable to sleep; the distress is very great and increases until the abscess is opened or bursts, when a feeling of relief quickly follows. The same person often experiences repeated attacks of this disease at intervals of a few months or one or two years.

TREATMENT.

Sometimes it may be aborted by the early application of turpentine to the throat externally. The tincture of iodine may be carefully painted over the inflamed tonsils internally, or a solution containing twenty grains of nitrate of silver in an ounce of water. These remedies should be used early in order to render the attack abortive.

A full dose of quinine taken early has been known to abort this distressing disease. The chlorine mixture as recommended in diphtheria is an appropriate and excellent gargle.

When the process continues or the inflammation has become well established before the use of the abortive treatment, other remedies will be required, such as aconite in drop doses for the fever and a Dover's powder for the pain.

The following gargle is highly recommended by good authority.

℞ Tinct. guiac ammoniated   one ounce
   Tinct. cinchona comp.   one ounce
   Clarified honey   three ounces
   Chlorate of potash (saturated solution)
                    q. s. for a one pint mixture

This is to be gargled freely every hour or half hour and a teaspoonful taken internally, by an adult, every two hours.

When the case goes on to suppuration hot fomentations will aid the process and afford some relief; also inhalations of hot steam from water, hops or vinegar and water. When the abscess is ripe the patient may be quickly relieved by lancing the suppurating tonsil, and this may save hours of suffering.

The bodily strength should be maintained by the use of nourishing broths. Stimulants are rarely needed.

Persons subject to attacks of tonsilitis should avoid exposure as wet clothing, wet feet and currents of air when heated. They should be suitably protected from the changes of temperature and give attention to any early symptoms of the disease, when the methods already suggested will usually succeed in warding it off.

CHAPTER XVIII.

THE TRACHEA, OR WINDPIPE AND LUNGS.

I.—THE TRACHEA. II.—THE LUNGS. III.—ASTHMA. IV.—BRONCHITIS. V.—CAPILLARY BRONCHITIS. VI.—PLEURISY. VII.—PNEUMONIA. VIII.—CONSUMPTION. IX.—THE PREVENTION OF CONSUMPTION.

I.—THE TRACHEA.

THE trachea is a hollow tube made up of cartilaginous rings and lined on the inside with mucous membrane. It extends downward from the larynx toward the lungs, and in the adult is about four and one-half inches in length and about one inch in diameter. It is situated in the front and middle of the neck and just behind it lies the œsophagus. The cartilaginous structure of the trachea keeps it open permanently as it is in constant use. The lower end of the trachea divides into the right and left bronchi, one of which enters the right and the other the left lung; further on it divides up like the limbs of a branching tree in order to reach and carry the air to every portion of the lungs. The trachea is of unusual interest because a sudden cold, congestion or inflammation of the mucous lining is often attended with great danger to life. In an infant or young child the trachea is small and even a slight obstruction may threaten serious results. It is sometimes necessary when the trachea is nearly obstructed and the respiration is greatly hindered to make an opening, tracheotomy, into the windpipe and insert a tube, to facilitate the passage of air into the lungs. This delicate operation has sometimes saved a life when hope had well nigh fled.

This operation may also be required for the removal of a foreign body from the trachea as a shoe button or a peanut, which has been accidentally drawn into the larynx and lodged at the bifurcation. Through this opening the foreign body may be extracted. Tracheotomy requires great skill and much attention to details to secure success.

II.—THE LUNGS.

The lungs are two cone-shaped organs situated, one on each side of the chest, and held in position by ligaments known as the roots of the lungs. The right lung is larger than the left. They are divided by natural fissures into lobes, the right lung possessing three, while the left has only two. The outside is covered by a thin, transparent membrane, which is a continuation of the pleura or covering of the inside of the chest walls.

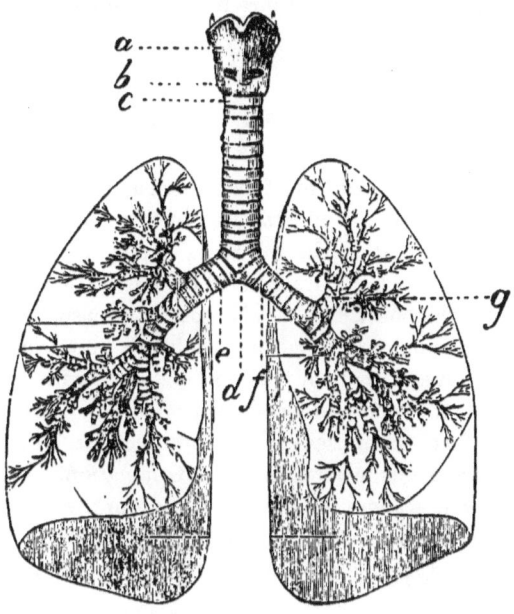

The larynx, trachea, bronchial tubes, outline and internal structure of the lungs: a, thyroid cartilage; b, cricoid cartilage; c, first cartilage of the trachea; d, bifurcation of the trachea; e, f, right and left bronchus; g, bronchial tube.

The lung substance is light, porous, spongy and elastic, floats in water and contains air in its spaces. The lungs contain a vast number of air cells which are the termination of the bronchial tubes. The renewal of air in the lungs is accomplished by the act of respiration which takes place in a normal condition about eighteen times a minute. A large amount of oxygen is consumed and the air is rapidly vitiated by the act of respiration, hence the importance of ventilation.

III.—ASTHMA.

Asthma is a spasmodic contraction of the circular muscular fibers of the trachea and bronchi. It is due particularly to a disturbance or irritation of the nerve filaments in the air passages, which produces the spasmodic condition. It renders the breathing labored and difficult for a varied length of time. Attacks may occur at intervals near or remote. The exciting causes which produce asthma are various, as indigestion, the inhalation of dust, certain odors and the pollen of plants. Exposure to cold and dampness favors an attack.

SYMPTOMS.

It may come on suddenly or after catarrh and bronchial irritations. The breathing is labored and attended by wheezing; the expression is anxious, and so great is the effort to obtain air that the face is sometimes bathed in perspiration. There is a peculiar feeling of tightness about the chest. In a characteristic case the patient sits and elevates his shoulders by resting his hands upon the knees, or he stands, leaning over a chair or some other article with the shoulders raised, the back rounded and sweating profusely. There is a dusky hue about the face, the pulse is small and quick and the extremities chilly. This disease is in no sense an inflammation. It is simply a nervous affection. There is no inflammation in the lung or air passages and when the paroxysm of asthma lets up the patient is immediately relieved and goes about apparently as well as ever.

TREATMENT.

Relief may be afforded by dropping a little nitrite of amyl upon a handkerchief and inhaling it, but relief from this source is uncertain. The inhalation of a little chloroform will modify or break up an attack but such a remedy is unsuitable to use except in severe cases and with the utmost caution. The most efficient remedy known to give relief is the fourth of a grain of morphia hypodermically administered, or twenty grains of chloral dissolved in sweetened water and taken by the stomach. The two remedies may be combined to advantage as in the following prescription:

℞ Morphia   one grain
    Chloral   four scruples
    Syrup of orange peel   half an ounce
    Cinnamon water   half an ounce

Mix. Dose a teaspoonful, and repeat in two or four hours if needed.

The tincture of lobelia is a valuable remedy, given in ten drop doses every fifteen minutes until nausea is produced. The following prescription is a good one. The author cannot recall a case that it has not either relieved or permanently benefited.

℞ Iodide of potash   two drams
    Extract grindelia   two drams
    Extract elecampane   half an ounce
    Tinct. of lobelia   half an ounce
    Syr. senega   one and one-half ounces
    Wintergreen water   q. s. to make four ounces

Mix. Dose a dessert spoonful as needed for an adult.

The following is said to afford relief:

Pulv. lobelia leaves   two drams
Pulv. stramonium leaves   two drams
Pulv. belladonna leaves   two drams
Nitrate of potash   three drams

Mix. Put some of this into a clean clay pipe and smoke for ten or fifteen minutes at intervals during an attack.

IV.—BRONCHITIS.

This is an acute inflammation of the bronchi or the mucous lining of the air passages. It may be local and involve only a few of the bronchi or extensive, and involve the whole of them. Sometimes the inflammation extends upward into the trachea or downward into the terminal air cells of the lungs. When the air cells are involved the disease is of great gravity, and is known as capillary bronchitis.

CAUSES.

The causes of this disease are a damp climate, cold, damp winds, sudden changes of the weather, wetting the feet, changing the under clothing too early in the spring, or taking cold. Bronchitis attacks those of feeble vitality, and hence old people and children are especially liable to it. Any depressing influences which unfavorably affect the health condition renders one liable to attacks, and it is often a complication of other diseases.

SYMPTOMS.

The first symptoms are usually a cold in the head with a watery discharge from the nose and eyes and frontal pain. This cold appears to travel downward toward the throat and chest. The patient complains of feeling chilly; has a slightly inflamed or sore throat, a feeling of soreness in the chest, and complains of a disagreeable smarting in the air passages and lungs. At first the cough is dry and hoarse—more troublesome toward evening, but later the mucous linings secrete an abundant amount of fluid, which soon becomes thick and viscid. Smarting of the lungs continues. The disease may last four or five days; it may continue much longer, or even become chronic. There is usually a marked amount of bronchitis in measles and typhoid fever. The breathing is not so much obstructed as in pneumonia. It is often a very serious disease for aged or debilitated persons and very young children.

TREATMENT.

The patient makes a more satisfactory recovery if confined to the bed. In the early stages foot baths of hot mustard water and hot drinks afford a measure of relief. Flaxseed tea and hot lemonade are good. If the mouth and throat are dry tablets of tartar emetic may be given in doses of one-twentieth of a grain or Hive syrup in doses of fifteen to twenty drops every two hours. A mustard plaster over the chest affords no little relief. If there is much fever the tincture of aconite may be given in drop doses and repeated every hour until the skin is moistened. Carbonate of ammonia is an excellent remedy in these cases. It may be given as follows:

℞ Ammonia carbonate	two drams
Morphia acetat	one grain
Syr. ipecac.	half an ounce
Glycerine	one ounce and a half
Anise water	one ounce

Mix. Dose teaspoonful every two or four hours.

The cough is necessary to clear the lungs. Stimulants are sometimes required in some debilitated cases of old people. If necessary as a stimulant brandy can take the place of the glycerine in the above prescription in the same amount.

For the restlessness of children do not give morphia but chloral in single grain doses will assist in relieving the overloaded air tubes.

The following prescription for children is excellent:

℞ Hydrate of chloral	sixteen grains
Syr. ipecac.	two drams
Syr. Tolu	one ounce
Anise water	six drams

Mix. Dose a teaspoonful every two or four hours.

V.—CAPILLARY BRONCHITIS.

This disease is also called broncho or catarrhal pneumonia. It is an acute inflammation in the small bronchial air passages which extend to the air cells of the lungs. It is chiefly confined to the extremes of life, infancy and old age. It is similar to bronchitis but a much more dangerous disease. It results from taking cold and from the same general causes as bronchitis. It is liable to follow measles, whooping cough, diphtheria and croup.

SYMPTOMS.

The symptoms closely resemble those of bronchitis, except that they are more severe. The respirations are short, superficial and greatly increased in number. The patient is restless, fitful, exacting, and not easily satisfied with constant attention. There is a high grade of fever and a troublesome cough. The disease has no definite course, it may be protracted for weeks or till the approach of warm weather. There is a constant tendency to relapse and to a chronic condition.

The restoration of the lung which attends recovery often requires several weeks under the best treatment.

TREATMENT.

The temperature of the sick room should not be over seventy or seventy-two degrees. Moisture in the air is desirable and should be supplied by a kettle of water constantly boiling. An emetic of the syrup of ipecac. is frequently needed to free the lungs of mucous. No attempt must be made to suppress the cough, as it is the only hope of keeping the air cells open and preventing collapse of the lungs. The patient's strength should be maintained by good nourishment frequently administered. The following is an excellent prescription:

> ℞   Carbonate of ammonia   one dram
>   Brandy   half an ounce
>   Syr. of liquorice   one and one-half ounces
>   Anise water q. s. to make four ounces

Mix. Dose one teaspoonful and repeat as often as the condition requires. This prescription is intended for a child one year old. Older children may take a proportionate quantity.

Cod liver oil favors recovery.

VI.—PLEURISY.

Pleurisy is an acute inflammation of the pleura, a membrane which lines the inside of the chest and which is reflected over the outside of the lungs. It is characterized by peculiar pain and by fluid in the chest cavity which is the chief element of danger in this disease.

The inflammation is usually confined to one side but in a small proportion of cases extends to both. In occasional cases only a small and limited portion of the pleura is involved and the character of the disease is correspondingly modified.

The cause of pleurisy is somewhat obscure. It is liable to occur in those who are somewhat debilitated. It occurs most frequently in the winter and spring and is usually attributed to taking cold. Aged persons and children are more subject to this disease than others because they possess less power to resist it. Pleurisy occasionally results from injuries as a fractured rib or extensive burns and scalds. When it results from such a cause it is known as traumatic pleurisy. It frequently complicates pneumonia and is then called pleuropneumonia.

SYMPTOMS.

It generally comes on suddenly sometimes with a slight chill or chilly sensations, but the most marked symptom is a sharp, cutting pain in the right or left side, which will not permit of taking a long breath. The breathing is short, shallow and difficult. The patient prevents the movements of the chest as much as possible for every breath when it reaches about such a point catches the sufferer with severe pain. The respirations reach forty or fifty a minute, the patient tries not to breathe but is unsuccessful in the attempt. The temperature may reach an elevation of 102 or more degrees. The patient has a pinched countenance and wears an expression of suffering.

In the early stages of the disease the ear placed over the chest in the vicinity of the pain, detects the characteristic friction sound, which is caused by the inflamed surfaces grating against each other. The inflammation at first checks the secretion of the pleural fluid and two sore surfaces grate upon each other, causing a cutting and agonizing pain. Sometimes the disease does not complete its full course, recovery taking place quickly. Such an attack is called dry pleurisy. Usually, however, after a little time, an abundant quantity of serum or fluid is poured out into the cavity about the lungs. This fluid may be so abundant as to cause a bulging out of the spaces between the ribs. The heart is crowded away from its place and the lung is pushed up into the apex of the chest, the pressure sometimes becoming so great as to drive all the air out of the lung and cause it to collapse.

Pleurisy has some symptoms in common with pneumonia but there is a marked difference in the character of the breathing, the pain and the expectoration. In pleurisy the pain is cutting, the cough is short and suppressed and brings up no expectoration. In pneumonia the sputa is rust colored and the pain constant.

TREATMENT.

In the early stage the patient should go to bed. Hot applications as a flaxseed poultice containing a little mustard, sufficient to redden the surface, should be applied. Tincture of aconite in half drop doses every half hour to allay fever may be used. Moving about is to be avoided on account of the pain. Mild remedies should be administered to produce rest and sleep. Food should be nourishing and easy of digestion. Twenty grains of quinine may be given in the beginning of the attack in divided doses of five grains each, one every two hours.

After removing the flaxseed and mustard poultice if the trouble continues, the patient should put on a cotton batting jacket covered on the outside with oiled silk. This is to remain on until after recovery. A five or ten-grain Dover's powder may be given to relieve pain and produce rest, and may be repeated every four hours. Simple cases tend to recovery, but severe cases may require other means to save life.

The fluid in the pleural cavity may be absorbed. This is the most common and favorable result that can take place. It may fail to be absorbed and changed to purulent matter, when it will have to be removed. If left to itself it may affect a passage by ulcerating into the air tubes or bronchi, when it is raised through the mouth. It sometimes works a passage through the chest walls and drains away, but as these conditions of discharge are dangerous and liable to become chronic, it is better to puncture the chest cavity and draw off the purulent material without waiting for these more tedious and debilitating results. The operation requires considerable surgical skill and its details can well be omitted. It is better to operate as soon as the temperature indicates a change to pus and not wait for the tedious and destructive process which nature is obliged to pursue.

Pleurisy, after recovery, usually leaves behind the proof of its former existence in adhesions formed between the lungs and chest wall.

VII.—PNEUMONIA, INFLAMMATION OF THE LUNGS OR LUNG FEVER.

Pneumonia is an acute inflammation of the lung tissues which causes serious embarrassment of the circulation and respiration. The real cause of pneumonia is disease germs. It is popularly and erroneously supposed to be occasioned by taking cold.

There are certain predisposing causes, and taking cold, as well as climatic changes or the debilitating effects of cold weather, may be included among them. Persons recovering from serious illness or suffering from the debilitating effects of malaria, habitual drinkers and such classes, are more liable to attacks of pneumonia than the vigorous and temperate. Whatever, then, debilitates the system and taxes the vitality, may be regarded among the predisposing causes.

Of all the mortality among aged people occasioned by acute disease, four-fifths is due to pneumonia, and this ratio increases as age advances. That pneumonia is due to a specific germ has been fully established.

SYMPTOMS.

The onset of pneumonia is usually sudden. The patient is taken with a chill, headache, pain in the back and limbs. The chill is soon followed by fever, pain in the chest, shallow, rapid and painful breathing, a short, hacking cough, and later on a rusty, blood-stained expectoration. If the ear is placed over the chest a crackling sound is heard, similar to that produced by rolling a hair between the thumb and fingers. All the symptoms do not appear at the same time, but one set of symptoms succeed another. The portion of lung first invaded is congested with blood. This condition lasts about two days, when the congested portion takes on a condition of solidification and resembles a piece of liver. The temperature is now high, ranging from one hundred and two to one hundred and five degrees. The urine is scanty and high colored. The patient's condition is one of anxiety and distress. The respirations increase and may reach from forty to sixty a minute, indicating that the functions of the lung are very much disturbed. This condition lasts from two to three days.

Should the case pursue a favorable course the solidified portion of lung begins to soften, the temperature falls rapidly, the fever declines, moisture appears upon the surface of the body and the patient begins to experience a sense of relief. This is the period of resolution, in which the lung returns to its normal condition. It occupies a period of from two to six days.

The disease does not always progress in the orderly way we have indicated, for frequently the process of inflammation extends from one portion of the lung to another, more and more of the lung tissue becoming involved from day to day. The disease, after traversing one lung, may pass over into the other, and is then known as double pneumonia. When the pulse advances beyond one hundred and twenty a minute and the temperature reaches one hundred and four degrees or more, the course of the disease is unfavorable, and is liable to terminate fatally.

When the tongue is dry and brown the disease is sometimes called typhoid pneumonia to indicate its severity. Should the patient complain of a sharp stitch in the side the probability of pleurisy as a combination ought to be considered. Abscess of the lung has been known to follow pneumonia and then the recovery is slow and tedious.

TREATMENT.

The treatment must be prompt and adequate to meet the symptoms as they arise. A poultice of ground flaxseed and mustard, of generous size, renders excellent service if applied early. It should remain until the skin is thoroughly reddened. Its removal may be followed by a stimulating liniment. The tincture of aconite is of especial service in the early febrile condition. It should be given in small doses repeated every half hour till it moistens the surface. Robust persons may take $\frac{1}{100}$ of a grain of tartar emetic every two hours. This is indicated only in the first stage.

In the second stage carbonate of ammonia is an excellent remedy; five or ten grains may be given to an adult every two or four hours in syrup. High temperature should be controlled by safe remedies. Demulcent drinks made from slippery elm and flaxseed are beneficial. Many other remedies of undoubted efficiency are known to the medical profession which are unsuitable for domestic practice. The patient should be supplied with pure air as no harm can come from proper ventilation. The diet should consist of milk, animal broths, beef extract, malt and other suitable nutrients.

VIII.—CONSUMPTION, PHTHISIS, OR TUBERCULOSIS.

We must consider this interesting subject in a general manner since it is not worth while in a work of this character to dwell on those features of a disease which could be appreciated only by medical experts. Consumption is a very common disease and very fatal to the human family.

Great progress in the study of this disease has been made in recent years. Late discoveries prove that but little was known of the causes of consumption even ten years ago. Consumption is now known to be a contagious disease caused by microscopic germs which are found to exist in the expectoration in great abundance. The reason that consumption was so long regarded as a hereditary disease is that certain tendencies are transmitted which are favorable to its development. The habits of life, the unfavorable localities in which men live, and their employment may contribute much to produce those conditions favorable to its development.

It is a very insidious disease, capable of deceiving the patient. When it progresses to a fatal termination it does so by undermining the powers of life, the appetite fails, digestion fails, the bodily weight diminishes, the muscular strength declines, fever is persistent, the pulse and respiration are rapid and the patient at last dies from exhaustion. In the latter stages purulent expectoration becomes abundant and the cough fatiguing; there is pallor and marked emaciation or waste; a consumption indeed not merely of the lungs but of all the tissues of the body.

SYMPTOMS.

These are at first a dry cough, which persists and increases until finally an irritation is produced, which is accompanied by considerable expectoration. Hemorrhage may occur early in the disease, and appears to afford in some cases a measure of relief. It may be profuse and fatal. The voice may be husky, hoarse or whispering; the pulse is quick and the temperature of the body is always slightly elevated. If the disease is progressing rapidly the disturbance of the pulse and bodily temperature will be well marked. When the fever is highest there is usually a bright red spot on each cheek and the eye is bright and glistening. Profuse night sweats are often a source of discomfort to the patient. The blood is impoverished and the appetite sooner or later fails. Diarrhœa is a common symptom and often attended by griping pains. The patient never ceases to expect and plan for recovery. The faculties of the mind are usually clear up to the last moment. In females the monthly flow usually ceases owing doubtless to anæmia and the poverty and emaciation of all the bodily tissues.

TREATMENT.

Many methods of treatment have been sprung upon the world as specific cures for consumption, but all of them have so far signally failed. Even the tuberculin of the celebrated Dr. Koch, which promised so much and created such universal interest in the press of the country, is now regarded as a failure. With our present knowledge it is impossible to administer or inhale any medicine which is strong enough to destroy the germ without harming the patient. The future may remedy the difficulty and produce a specific that will arrest this desolating disease.

Climate is a very important factor in the treatment of consumption. Medicine in this disease is scarcely of more importance than hygienic measures. A dry climate with even temperature and a pure atmosphere, combined with healthy and well-cooked food, well ventilated apartments and abundant outdoor exercise such as riding, driving, fishing and hunting with agreeable companions will benefit the patient if the case is not too far advanced. A sea voyage has proved beneficial in some cases. That diverse employment, out of doors, should be sought after, which will increase the appetite, improve digestion and increase the bodily weight.

Inability to take sufficient food to maintain the bodily condition is unfavorable. Among the numerous articles of diet suitable for such a patient are milk, cream, koumiss, buttermilk, eggs in liquid form, meats, beef, mutton, lamb, chicken or quail; and if the digestion is unimpaired any other healthy food which is relished and especially fattening foods.

Medicines are given in this disease to improve the appetite, aid digestion and nutrition and to relieve any unfavorable symptoms. With respect to the use of alcoholic drinks the advice of an intelligent and conscientious physician should be sought and his direction followed. In many cases they are not essential while in others milk punch or egg-nog are considered advantageous.

No remedy at the present time is yielding so good results as beechwood creosote. It can be inhaled and taken internally. It has been injected into the diseased tissues with decided benefits. One-half to one grain should be taken in pill form three times a day; its use ought to be continued until the health is well established.

Nearly all cases are benefited by small doses of arsenic, as $\frac{1}{40}$ of a grain in tablet form three times a day. It is the most efficient known remedy to prevent destructive waste of tissues.

When the cough is so annoying as to prevent sleep sedative remedies are required. The following are old but efficient remedies:

℞	Extract of hyoscyamus fl.	one and one-half drams
	Spirits of chloroform	two drams
	Syr. of lactucarium	two ounces

Mix. Dose a teaspoonful every two or four hours.

Should hemorrhage occur suddenly use a strong solution of common salt until the following can be obtained.

℞	Extract of ergot fl.	one ounce
	Syrup of orange peel	one ounce

Mix. Dose one teaspoonful, frequently repeated until the hemorrhage subsides.

Night sweats may be relieved by taking at night a tablet containing $\frac{1}{100}$ of a grain of atropia. This remedy will also have a favorable influence upon the tendency to cough.

IX.—THE PREVENTION OF CONSUMPTION.

From reliable statistics we learn that consumption causes the remarkable mortality of about ninety thousand persons every year in the United States. Such a mortality indicates an amount of suffering, distress and heartache on the part of patients and friends as to exceed the power of thought or imagination. The importance of preventing this singularly fatal disease ought to awaken everywhere the most enthusiastic interest.

It is now known that consumption is caused by a rod-shaped disease germ or bacillus. The contagion is not communicated by the breath, for the sick and the well have often lived and slept together without its being contracted by the latter. It is always the sputa or expectoration which contains the germs in great number, and consequently this is the source of danger. If the expectoration is promptly disinfected and destroyed the danger is averted.

When such precaution is not taken the germs are found clinging to the walls of a room which has been occupied by a consumptive patient, or upon the windows where they have been carried by the common house fly, which delights to feed upon such material.

Expectoration upon the street is perilous to the healthy, for when it becomes dry the living germs are wafted about everywhere like dust or the seeds of the thistle.

When we consider the carelessness of the people or their lack of knowledge upon this subject it is a wonder that every person, whether strong or weak, does not contract this terrible disease. That many do not proves that nature is strong to resist and destroy disease producing germs.

The expectoration of consumptives ought to be disinfected and destroyed while it is moist. It should be discharged into cups containing a solution of corrosive sublimate, or upon paper or old pieces of muslin and burned up as soon as convenient.

There are also other possible sources of contagion as infected milk or meat, for cattle are subject to this disease and no public system of inspection exists at present sufficient to prevent all danger from these sources.

In a general way and in the line of prevention it may be said that a debilitated or consumptive mother ought not to nurse her infant. The milk fed to babies should be from healthy young cows kept in the country.

School children ought always to be supplied with a healthy and nutritious diet and special cravings for food may be regarded as a hint which ought to be gratified, for nature makes use of a large amount of material in building up a healthy body.

The importance of fresh air and sunlight are to be remembered as the means employed by nature for destroying contagious germs.

The apartments of sick persons should be frequently and thoroughly cleansed and as well ventilated as the welfare of the patient will permit.

Clothing ought always to be adapted to the climate and season in order to secure the comfort and well being of the patient.

Where many persons are employed in shops, mills and mines the employer should be compelled to provide the best modern methods of ventilation.

Some remarkable cases of recovery from incipient consumption have been correctly attributed to an abundant supply of fresh air and outdoor life without the aid even of medicine. Journeys on foot or on horseback, camping out in the vicinity of pine woods and long sea voyages have frequently resulted in restored health. If such means will cure this disease they will much more certainly prevent it.

In the line of prevention the importance of proper inflation and development of the lungs ought to be more fully recognized. Seeds cannot germinate in any soil where they are subjected to constant and daily agitation. Perhaps these germs of disease cannot effect a lodgement in the lungs if constantly agitated by the passing in and out of fresh air and an abundant supply of oxygen. We can at least see in this hint the necessity of standing erect and by forced inspiration fully expanding the lungs, so that there shall be no nook or corner quietly left as a breeding place for disease germs.

A narrow chest may be inherited, but a broad and full one can be successfully developed. The following rule is a good one for all to follow. "Throw your shoulders back and draw in through your nose all the pure air possible, meantime elevating the chest so as to increase its circumference. Do this several times daily and continue doing it till you acquire the habit of deep and correct respiration, and when you have acquired this habit persevere in it through life."

CHAPTER XIX.

THE ŒSOPHAGUS AND STOMACH.

I.—The Œsophagus and its Affections. II.—Description of the Stomach and Digestion. III.—Dyspepsia or Indigestion. IV.—Gastritis, Gastric Fever, or Inflammation of the Stomach. V.—Gastric Ulcer, or Ulcer of the Stomach. VI.—Nausea and Vomiting. VII.—Gastralgia, Stomach Ache, or Neuralgia of the Stomach. VIII.—Cancer of the Stomach. IX—Loss of Appetite. X. — Unnatural Appetite. XI. — Hiccough.

I.—THE ŒSOPHAGUS AND ITS AFFECTIONS.

THE œsophagus is a vertical canal or tube extending from the throat or pharynx to the stomach. Back of it lies the spine and in front the trachea. It is simply a tube for the transmission of food from the mouth to the stomach. Its length is about nine inches, in its course it crosses over the arch of the aorta, passes through the diaphragm and terminates by means of an opening in the cardiac end of the stomach. It has three layers of membranes, a muscular, a cellular and a mucous. The mucous layer contains a numerous supply of glands which secrete mucous.

The œsophagus is of considerable interest to the surgeon on account of its proximity to the aorta, the trachea, the pneumogastric nerve and other important tissues. It is not very liable to disease unless some caustic fluid is swallowed which may produce subsequent contraction or stricture. It is sometimes obstructed from the accidental swallowing of some foreign body as a set of plate teeth, a piece of bone or other substance.

When a stricture occurs it may be dilated by the careful and repeated passage of a bougie. A foreign body in the œsophagus as a piece of meat or fish bone, may be dislodged by an emetic or pushed down into the stomach or brought up by means of a bullet-pointed bristle probang. A foreign body so irregular as a partial set of plate teeth can be removed only by an operation which requires great surgical skill.

II.—DESCRIPTION OF THE STOMACH AND DIGESTION.

The stomach is an important organ of considerable size, situated below the diaphragm. Its position is transverse, the left portion is in contact with the spleen, and is much larger than the right. It is sometimes called the splenic or cardiac end. The right end tapers considerably in size and is known as the lesser or pyloric end.

The stomach has four distinct layers or coats, a serous, muscular, cellular and mucous. The serous coat is a layer of the peritoneum, the muscular layer has three sets of fibres, longitudinal, circular and oblique. The cellular layer connects the muscular and mucous and lodges the blood vessels. The internal or mucous layer is thick, soft and velvety.

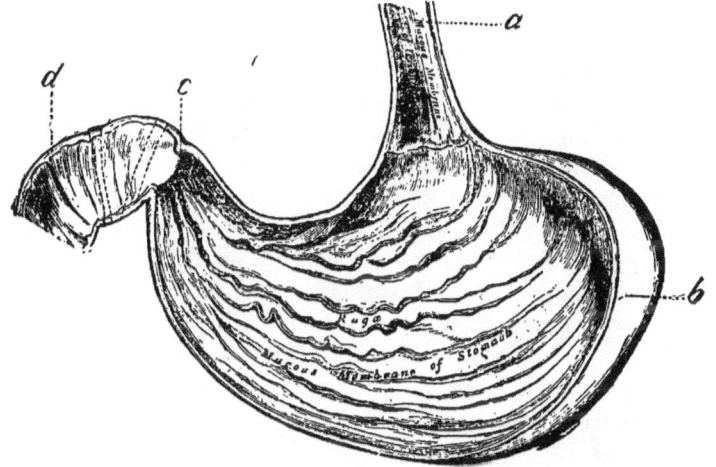

A view of the interior of the stomach, showing the ridges or folds called the rugæ and the mucous surface: a, œsophagus; b, cardiac end of stomach; c, pyloric end of stomach; c. junction of stomach and duodenum; d, duodenum.

The stomach is much larger when distended with food than when empty. In the latter state it contracts and the mucous coat is thrown into longitudinal ridges or folds. It is liberally supplied with blood from the gastric, hepatic and splenic arteries, and with nerves which are branches of the pneumogastric and the sympathetic. The mucous membrane is liberally supplied with mucous and peptic glands.

It is held in position by bands of omentum and a fold of peritoneum. During digestion its muscular walls institute a sort of churning motion which mixes the food with the secretions of the glands. The stomach is the receptacle for food during the early process of digestion, to which process it renders important aid.

The first act of digestion is the mastication of food in the mouth where it is crushed by the teeth and mixed with the saliva. The more thoroughly this preliminary work is performed in the mouth, the more promptly and efficiently will the digestive ferment act upon it when it reaches the stomach. The process of mastication in the mouth consequently becomes very important. Starchy foods in contact with the saliva are soon converted into a sweet substance called glucose

The saliva of the mouth is secreted and poured out abundantly by glands during mastication. The food after being thoroughly crushed, moistened and mixed with it is swallowed and forced onward into the stomach.

The stomach is liberally supplied with glands which secrete a fluid which is essential to the digestion of food, namely, the gastric juice. This is a complex fluid composed of water, acid, common salt and traces of lime, magnesia, potash, ammonia, iron and a large amount of pepsin. The most important ingredient of the gastric juice is pepsin. Pepsin possesses the power of preventing putrefaction. It also arrests putrefaction after the process has begun to take place. Pepsin must be combined with acid in order to act efficiently upon the food and in nature such combination always exists. Warmth aids the process of digestion, but too great heat as in boiling destroys the digestive power of pepsin. The properties of pepsin are destroyed by coming in contact with the secretions of the liver, especially bile, and this explains why digestion is so completely disturbed when an excess of bile enters the stomach. Food is then loathed and nausea and vomiting are persistent.

The glands of the stomach act energetically, secreting and pouring out gastric juice rapidly after food has been taken, but their activity entirely ceases after the stimulus of food has been removed.

The pyloric end of the stomach opens into the upper part of the intestines, the portion known as the duodenum. This opening is guarded by a valve-like arrangement which prevents the food from escaping from the stomach too soon. A very important part of digestion, however, takes place in the intestines.

It is well known that disturbance of the nervous system interferes with the production of gastric juice and is often an important matter to be considered in connection with the affections of the stomach.

Alcohol interferes temporarily with the process of digestion; it precipitates the pepsin but does not destroy its properties and when diluted sufficiently with water it again becomes active.

After eating it is a good rule not to think too much about the process of digestion. The stomach is exceedingly sensitive and resents being watched and distrusted. After eating it is a good idea to occupy the mind in a pleasant way or take a nap.

III.—DYSPEPSIA OR INDIGESTION.

Owing to irregular methods of living and excessive mental work or worry, dyspepsia is a common disorder. It is ordinarily a symptom of gastritis, and can hardly be called a disease unless it has become chronic and habitual.

CAUSES.

It is due to a functional disturbance of the digestive forces, hence whatever interferes with the complex process of digestion sooner or later brings on dyspepsia in some form, but at first it is usually mild.

The constant influence of the nervous system upon all the processes of life must be remembered. The faithful fulfillment on the part of the nerves of their full share of work is essential to all vital processes and to the performance of every animal function.

Strong emotions and mental overwork check the glandular secretions, and may be the means of arresting the process of digestion. Indigestion is chiefly due to a disturbed condition of the nervous forces of the stomach. Every one has observed how quickly some slight shock of the nervous system, as fright or bad news, will destroy the appetite, and even produce nausea or vomiting. The excitement of preparing for a journey on the part of children or those unaccustomed to travel, often destroys the relish for food, which if taken in such a condition could not be digested.

The great mental activity so characteristic of American life, the results of competition, haste to get rich, political and social ambition, success and failure, are all prominent in disturbing the physiological equilibrium which is so essential to healthy animal existence.

Whatever depresses the vitality or disturbs the relation of the fibers of our organism may be reckoned among the causes of dyspepsia. Warm weather is debilitating and the stomach is foremost in experiencing its effects. Little children who have been healthy from birth, at the first approach of hot weather are often unable to digest their food and such indigestion is the usual beginning of diarrhœal complaints and that dread disease, cholera infantum.

People who live in hot countries are obliged to discard to a great extent fat meats and hearty food, and live upon rice and fruit. This is not always from choice but in the interest of health.

A tendency to dyspepsia may be hereditary and when this is the case it usually manifests itself at an early age.

Among the more common causes of dyspepsia should be emphasized the imperfect and hasty mastication of food. In the mouth it is moistened with saliva and the starch begins to be changed into sugar by its chemical action. This process is essential. It takes time to do it. In our haste we drink water freely, swallow our food hastily and pay the penalty reluctantly, which is dyspepsia. Bolting the food, as it is called, is a vicious practice so far as health and longevity are concerned.

Indigestible and unwholesome foods are commonly regarded as prominent causes of dyspepsia; also excesses either in eating or drinking. It is reasonable to suppose that the introduction into the stomach of food in excess of the requirements of the body disturbs the balance between supply and demand and may cause sickness.

Indigestible, unwholesome or badly cooked food, must of necessity disturb the terminal nerve filaments, having in charge the important process of digestion reacting unfavorably upon the disposition.

Irregular methods of eating, as the taking of food at all hours, is detrimental and disarranges the functions of the stomach. Cooks from the habit of nibbling or tasting food constantly often lose their appetite for a hearty meal.

The use of alcoholic liquors is a common cause of the very worst forms of dyspepsia. It produces chronic catarrh of the mucous coat of the stomach, while it disturbs the functions of the other digestive organs, as the liver and pancreas.

The nervous forces weaken with old age. The stomach shares largely in this debility. The activity of the peptic glands is diminished, and but little gastric juice is secreted. Old people, therefore, should eat less food and of a more simple kind than those whose mental and muscular efforts are vigorous.

SYMPTOMS.

These are, in brief, a sense of discomfort and fullness after meals, acid eructations, flatulence, regurgitation of food, and what is popularly called "heart burn," which is merely distress of the stomach. Dyspepsia seldom causes acute pain, only uneasiness. Other symptoms may be dizziness, languor, drowsiness or inability to sleep, irritability, anxiety and despondency.

Skin diseases, as eczema and urticaria are often among the many symptoms of dyspepsia. Constipation may also be experienced.

TREATMENT.

This should be largely preventive. Use wholesome and digestible food. Avoid raw vegetables, pastry, fried fish or steak and rich or greasy articles of diet. Avoid fresh bread, hot biscuit, heavy cakes and take time to masticate the food thoroughly.

Those who tend to obesity should use potatoes, rice and other starchy foods, also cream and fat meats sparingly.

Beef roasted or broiled, mutton, chickens, game and eggs, with bread a day or two old are good articles of food. Avoid despondency and every grade of worry so far as possible, for all morbid conditions affect the stomach and its work unfavorably. Avoid the excessive use of medicines and drugs. They are very seldom necessary in the intelligent treatment of this complaint. Improve the general health by such exercise in the open air as horseback riding, foreign travel and other suitable means.

Koumiss and peptonized milk are excellent articles for a weak stomach. In prolonged and aggravated cases medicines may be needed to promote nutrition. Of the simple vegetable bitters which improve the appetite, gentian and nux vomica are worthy of favorable mention. The latter is a very valuable remedy in cases of debility, impaired nutrition and resulting anæmia. Five to ten drops of the tincture taken in water three times a day after meals, is a suitable adult dose. When there is partial arrest of the gastric secretions one or two grains of pure pepsin may be taken with or after each meal. Mineral waters may be beneficial in some cases. Benefit is sometimes derived from the administration of bismuth, iron and the mineral acids. Chief reliance should be placed, however, not upon such remedies but upon appropriate food, correct habits, taking care to avoid overwork and prostration, either mental or physical. Individual limitations should not be lost sight of as they are important guides in the treatment of this common affection.

IV.—GASTRITIS, GASTRIC FEVER, OR INFLAMMATION OF THE STOMACH.

Gastritis is a common affection, and in addition to the above names it is sometimes called catarrh of the stomach. The inflammation usually affects only the mucous lining, but sometimes the deeper tissues are involved. There are two forms of this affection, the acute and chronic.

CAUSES.

Various causes are assigned, but the more common are errors of diet or the abuse of alcoholic stimulants. Perhaps the use of substances too cold, or too hot, or the immoderate use of such articles as pepper, mustard and horse-radish, are worthy of consideration as possible causes.

The stomach is weakened and made sensitive to inflammatory conditions by habits that are debilitating. It is especially sensitive to all the irregularities and exhaustions of modern life. It is often the first organ to disclose approaching sickness, as acute fevers, and frequently the most unpleasant symptoms in acute disease is the irritability of the stomach.

SYMPTOMS.

The appetite is diminished or wholly lost. If food is taken digestion is labored, causing flatulence and other distresses. There may be much nausea and an intense loathing of all articles of food, together with pain in the region of the stomach, headache, vertigo and restlessness, with considerable fever and great thirst. There may be constipation or diarrhœa, faintness, hiccough, a coated tongue, foul breath and low spirits, but the most characteristic symptoms are persistent vomiting and thirst.

TREATMENT.

Pieces of ice may be held in the mouth to allay thirst. Ice-water containing a small amount of brandy may be allowed. It should be taken often in teaspoonful quantities. Minute doses of ipecac or tartar emetic may be administered with benefit, the latter in doses of $\frac{1}{1000}$ of a grain. Lime water added to milk may be retained by the stomach. Two or three drops of pure carbolic acid may be added to half a glass of water and thoroughly mixed with it; this mixture may be taken in teaspoonful doses and is very efficient to arrest fermentation and allay vomiting. For chronic cases bismuth in doses of fifteen grains or pure pepsin in doses of one or two grains are excellent remedies. Dilute muriatic acid in ten drop doses, well diluted with water, is often beneficial. Tincture of nux vomica in five drop doses is one of the best tonics in the chronic stage of this disease. When gastritis is due to the abuse of alcoholic stimulants it is necessary to abandon their use. The following prescription is a good one for chronic cases due to alcoholism.

℞	Tinct. of camphor	two drams
	Tinct. of capsicum	one dram
	Tinct. of nux vomica	four drams
	Peppermint water q. s. to make	four ounces

Mix. Dose one teaspoonful in water every four hours.

V.—GASTRIC ULCER, OR ULCER OF THE STOMACH.

Among the several diseases of the stomach ulcer takes a prominent place, from the fact that it is a common affection of this organ.

The causes do not seem to be determined, and whether it is in any way due to indigeston appears to be undecided. Some obstruction to the circulation or blood supply appears to be the immediate cause, but why there should be such obstruction in the interior surface of the stomach rather than in other portions of the body is not easy to explain.

SYMPTOMS.

The most prominent symptom is hemorrhage, soon followed by vomiting of blood and exhaustion. If from a large vessel it may prove fatal. If the ulceration involves the deeper tissues there may be perforation of the stomach, followed by peritonitis collapse and death.

TREATMENT.

The treatment demands quiet, so that rest in bed should be insisted upon, and the preferable position for the patient is lying upon the back. Cold may be applied over the stomach in the form of ice water or ice. If a condition of collapse or extreme exhaustion exists the cold had better be omitted, bits of ice may be swallowed and warmth applied to the extremities. Brandy may be given in ice water if the condition demands a stimulant. Liquid food only should be administered, as milk and beef tea. Milk is preferable to all other articles of diet; it does not irritate. Lime water may be added to the milk with advantage. Suitable medicines for this affection are Fowler's solution in one, two or three drop doses three times a day after meals. It must be well diluted in water. Nitrate of silver in one-fourth grain doses three times a day is an efficient remedy. It should be given in pill form. It forms an albuminous coating over the ulcer and facilitates the process of healing underneath. Bismuth in doses of fifteen grains is another remedy of great value. Rectal alimentation is sometimes necessary in order to give the stomach perfect rest. A case requiring such careful methods ought to be in the hands of a physician whose judgment must decide as to appropriate measures.

VI.—NAUSEA AND VOMITING.

Various minor affections of the digestive apparatus may be treated here appropriately. Some of them are not diseases but simply symptoms so common as to deserve a few words of special notice.

Nausea and Vomiting.—These are symptoms in many diseases, and often quite troublesome to manage. They accompany sea sickness and are caused by the motion of the vessel, which affects the brain and pneumogastric nerve. Many remedies have been suggested, and most of those tried have been more or less disappointing.

A few of the more reliable remedies are the effervescing citrate of magnesia or hydrobromate of caffeine, the hydrate of chloral, lemon juice, carbonic acid water, champagne, cocaine in doses of one-tenth of a grain, and the hypodermic injection of morphia.

For nausea and vomiting of pregnancy see diseases of pregnancy.

When blood is vomited it should be remembered that this is a prominent symptom in ulcer or cancer of the stomach. Falls, causing concussion of the brain, are followed by vomiting. Nausea and vomiting are common with the onset of scarlet fever. Vomiting occurs in digestive derangements and in functional disturbances of the liver.

Obstruction of the bowels is followed by persistent vomiting, in which the contents of the bowels above the obstruction may at length appear in the vomited matter. Vomiting is a characteristic symptom in many varied affections.

An emetic of warm salt water or mustard water to empty the stomach is proper in some varieties of vomiting, but would be inappropriate in other forms.

Vomiting is very weakening and distressing when long continued, and for this reason it often demands special attention. It requires attention in cholera morbus and cholera infantum, and may be allayed by carbolic acid or creosote in doses of a fraction of a drop well diluted with water, or by rectal injections containing a mixture of starch water and laudanum. Some physicians are fond of calomel in small doses to allay vomiting. One-tenth of a grain may be given as often as necessary until eight or ten doses have been administered.

VII.—GASTRALGIA, STOMACH ACHE, OR NEURALGIA OF THE STOMACH.

This is a painful affection of a paroxysmal type, due to irritation of the terminal nerves of this organ, and familiarly known as stomach ache. When the nerves of the stomach are sufficiently irritated there arises painful contraction or spasm of the muscular fibers.

The causes generally enumerated are indigestion, excessive acidity, stale or unsuitable foods, too rich food, delayed digestion, gas from fermentation of food, eating when exhausted, and anything which can derange the functions of the stomach.

The chief symptom is pain, which is not constant but paroxysmal, and is relieved by pressure and lessened by walking.

TREATMENT.

Hot drinks often relieve, as ginger tea, a teaspoonful of the spirits of lavender compound in water, a few drops of the spirits of camphor, or five drops of oil of cajuput upon a lump of sugar, or two or three drops of choloform in glycerine, or a simple cup of hot water may afford relief. When the pain is very severe and is described by the patient as cramps, a teaspoonful of the spirits of chloroform may be given in water, or if these fail to afford relief the hypodermic injection of an eighth of a grain of morphia may be administered. Hot applications or a mustard poultice may be applied to the stomach. The after treatment consists in regulation of the diet.

VIII.—CANCER OF THE STOMACH.

This common, and at length fatal disease, can be dismissed with few words. The stomach is more liable to be the seat of cancer than any other of the internal organs. The more common situation of this affection is about the pyloric orifice. It seldom occurs under forty years of age and terminates fatally, for no treatment can avail for its cure.

The symptoms are pain, tenderness, vomiting of bloody mucous, indigestion, constipation, a sallow complexion and emaciation. Pain, though a common symptom, is not always experienced.

TREATMENT.

The diet should be regulated so as to be nourishing without irritating the stomach or aggravating the trouble, and should consist of liquid food.

The pain should be relieved by hypodermic injections when necessary or anodynes in a suppository, the dose varying with the amount of pain.

For the vomiting creosote in one-half drop doses, given in some suitable syrup as acacia or glycerine, will be beneficial. Fowler's solution in doses of one to three drops three times a day is believed to retard the growth of this affection more certainly than any other remedy.

IX.—LOSS OF APPETITE.

In health the demand for food is quite regular; the thought of food adds to hunger, while the odor of savory articles causes an increase in the flow of saliva and gastric juice, and powerfully stimulates the appetite. In sickness the appetite is frequently impaired, and sometimes the odor or even the thought of food causes nausea and disgust.

Loss of appetite may be due to weakness or exhaustion, and it is usually very troublesome in consumption and other wasting diseases. It is to be expected in severe fevers and many acute diseases. The appetite returns with the recovery of health. If loss of appetite is protracted the patient is liable to lose more flesh and become more debilitated and anæmic, and recovery will be very much retarded.

When loss of appetite persists the patient's condition will be improved by exercise in the open air and the administration of bitter tonics as nux vomica. The following tonic prescription may be used after debilitating diseases to improve the appetite and the general condition.

  ℞ Quinnia sulph.   twenty grains
   Ext. nux vomica   five grains
   Hydrastin   ten grains
   Ext. gentian   twenty grains
   Piperin   five grains

Mix and make into twenty pills. Dose one after each meal three times a day.

If constipation exists add to the above prescription one grain of podophyllin.

X.—UNNATURAL APPETITE.

Sometimes instead of loss of appetite it becomes so unnatural, or ravenous as to exceed the ability of the stomach to digest the amount of food which is desired. This may occur in recovery from fevers and other acute diseases. In such cases caution must be used and good judgment exercised. Food should be given these cases at frequent intervals, and it must be of such a character as to be easily digested, else much harm may be done. Worms are frequently the cause of an unnatural appetite; they should be expelled by the remedies suggested.

In pregnancy the appetite is often abnormal and ravenous. In some conditions of the system there is a strong craving for certain articles of food, as vinegar, lemon juice or other acids. This craving is sometimes manifested for unwholesome or unnatural substances, as chalk, plaster, ashes, starch and other indigestible articles. When the craving indicates the want of some ingredient which is essential for the health of the individual it may be appropriately supplied.

XI.—HICCOUGH.

Hiccough, though not strictly a disease of the stomach, may be appropriately mentioned here. It is the result of a spasmodic action of the diaphragm. It is thought to be caused by too rapid eating or the eating of irritating substances, or over-eating or drinking, or indigestion. It is quite troublesome to infants, but ordinarily is otherwise of little account. Only when it is persistent and due to exhaustion, or when it results from severe nervous disorders, should it be regarded as an unfavorable symptom. If due to an over-distension of the stomach an emetic will afford relief. Sometimes a swallow of water will cause its disappearance. In some persistent cases it has been found necessary to control it with the hypodermic injection of morphia or the internal use of anti-spasmodics. In some diseases approaching an unfavorable issue, hiccough appears as a very annoying and persistent symptom, and seems to admonish that the end is not far away. In these cases no treatment avails.

CHAPTER XX.

THE LIVER, SPLEEN AND GALL BLADDER

I.—Description of the Liver and its Functions. II.—The Gall Bladder. III.—Diseases of the Liver in General. IV.—Congestion of the Liver. V.—Jaundice or Icterus. VI.—Cirrhosis or Hardening of the Liver. VII.—Gall Stones and Bilious Colic. VIII.—Other Affections of the Liver. 1, Abscess of the Liver; 2, Cancer of the Liver; 3, Fatty Degeneration of the Liver; 4, Amyloid Degeneration of the Liver; 5, Acute Yellow Atrophy; 6, Hydatid Disease of the Liver. IX.—The Spleen and its Diseases. 1, Inflammation; 2, Enlargement.

I.—DESCRIPTION OF THE LIVER AND ITS FUNCTIONS.

THE liver is a large organ situated upon the right side of the body below the diaphragm. It is, in fact, the largest glandular organ in the body, and weighs in the adult three or four pounds. The region occupied by the liver is known as the right hypochondriac. A portion of the liver, the left lobe, extends to the opposite side into the left hypochondriac. The lower border of the liver extends to about the margin of the ribs, where it may be felt by the practiced hand. The upper border is convex and fits into the concavity of the diaphragm.

The position of the liver is altered somewhat by change of position, as the rise and fall of the diaphragm in respiration, the distension of the stomach with food, and dropsical diseases of the chest and abdomen.

The liver is peculiar in shape and structure. It is made up of five lobes and five fissures, but since the liver of man is similar to that of other animals a familiarity with its appearance and structure may be assumed.

The liver is held in position by five ligaments, four of which are composed of folds of the peritoneum, the fifth being simply a remnant of fœtal life. The right lobe of the liver contains the bulk of its substance, it being six times larger than the left lobe.

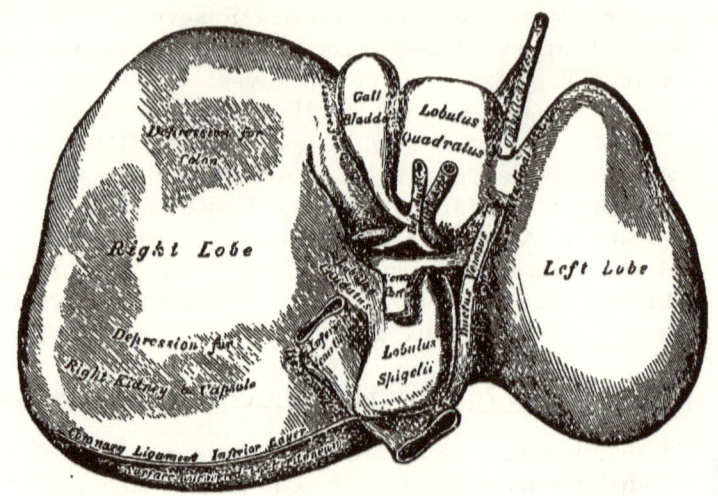

The Liver, under surface of.

The liver substance is made up of lobules held together by a mass of connective tissue and nourished and supplied by an extensive network of vessels. The blood vessels of the liver are peculiar. There are two sets, each supplied from a separate source. The first from the hepatic artery which furnishes the liver substance with nutrition, and the second from the portal vein, which carries to it a large supply of venous blood from the stomach, the spleen, the pancreas and the intestines. This venous blood traverses the liver substance and supplies it with the material out of which its secretions are elaborated.

The liver has several important functions to perform. These were formerly the cause of much speculation, but modern research has added light to this subject. It had long been known that the liver secreted a large amount of bile. It has also been known to medical men that the liver is an immense sugar factory where starchy material is converted into a sweet substance like sugar, known as glycogen. This is considered the most important function of the liver, and is known as the glycogenic.

It has been ascertained more recently that certain blood changes take place in the liver, such as the formation of white blood corpuscles and the destruction of red blood corpuscles, also that the formation of urea takes place in the liver. It is also agreed that the destruction of certain poisons which enter the liver through the portal circulation, and which are destroyed or prevented from entering the general system, is one of the many functions of this organ. According to recent, careful investigations, certain waste of nerve tissue is restored by the action of the liver.

From the foregoing it is not difficult to see that the functions of the liver are numerous, and that their healthy performance is essential to the well being of the individual. Derangement of the functions of this important organ may cause diabetes, rheumatism, gout, and a disease which to-day is attracting much attention, namely, lithæmia or lithuria, a condition in which lithic and uric acid are found in excessive quantities in the urine.

The liver when overworked may produce more bile than the system requires, and this excess may inaugurate a condition of congestion generally recognized under the head of biliousness.

The bile is a greenish colored viscid fluid, with a specific gravity of 1025. The quantity secreted by the liver begins to increase after a full meal. This fluid serves an important and essential purpose, although its full use is still somewhat obscure. It aids digestion by converting starch into sugar and fatty materials into an emulsion. It excites the normal action of the bowels, and is nature's great cathartic. It not only emulsifies fat but favors its absorption. The bile after performing these important functions is reabsorbed and again enters the circulation.

An excess of bile causes headache, stupor, nausea, constipation, irritability and other derangements which burden the kidneys, upset the stomach and the whole system in general.

When the sugar making function of the liver is deranged excessive quantities of sugar may enter the blood and appear constantly in the urine, causing that peculiar and fatal disease known as diabetes.

Other functional disorders of the liver are believed to be important factors in causing rheumatism, gout and other diseases caused by an excess of uric acid.

The liver contains a numerous supply of lymphatic vessels and an abundant supply of nerves. It also gives origin to a vast number of bile ducts, which collect and transport this fluid after it is secreted, carrying it on to the general reservoir for this fluid, namely, the gall bladder.

II.—THE GALL BLADDER.

The gall bladder is a pear-shaped sack about four inches long, attached to the under surface of the right or large lobe of the liver. It is a reservoir and capable of holding, when full, an ounce or more of fluid. It empties into the duodenum, the upper portion of the small intestines, by means of a duct, which joins another coming from the liver. The duct coming from the liver is called the hepatic, and that from the gall bladder the cystic; and after the two unite they form the common duct which is about two inches long and about the size of a goose quill. It transports the secretions of the liver to the intestines, and is also the outlet of the gall bladder.

The gall bladder, like the liver, is subject to a variety of diseases, both functional and organic. It is the frequent seat of catarrhal inflammation, the formation of calculi and of abscess. Calculi are formed from the solid constituents of the bile, the gall bladder becoming simply the receptacle where they may be retained. The duct may be obstructed so that the bile cannot flow out into the intestines. In such cases jaundice supervenes.

III.—DISEASES OF THE LIVER IN GENERAL.

The liver, until recently, has been rather of an obscure organ. It has been customary to blame it for many derangements, making it a sort of scape goat for ignorance and obscure affections.

Functional derangements of the liver are frequent and are generally classed under the indefinite term, biliousness. Since so much is said about this affection in medical literature and in the advertisements of patent medicines and nostrums, it is timely to notice what ought to be understood upon this subject. Many functional disturbances of the liver are due to the food supply, the process of digestion and absorption furnishing this organ with a direct and enormous supply of material and blood.

If the amount of food is too rich and abundant to satisfy the demands of nature the liver is likely to suffer from over nourishment, overwork and congestion, leading to a series of important derangement, which will be more fully noticed in the following pages. It is to be remembered that in all affections of the liver the diet is of great importance.

IV.—CONGESTION OF THE LIVER.

This affection, as already intimated, is known in common language as biliousness. It indicates that the liver is embarrassed by receiving too large a supply of material and blood, or in other words, that the food supply has been too abundant or not rightly proportioned. The food may contain an excessive amount of sugar, starch or fat, or may be otherwise too rich and abundant.

The causes of congestion of the liver are habitual excess in the eating of foods too concentrated or too stimulating. This condition is more liable to occur where high living is coupled with the use of alcoholic stimulants and sedentary habits.

Hot climates, malarial districts and disturbance of the nervous system, are factors which emphasize the frequency and importance of this affection. In certain fevers and affections of an inflammatory character the liver may be congested. Certain diseases of the lungs and heart may obstruct the circulation to such an extent as to cause a congestion of the blood vessels of the liver.

SYMPTOMS.

These are in general a coated tongue, loss of appetite, nausea, headache, pain, dullness or a sense of fullness upon the right side, bitter taste in the mouth, rise of temperature, and sometimes jaundice of a mild type or a sallow appearance of the skin. The urine is usually highly colored, and a deep breath causes discomfort or pain.

TREATMENT.

Rest of the digestive organs is important. The diet should be carefully regulated and a few simple directions followed which will often enable nature to afford relief without the aid of medicine. Saline mineral waters are sometimes helpful to cleanse the clogged and over burdened system. Epsom salts may be used for this purpose, in dessert spoonful doses dissolved in water or coffee. Podophyllin in doses of one-tenth of a grain continued for several days, arouses a sluggish liver and assists in regulating its functions. A pill composed of the following remedies, works well in chronic cases:

℞	Podophyllin	one grain
	Extr. of nux vomica	two grains
	Euonymin	ten grains
	Irisin	ten grains
	Ipecac.	four grains
	Extr. of hyoscyamus	two grains

Mix. Make into twenty pills.

Dose one or two pills each night for two or three weeks. This will usually relieve the most chronic and obstinate cases.

V.—JAUNDICE OR ICTERUS.

Jaundice though not a disease of itself, is yet so important as a symptom as to demand special notice. It may result from a large number of causes such as catarrhal inflammation of the gall bladder and gall ducts, an accumulation of gall stones causing obstruction or any pressure upon the liver and bile ducts which prevent the outflow of this secretion.

The development of a cancer or other tumor or even pregnancy may cause obstruction of the bile ducts. In some diseases of the liver as acute yellow atrophy, jaundice is a well marked symptom. When there is obstruction of the bile ducts, the bile is absorbed into the general system when it enters the blood and changes its character. It also affects the nervous system.

In the bowels the bile aids digestion, absorption, and stimulates them to a healthy action, but when taken into the blood it acts as a poison.

SYMPTOMS.

The bile out of place creates much general disturbance. The coloring matter which it contains permeates all the tissues of the body and gives to them a yellowish, or in some severe cases, more of a greenish hue. This coloring of the tissues is usually most noticeable in the whites of the eyes. It can not be so well observed by lamp light as in daylight. The urine is highly colored and the perspiration stains the linen yellow. When the obstruction is so complete that no bile passes into the intestines, the stools lose their natural color and resemble chalk or clay and the bowels are usually obstinately constipated. The disposition is affected, the patient is usually irritable, low spirited and despondent.

Digestion is disturbed, the appetite is poor, and food causes flatulence. The pulse is slow and the patient feels wanting in ambition and is not inclined to labor. The skin is yellow, dry and itchy, the mouth is dry and the tongue coated. There is often nausea and vomiting, there may be chills, alternating with fever, pain in the abdomen and pain extending into the right shoulder.

When delirium and stupor occur the case is usually critical, although delirium in the hot stage following a chill is not to be regarded as an unfavorable symptom.

TREATMENT.

The treatment consists in regulating the diet. Foods composed of starch, fat and sugar should for the most part be avoided. Medicines are needed to stimulate the eliminative functions so as to get rid of the excess of bile as speedily as possible.

Podophyllin in doses of one-twentieth to one-tenth of a grain two or three times a day does its work well, and in most cases improves the action of the liver. Sometimes a brisk cathartic is needed.

Excess of bile is eliminated also by the kidneys and to aid them in their important work diuretics such as cream of tartar water is beneficial. Acid drinks, as cream of tartar lemonade, are refreshing and grateful to the patient. A decoction of barberry bark and sour cider had considerable reputation formerly in domestic practice, and no doubt was often beneficial, but the cream of tartar lemonade is preferable for several reasons.

A mustard poultice placed over the liver externally, is beneficial and a fly blister is of decided advantage in very obstinate cases. The treatment of jaundice depends largely upon its cause, when it is due to functional disturbance it yields readily, but when due to organic diseases it is often very obstinate and persistent.

Jaundice of malarial origin is benefited by bitter tonics the best of which is probably quinine, cinchonidia, or chinoidine. The following prescription cures jaundice of malarial origin usually in a short time:

℞	Cinchonidia	forty grains
	Podophyllin	one grain
	Euonymin	ten grains
	Extr. of taraxacum	forty grains
	Oleo-resin of ginger	ten drops

Mix. Make twenty pills or capsules.

Dose one three times a day until recovery ensues.

When jaundice is caused by a catarrhal condition of the bile duct the phosphate of soda may be used with benefit in doses of twenty grains three times a day. This remedy can be taken agreeably in milk. The drinking of hot water and the use of hot baths are often beneficial.

VI.—CIRRHOSIS, OR HARDENING OF THE LIVER.

This disease takes its name from the fact that the liver becomes contracted and hardened. It is also called hob-nail liver or gin-drinkers' liver. It is a chronic affection and caused chiefly by the excessive use of alcoholic liquors. This disease rarely appears before adult life, and more frequently in the male sex. Those who drink strong alcoholic liquors without diluting them with water are the most liable.

SYMPTOMS.

The early symptoms are liable to be overlooked or confounded with dyspeptic troubles. This is unfortunate, for there is no permanent help for this affection when it has reached a chronic condition.

In the first stages the symptoms are identical with those of congestion of the liver and are mistaken for indigestion and biliousness. The liver is enlarged and pressure over it reveals tenderness and pain. Following the stage of enlargement is the opposite condition of contraction and induration. When contraction of the liver ensues it becomes nodulated, the circulation is obstructed and another class of symptoms present. When the circulation of the liver is thus interfered with the spleen becomes enlarged, piles are troublesome and the blood vessels on the surface of the abdomen become large and prominent. Dropsy of the feet and ankles is noticed which tends to extend up to the abdomen, and jaundice, though not a regular symptom, may occur.

The whole digestive apparatus is disordered, the appetite is poor, food occasions distress, gas and acidity of the stomach are troublesome and the bowels may be constipated. The patient loses strength and has a waxy and sickly appearance. The general condition is that of sallowness and emaciation, with well marked dropsical tendencies. The disease may last two or three years before the death of the patient occurs.

TREATMENT.

The only hope for these cases is in their early treatment during the stage of congestion and before induration has taken place. The diet ought to receive appropriate attention. Foods highly seasoned or rich in starch, sugar or fats, must be used very sparingly or abandoned and the use of alcoholic liquors regulated or prohibited. Congestion of the liver at this stage needs to be relieved by the use of alkaline waters, or podophyllin in small and repeated doses.

The functions of the skin and kidneys should receive attention. When the disease has advanced to a hopeless stage, but little can be done except to combat the unfavorable symptoms and such means must be employed as the condition of the patient demands. Flannel should be worn next to the skin. Hot poultices may be applied over the liver and tapping may be essential to draw off an excess of fluid from the abdomen.

The suffering which this lingering disease entails, should cause every one to contemplate the use of alcoholic drinks with alarm. No organ is more directly or more unfavorably affected by the continued use of alcohol than the liver. Next to this organ the spleen and kidneys feel the unfavorable force of this widespread habit. See chronic alcoholism.

VII.—GALL STONES AND BILIOUS COLIC.

These are due to a solidification of the constituents of the bile and just why this should take place it is difficult to determine. A second attack of gall stones is usually much dreaded by those who have experienced a previous one, for in passing through the duct they cause excruciating pain.

They vary in colors and in numbers. In some cases only one calculus exists, in others many, and in still others they are so numerous as to completely fill and distend the gall bladder. Their average size is about that of a small pea, but in this respect there is also great variation.

SYMPTOMS.

These are severe pain, nausea, vomiting, flatulence, and sometimes diarrhœa. The pain is called bilious colic and is accompanied by an expression of great anxiety. It is felt in the right side over the region of the liver and sometimes extends to the right shoulder. At times it is agonizing with clammy skin, weak pulse, and other symptoms of prostration. An attack may last a few minutes or several hours. The pain usually calls loudly for relief.

TREATMENT.

Such applications externally, as the hot pack and mustard plasters often afford a measure of relief. Ether may be inhaled carefully or anodynes administered, but the most efficient means is the administration of morphia hypodermically. Sweet oil in large doses has been much lauded as an effective agent for the removal of gall stones. It produces better results when combined with castor oil. The dose should be large and frequently repeated for one or two days.

After the subsidence of the pain, the gall stones may be found in the stools. After a person has once suffered from an attack of gall stones, much attention should be given to the general health to prevent subsequent attacks. The diet ought to be carefully regulated and rich food eliminated. Exercise in the open air is important and the bile may be rendered thinner and less likely to solidify by the use of appropriate mineral or alkaline waters.

VIII.—OTHER AFFECTIONS OF THE LIVER.

There are several other affections of the liver which are either too rare or of insufficient interest to engage general attention except to a very limited degree.

Abscess of the Liver.—This occurs as the result of blood poisoning, pyæmia, or it may be due to the debilitating effects upon the system of a tropical climate. In temperate regions it is a disease of rare occurrence. Injuries have sometimes been followed by an abscess of the liver. The symptoms of hepatic abscess are obscure in the early stages, but later they are prominent. The first symptoms are of a general character, such as a chill, pain in the back and limbs, headache, coated tongue, nausea, vomiting, local pain and rise of pulse, with rise of temperature. The duration of this affection is irregular and uncertain. When left to itself the abscess will rupture and recovery may ensue. Should it rupture into the peritoneal cavity it would be likely to cause collapse and death. Surgical interference may be called for, and may result in saving the patient's life. An abscess of the liver requires careful watching and skillful treatment.

Cancer of the Liver.—This is of comparatively frequent occurrence. Its cause is obscure. The symptoms are similar to those of cancer of the other internal organs. They are local uneasiness in the region of the liver, pain, emaciation, low spirits, dropsy, and the peculiar waxy look which is characteristic of cancerous disease.

The treatment must palliate the symptoms, as no cure can be expected. The diet should receive attention, the pain should be relieved and the patient should be made comfortable.

Fatty Degeneration of the Liver.—In this disease the liver substance seems to have changed to fat and the organ is enlarged, smooth and soft. It is not tender upon pressure and jaundice and dropsy which call attention to the liver so frequently are wanting, hence there are few symptoms to give rise to the suspicion that the disease exists.

In the treatment an effort should be made to improve the general condition. Medicines are of but little service except tonics, to improve the appetite and strength. A tendency to the accumulation of fat should be obviated by the means recommended for the treatment of obesity.

Amyloid Degeneration of the Liver.—This disease is so called because material resembling starch, is deposited in the tissues of the liver which, in consequence, becomes much enlarged. It is also known as lardaceous or waxy liver. It is due to prolonged suppuration and bone disease, necrosis. Syphilitic and malarial affections have been suggested as causative factors. The functions of the liver are much disturbed. Well marked cases do not recover, and no appropriate line of domestic treatment can be suggested.

Acute Yellow Atrophy.—In this disease the entire liver is involved. It is rapidly diminished in size and a destruction of the cells takes place. There is nausea, vomiting, severe pain, and jaundice which is always present. The spleen is also enlarged. It sometimes, though rarely, occurs during pregnancy, and hereditary syphilis, has been suggested as a cause. Medicine is powerless to improve the general condition, or to arrest the intensity of the disease, but should be used as needed, to relieve pain and add to the patient's comfort.

Hydatid Disease of the Liver.—This disease is prevalent in some portions of the globe. It is due to a parasite, the eggs of which may be contained in the fæces of the dog. Those who live in filthy habitations, surrounded by animals, as do the inhabitants of Iceland are subject to this undesirable affection. Cleanliness and care in associating with dogs, is a means of prevention. Medicines taken internally have little or no effect. Surgical means are sometimes essential and successful.

IX.—THE SPLEEN AND ITS DISEASES.

The spleen is a small organ or gland, ordinarily weighing only about seven ounces. It is situated at the left end of the pancreas and near the cardiac end of the stomach. Its substance is dark red in color and quite brittle. It is very liberally supplied with blood. Its outer surface is convex and its inner concave. It is only about an inch to an inch and a half in thickness. It is held in position by ligaments formed from folds of the peritoneum. Its size is increased by the taking of food. It is also larger in the well fed than in those poorly fed or suffering from hunger. Its size is diminished in old age. Its minute structure is of interest only to the student of anatomy or the medical practitioner.

In intermittent fevers and in diseases of the liver it is liable to be congested, and sometimes it attains an enormous size. In malarial regions it has been known to enlarge until its weight reaches eighteen or twenty pounds, distending the abdomen to an unusual degree.

The functions of the spleen are somewhat obscure, but when it is disturbed by disease the quality of the blood in the body appears to be correspondingly affected, its specific gravity becoming reduced and its condition becoming thin and watery. There is also a disturbance of the relative quantity of the white and red blood corpuscles, the patient feels weak and there is a tendency to a dropsical condition. From these facts we may infer that the function of the spleen is to assist in maintaining the normal condition of the blood, and the proper proportion between the white and red blood corpuscles.

Inflammation of the Spleen.—With regard to diseases of the spleen, there is but little that needs to be said. It may be inflamed by injury, or perhaps from other obscure causes. When this condition is suspected, the bowels should be moved with saline cathartics, and generous doses of quinine administered.

Enlargement of the Spleen.—In malarial sections, this condition is common. In its treatment the most satisfactory results are obtained from the administration of quinine, used in connection with doses of Fowler's solution, three or four drops of which well diluted with water, are to be taken after each meal.

Diseases of the spleen except excessive enlargement are recognized with difficulty, and their management is similar in principle, to diseases of the liver, owing to the intimate relation of the two organs. The tincture of iodine painted over the region of the spleen may be of some benefit in enlargement of this organ. The syrup of hydriodic acid in teaspoonful doses, is likely to be of benefit. It should be taken in a little water.

CHAPTER XXI.

THE HEART, CIRCULATION, PERICARDIUM, BLOOD VESSELS, AND THEIR DISEASES.

I.—DESCRIPTION OF THE HEART AND ITS VALVES. II.—THE CIRCULATION. III.—OVERWORK OF THE HEART, OR HEART STRAIN. IV.—THE PERICARDIUM, OR HEART SAC. V.—INFLAMMATION OF THE HEART SAC, OR PERICARDITIS. VI.—VALVULAR DISEASE OF THE HEART, OR ENDOCARDITIS. VII.—ANGINA PECTORIS, OR NEURALGIA OF THE HEART. VIII.—PALPITATION. IX.—VARIOUS OTHER DISEASES OF THE HEART. 1, HYPERTROPHY, OR ENLARGEMENT OF THE HEART. 2, FATTY DEGENERATION. X.—THE BLOOD VESSELS, AND THEIR DISEASES. 1, ANEURISM; 2, VARICOSE VEINS.

1.—DESCRIPTION OF THE HEART AND ITS VALVES.

THE heart is a powerful muscular organ, placed between the lungs somewhat obliquely in the left side of the chest above the diaphragm; where its motion can be felt by the hand and its sounds heard by the ear.

The great function of the heart is to maintain the circulation of the blood. It performs this work with marked fidelity, from birth to the close of life, never stopping to rest for a single instant, day or night. It beats, on an average, seventy-two times a minute in an adult, and about one hundred and twenty times a minute in a newly born infant.

The shape of the heart is that of a cone, with the apex downward, the base upward, and from one to the other, the distance is about five inches. The diameter of the base is about three and one-half inches; its average weight is from ten to twelve ounces, depending upon the size of the individual.

The heart is composed chiefly of muscular fibres, arranged in layers which interlace each other. Many of these fibres are circular, and in contracting, squeeze the blood out of the internal hollow cavity in which it is allowed to remain scarcely for an instant.

The contraction of the heart is known as the systole, and its relaxation the diastole, the one movement alternating with the other.

The heart is divided by a muscular partition into two halves, known as the right and left heart or sides. The right heart is known as the venous side because it receives and transmits the venous blood. The left heart is the arterial side, and receives and transmits the arterial blood.

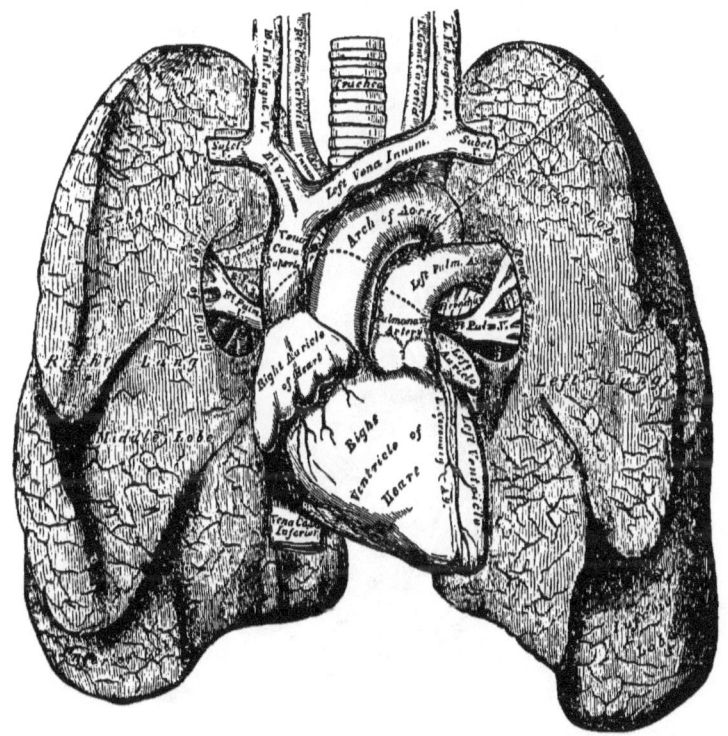

Front view of heart and lungs. The borders of the lungs have been turned back to show relation of heart and its vessels.

The muscular walls of the left side are thicker and stronger than those of the right owing to the greater force required to send the arterial blood thoroughout the body. Each side of the heart is further divided into apartments, an auricle and a ventricle, four cavities in all, two auricles and two ventricles. The necessity for this arrangement can be seen when we come to understand the circulation.

The heart muscle receives its nourishment from two small arteries, the right and left coronary, the first branches of the aorta just outside of the semilunar valve. Its nerve supply is abundant from the sympathetic and cerebro-spinal system.

The valves of the heart are an ingenious arrangement permitting the blood to flow freely only in the direction in which it ought to go, and by closing at the right instant they prevent the blood from flowing in the wrong direction. If from any reason the valves of the heart do not close tightly, a portion of the blood flows back after each stroke, a condition common in valvular disease.

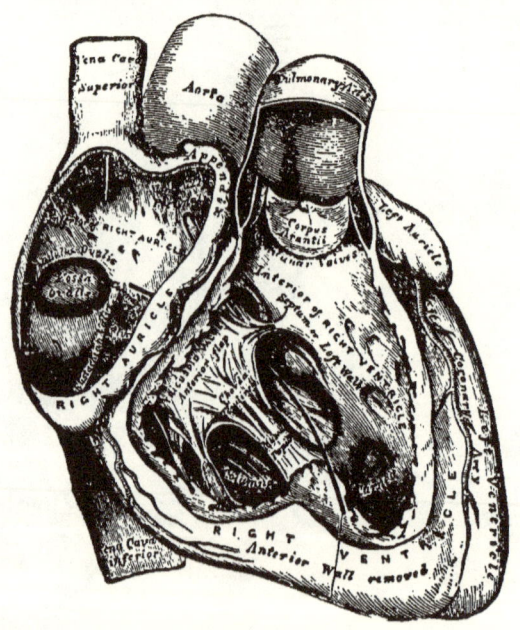

The heart with the right auricle and right ventricle laid open to show the interior structure.

The valves between the left auricle and the left venticle are known as mitral; the valves which guard the outlet of the left ventricle are known as the semilunar. The mitral and semilunar valves of the left side are much more liable to be disabled and suffer from disease than the valves of the right heart, because the left ventricle is larger and stronger than the right and contracts with greater force. Hence these valves are subjected to a powerful and constant strain. The valves of the right heart are the tricuspid and semilunar. The tricuspid guard the opening between the right auricle and the right ventricle, and the semilunar guard the opening of the pulmonary artery. The left ventricle is obliged to contract with sufficient force to keep the blood current moving throughout all parts of the body, while the right ventricle is obliged to contract only with sufficient force to accomplish the pulmonary circulation.

II.—THE CIRCULATION.

In order to understand the work of the heart in maintaining the circulation, it is necessary to follow the blood current passing out from the heart, until it returns again. The left auricle receives the blood coming from the lungs, where it has been oxygenized. It is bright red, arterial blood, and passes from the left auricle to the left ventricle, when the left ventricle instantly contracts, it is prevented from flowing back into the auricle by the mitral valves which instantly close; simultaneously with their closure, the semilunar valves open, allowing this blood current to be forced into the aorta, after which they instantly close and prevent its returning, and this process is constantly repeated. The blood forced into the aorta is now pushed forward by each heart stroke, a small portion of it entering the coronary arteries, to nourish the heart, and every other branch in turn throughout the whole body. These branches are numerous, and the size of the arteries is constantly diminishing, until they become so small that they are scarcely visible to the naked eye.

These little minute vessels form a net work throughout the tissues of the whole body, and are called capillaries. By the time the blood current has reached these little vessels, it has lost the spurting character imparted to it by the heart beat, and flows in a steady, minute stream, giving nourishment to every organ, tissue, and part of the body, and receiving in turn worn out products, which must be eliminated by the liver, kidneys and skin.

After the blood has passed through this extensive capillary network it emerges into larger tubes called veins, which converge toward the heart. The blood has now become changed in color and character and is known as venous blood. It comes from every direction and enters the right auricle of the heart, through the superior and inferior vena cava.

It passes from the right auricle into the right ventricle. Instantly the right ventricle contracts, the tricuspid valves close, the semilunar valves open, and the blood is forced into the pulmonary artery. It ought to be observed at this point that the pulmonary artery transports venous blood, and the pulmonary vein arterial blood.

By the repeated contraction of the right ventricle the venous blood is forced through the pulmonary artery until it reaches the lungs, where it comes in contact with the oxygen of the air, the blood and the air being separated from each other only by a very thin, moist membrane. Through this thin membrane the carbonic acid gas which the venous blood contains passes out, and oxygen from the air passes in. Thus the color of the blood is again changed or oxygenized. After this process has taken place it is rapidly forced on into the pulmonary veins and flows into the left auricle. This completes the circuit and process called the circulation.

It may be observed that this process is a double one, the left heart maintaining the circulation of the body and necessary for its nourishment; the right heart maintaining the circulation of the lungs and necessary for the purification of the blood. The heart, then, is a double pump maintaining a systemic and a pulmonary circulation.

The circulation is an interesting, though complex process. While it is taking place, urea and other waste products are being eliminated from the blood by the kidneys; other products are being eliminated by the liver, carbonic acid gas escapes and other waste products pass out through the sweat glands. Thus nature is making a constant and heroic effort to keep the life giving current pure.

Because the arteries were empty after death, they were once supposed to be hollow tubes, through which only air was conveyed. In order to understand the circulation, it is necessary not only to follow the blood in its course through the body, but to observe the changes which take place in it as it comes from the kidneys, liver and lungs. Nor is this all. The blood is constantly being influenced by forces coming from without; as the food which we eat, by means of digestion and absorption, is conveyed into the circulation, to enrich and maintain the blood supply. The circulation is intimately related to the process of respiration, digestion, absorption and elimination. For all of these processes the heart simply supplies the force, and without its action there would be immediate stagnation and death.

Before the lungs are expanded with air, only sufficient blood is sent to them for their nutrition, but when their inflation takes place, the blood must be sent to the lungs, and oxygenized. Hence a remarkable change takes place in the circulation at birth. Prior to birth, there is an aperture or opening between the two auricles, through which the blood passes, and the pulmonary circulation has not yet been established. At birth, this direct opening between the two auricles is closed up, and adult circulation takes place.

III.—OVERWORK OF THE HEART, OR HEART STRAIN.

There is no organ in the body, more liable to overwork than the heart. Its activity is constant. When the body is in a state of repose, the heart must continue its work. If increased effort or greater activity is rendered necessary, as in running or severe labor, the heart beats more rapidly in order to supply the requisite force. When extreme effort is carried too far from overwork or protracted effort, the stomach becomes feeble, the limbs tremble, the muscles lose strength, the face is care-worn, the skin is shriveled, the memory falters, and the signs of old age appear, even though years do not indicate the autumn of its approach. There is no excitement, emotion or over-exertion which does not perceptibly touch and affect the heart. Therefore it is wise to avoid violence to this all important organ.

IV.—THE PERICARDIUM, OR HEART SAC.

The heart is surrounded by a membranous sac called the pericardium, which is a reflection of its outside covering. It also surrounds the great vessels which arise from the heart for a distance of two inches. It is composed of two layers, an external or fibrous, and an internal or serous. The serous layer covers the external surface of the heart and the internal surface of the sac. It is smooth and glistening. It secretes a lubricating fluid about the consistency of glycerine, which keeps the membrane moist and prevents friction and disturbance, as a result of the incessant motion of the heart. In health there is always a small quantity of this fluid contained within the sac. In disease it may be deficient, excessive, or its character may be altered.

Inflammation of this membrane is known as pericarditis, of which there are several varieties. The function of the heart sac is the protection of the heart and other organs separating it from those which it might otherwise disturb.

V.—INFLAMMATION OF THE HEART SAC, OR PERICARDITIS.

Pericarditis is an inflammation of the heart sac. It is characterized in general by an effusion of fluid which displaces the heart and is liable to be mistaken for pleurisy. The disease may be of a mild or violent type.

CAUSES.

The causes are somewhat obscure, but are believed to be changes of temperature, such as result from taking cold, the inflammation of neighboring tissues as in pneumonia and pleurisy, or as secondary to some febrile condition, as scarlet fever, or more frequently rheumatism. It is sometimes a complication of Bright's disease.

SYMPTOMS.

The first symptoms are a chill, followed by fever, accelerated pulse, loss of appetite, nausea, vomiting, and pain with tenderness about the chest in the region of the heart. The pain may be slight or severe. The features usually express an anxious and suffering condition. The respiration is labored and attended with a short hacking cough. The pulse is weak and irregular.

After the acute stage is passed, an effusion of fluid takes place in the heart sac, sometimes so abundant, as to alter the position of the heart. Before the effusion takes place, friction sounds may be heard, which are often mistaken for pleurisy, unless the patient holds his breath for the listener. After the effusion, the friction sounds disappear and the natural sounds of the heart are heard with difficulty.

TREATMENT.

This is a dangerous disease, liable to be protracted, and requires skillful treatment. Exertion should be prevented as far as possible and rest maintained. Pain should be relieved by anodynes. When there is an excessive quantity of fluid, it may be justifiable to withdraw it with an aspirating syringe. This is a delicate operation, and care must be exercised not to puncture the heart. Stimulants are sometimes required in this disease, after the acute symptoms have subsided. The carbonate of ammonia answers an excellent purpose. It is impossible to map out a definite line of treatment, as the different stages of the disease and the varying degrees of its severity require a separate treatment for each case.

In all cases the vitality should be sustained by appropriate nutrients, as milk, beef tea and other simple food. Physical and mental excitement should be avoided by the patient, until recovery has fully taken place.

VI.—VALVULAR DISEASES OF THE HEART, OR ENDOCARDITIS.

The interior surface of the heart is lined by a thin membrane which is reflected over the valves and forms their external surfaces. The valves of the heart are thin and glistening in health, but in disease they become rough, thickened, and lose their shining character. Little vegetations may develop on their borders, sometimes as large as a pea, and prevent the perfect working of the valves. This allows some of the blood to return which has been forced by them. In other words, the valves may leak and cause a murmur known as mitral insufficiency and aortic regurgitation.

The principal cause of valvular disease is rheumatism or rheumatic fever. It is sometimes associated with Bright's disease.

A heart murmur may be caused by anæmia. This is not an organic affection.

Severe attacks of rheumatism may leave the heart valves in such a condition as to prevent their perfect closure and permit the blood to flow back after it has been forced out. This embarrasses the heart and adds to the work it is obliged to perform.

When the valves leak the heart is compelled to beat faster and work harder in order to compensate for the loss. In the same manner as a pump when it is so out of order that the valves leak you must pump harder and longer in order to get a pail of water. The increased work which the heart has to do in valvular disease usually causes a multiplication of the muscular fibres and an increase of heart tissue, which is known as enlargement of the heart or hypertrophy.

Sometimes instead of increase of the fibres the walls of the heart become stretched. This is known as dilitation of the heart, a process which may extend until the walls become so weakened as to rupture. When the valves of the heart are affected recovery may take place and no trace of the disease remain, or the affection may become chronic, remain stationary, or advance from bad to worse.

Ulceration of the valves and other chronic changes sometimes occur. Ulcerative endocarditis is a severe but fortunately unfrequent affection.

A mere roughness along the borders of the valves may work mischief by entangling the fibrin of the blood and forming little clots, which may be swept into the circulation and obstruct some distant and minute vessel of the brain, kidneys, lungs or other organs. When the arterial supply of any portion of the body is thus cut off death of the part may result, or an abscess may form or some irreparable mischief.

Thrombosis.—This is the technical designation of a clot which forms in the heart, arteries or veins. When it is swept along to some distant point and plugs up a vessel it is called in this new location an embolus. Should an embolus cut off the circulation of a portion of the brain, softening of that portion would soon follow, and also paralysis of those parts of the body controlled by that portion of the brain. The plugging up of an artery in the lower extremities is the cause of gangrene. Embolus of the pulmonary artery may cause sudden death. The valves on the left side of the heart are the ones most usually affected.

SYMPTOMS.

When the valvular affection is slight, the disturbance it causes is likely to be slight; but when it is of a high grade, the disturbances are often well marked and accompanied by severe symptoms, as labored respiration, anxiety of expression, severe pain, disordered digestion and dropsy. When the trouble is with the semilunar valves of the aorta pain and difficulty of respiration are prominent symptoms. The tendency of such affections is usually progressive. Persons often live for years with some defect of the heart valves if the amount of regurgitation is small and does not result in the formation of an embolus or the plugging up of some distant arterial canal.

Pain about the heart is often due to indigestion, and care must be taken not to be misled in this direction. The most reliable symptom in diagnosis is an abnormal sound of the heart or murmur, and yet it must be remembered that a murmur may be caused by weakness as well as by valvular disease. A constant difficulty in breathing may be the most reliable symptom and the one which threatens danger.

TREATMENT.

Full treatment for all the varying phases of valvular disease could hardly be outlined in a condensed work for domestic use. Persons with valvular disease should avoid excitement or exertion, as the climbing of stairs or hills, running, lifting and severe muscular exercise. It is perhaps needless to say that ball playing, boat racing and similiar efforts of an exciting character should be scrupulously avoided. In some cases, where there is a tendency to dropsy, and the action of the heart is feeble and irregular, digitalis and caffein make a fortunate combination. The following may be used.

℞ Pulv. digitalis   thirty grains
   Caffein   forty-five grains

Mix. Make into thirty pills.
Dose one before each meal for an adult.

When tea, coffee or tobacco unfavorably disturb the action of the heart, their use should be abandoned. Strychnia, in doses of $\frac{1}{100}$ of a grain three times a day, is an excellent tonic for a weak heart. It also improves the respiration.

Dropsy is often troublesome in the last stages of heart disease. It causes shortness of breath and marked discomfort when the patient attempts to lie down. It begins first with swelling of the ankles and its progress is onward, making the demand for skillful attention imperative.

VII. ANGINA PECTORIS, OR NEURALGIA OF THE HEART.

This is a nervous affection or neuralgia, which comes on suddenly and is characterized by intense pain in the region of the heart, extending to the left arm. The attacks are attended by alarming symptoms, as paroxysmal pain, anxiety and distress. It may be brief or last several hours, or the attack may prove fatal.

CAUSES.

It results from such organic disease of the heart as fatty degeneration of the muscular fibres, ossification of the aorta or coronary arteries, and valvular disease. Gout predisposes to this affection. Sometimes it is only a neuralgic affection, there being no organic disease whatever, and in these cases the pain may be due to indigestion or neuralgia of the stomach.

SYMPTOMS.

The pain attending this affection is spasmodic and peculiarly severe. It demands prompt measures for its relief The face is pale and anxious, the patient is weak and restless, and feels and appears as if death was near.

TREATMENT.

A hot mustard plaster of full strength and generous size may be placed over the seat of the pain. Ether may be carefully inhaled or morphia given by the mouth or hypodermically, and repeated until relief is obtained. Three or four drops of nitrite of amyl may be inhaled from a handkerchief, and the process frequently repeated. Nitro-glycerine in doses of $\frac{1}{100}$ of a grain or the aromatic spirits of ammonia in teaspoonful doses may be given if the action of the heart is weak. When attacks recur, caused by gout, the wine of colchicum seed in doses of ten or fifteen drops three times a day is a remedy of remarkable efficiency.

VIII.—PALPITATION.

This is not only a disturbed, but an excited action of the heart which may be due to a great variety of causes or to some functional or organic trouble.

When palpitation is functional, it may be due to dyspepsia, to anæmia, to some fault in the diet, to intemperate habits, or to some disturbed condition of the nervous system. This trouble is frequently a source of great discomfort to the patient and sometimes alarming. It is important in each case to ascertain the cause before appropriate treatment can be intelligently employed. In some cases nerve tonics, as the phosphate of iron and strychnia, are beneficial.

When due to anæmia, remedies should be used which improve both the quality and quantity of the blood. (See anæmia.)

When this affection results from the use of strong tea, coffee, tobacco, alcoholic drinks, or any debilitating habits, their use should be discontinued and correct habits vigorously enforced. When palpitation exists in connection with dyspepsia, outdoor exercise should be enjoined, and the diet receive suitable attention. (See indigestion.)

Palpitation resulting from enlargement of the heart or other organic affections demands a line of skillful treatment.

IX.—VARIOUS OTHER DISEASES OF THE HEART.

There are quite a number of diseases of the heart in addition to those previously mentioned. These diseases are for the most part organic, and are of great importance to the medical profession, but as they are recognized with difficulty they could hardly be intelligibly treated in domestic practice, and for this reason they require only a brief notice.

Hypertrophy or Enlargement of the Heart.—This is usually caused by over-action of the heart especially in valvular disease. It may result from stenosis of the aorta, from Bright's disease, and from other obstructions to the circulation, as in some form of lung trouble. It is an organic disease of chronic character.

Mental excitement and physical exertion should be moderated. The habitual use of stimulants aggravate this trouble and should be avoided.

Persons who have enlargement of the heart are especially liable to apoplexy.

Fatty Degeneration.—Fatty degeneration of the heart muscle occurs from the lack of nutrition, due to various wasting diseases, as consumption, scrofula, cancer and others which entail immense drain upon the system. It may result from compression of the coronary arteries which supply the muscles of the heart with blood.

There is a change in the structure of the muscles of the heart, and fat, more or less, takes the place of the fibre. The heart consequently is weak and its contractions feeble, the pulse is weak and irregular. The breathing is especially liable to be effected as the result of exertion. Pain in the region of the heart causes anxiety and failure of the heart's action threatens.

Medicine should be used to enrich the blood and improve the general condition. The following prescription is appropriate in many cases.

℞ Elix. phosphate iron, quinine and strychnia   four ounces

Dose one teaspoonful in water after each meal.

In some cases, where a tendency to dropsical effusions exists, the following is especially appropriate:

℞ Pulv. digitalis   twenty grains
    Citrate of caffein   thirty grains

Mix. Make into twenty pills or powders.

Dose one three times a day.

It is well to emphasize the remark that death may result in these cases from some unnatural strain or exertion.

X.—THE BLOOD VESSELS AND THEIR DISEASES.

The blood vessels include the arteries, the capillaries and the veins. The arteries are strong elastic tubes for the purpose of transporting the blood. The large arteries are strong, thick, and admit of great strain. They are composed of three coats, an internal or serous, a middle or muscular, and an external or cellular. The arteries, except those of the cranium, are contained in a loose, fibrous sheath. They diminish in size as branches are given off until the capillaries are reached.

The capillaries are very minute vessels, averaging in diameter not more than $\frac{1}{3000}$ of an inch. The capillary circulation is very extensive and reaches every part of the body, furnishing nutrition to all of its organs. The more active the functions of an organ the more numerous are the capillaries to supply the increased demand for nutrition.

The veins, as well as the arteries, have three coats, the middle one of which is less firm, so that an empty vein falls together, whereas an empty artery retains always its circular form.

Most of the veins are supplied with valves which favor the onward movement of the blood toward the heart.

While the arteries may be attacked by inflammation, dilatation and other forms of degeneration, fortunately these diseases are rare.

Aneurism.—The most frequent affection of the arteries is aneurism, due to a dilatation of the coats or layers of the vessel. The treatment of this affection is for the most part surgical. Aneurism of the aorta is beyond the reach of treatment, but those of more superficial arteries may be cured by ligation, by pressure and other appropriate means.

The rupture of a large internal aneurismal tumor is usually fatal. Fatty degeneration of the small arteries of the brain may occur, and when these arteries are so weakened as to rupture apoplexy results.

A calcareous degeneration of the arteries may occur in advanced life. In this affection the walls of the arteries lose their elasticity and the circular tubes become hard, resembling bone. Such changes in the arteries are known as ossification or atheromatous degeneration.

Most of the affections of the blood vessels are due to injury, old age, the action of alcohol or the result of syphilis. (See chronic alcoholism.)

Varicose Veins.—The most common affection of the veins is due to their dilatation and to the breaking down or rupture of the valves. This condition occurs frequently in the veins of the lower extremities, and is known as varicose veins. This condition may be caused by any occupation which requires standing constantly upon the feet. Childbearing, however, is the most frequent cause. Chronic constipation may be regarded as a factor of some importance in the production of this trouble.

From varicose veins may result swelling of the limbs, ulceration and hemorrhage.

The affected limb is purple about the ankle, shin or under the knee, the discoloration extending upward sometimes to the thigh, involving more or less extent, according to the severity of the case. The veins are distended, more or less twisted and knotted, and give to the limb a characteristic discoloration.

Varicose veins require external pressure and support by means of bandages or the elastic stocking. Rest and elevation of the limb favors the circulation, especially if the limb is raised higher than the head while in a reclining position.

CHAPTER XXII.

THE INTESTINES, RECTUM AND THEIR DISEASES.

I.—The Small Intestine. II.—The Large Intestine. III.—Diseases of the Rectum. 1. Congenital Deformity. 2. Injuries of the Rectum. 3. Fissure and Ulcer. 4. Rectal Abscesses and Fistula. 5. Itching about the Anus or Pruritis. 6. Piles or Hemorrhoids. 7. Prolapse of the Rectum. 8. Polypi. IV.—Other Rectal Affections. 1. Stricture. 2. Cancer. V.—Rectal Alimentation. VI.—Intestinal Catarrh. VII.—Dysentery. VIII.—Cholera Morbus. IX.—Cholera, Asiatic. X.—Inflammation of the Bowels, Obstruction and Appendicitis. XI. — Hernia. XII. — Peritonitis. XIII.—Colic. XIV.—Constipation. XV.—Worms.

I.—THE SMALL INTESTINE.

THE small intestine is a circular canal about twenty feet in length and leading from the stomach to the ileo-cæcal valve, where it joins the colon. It is folded upon itself and held in place by folds of the omentum. Its situation is within the abdominal cavity.

The small intestine is divided into three portions, the duodenum, the jejunum and ileum. The duodenum is the first portion and receives the contents of the stomach as they pass out from the pyloric orifice. The pancreatic duct and the common bile duct open into the small intestine three or four inches from its beginning. The small intestine is composed of four coats or layers. The muscular coat contains two layers of fibers, one taking a longitudinal and the other a circular direction. The mucous or internal layer contains numerous glands which open upon the surface and which secrete fluids abundantly to aid in completing the process of digestion. This process is complicated in the small intestine, for the reason that a variety of work is going on at the same time, as, for instance, the process of absorption, which is simultaneous with digestion.

The absorbent vessels take up and carry away the material which has been digested and changed into chyle. It is carried and poured into the circulation, and by the time the contents of the bowels have reached the colon both the process of digestion and absorption have thoroughly taken place.

In order to understand the process of absorption it is necessary to know that the small intestine is covered over on the inside surface by numerous little elevations, called villi, which give it a velvety appearance. These villi are very numerous, being estimated in each individual as several millions. They are the agents which carry on the work of absorption. They project out into the nutritious fluids and semi-fluids contained in the intestine very much as the roots of a tree permeate the soil. They drink into little microscopical mouths in a rapid and thorough manner the liquids prepared for their use. The process of absorption takes place throughout the entire length of the small intestine. The vermicular motion of the bowel serving to bring these little hungry and thirsty absorbents into contact with the contents of the intestine, so that nearly everything suitable to be taken into the circulation is appropriated, while the food is slowly passing from the stomach to the large intestine. The villi contain arteries, veins and lymphatic vessels, called lacteals, all of which are more or less engaged in the process of absorption.

It is interesting to follow the course of this nutritious material taken up from the small intestine and see how it is able to reach the general circulation.

That portion absorbed by the blood vessels is carried directly to the liver by means of the portal vein, where it is prepared to pass into the general circulation.

That portion absorbed by the lacteals is turned into the thoracic duct and passes onward to the left subclavian vein, where it flows into the venous blood current and mingles with it. Changes are constantly taking place in this nutritious fluid, so that by the time it has reached the lungs, it is simply rich blood and all traces of its previous character have disappeared. In this interesting manner the blood is constantly supplied with new and rich material from the food. The tissues of the body are rebuilt daily to some extent and destructive wastes are compensated for by the reception of new elements.

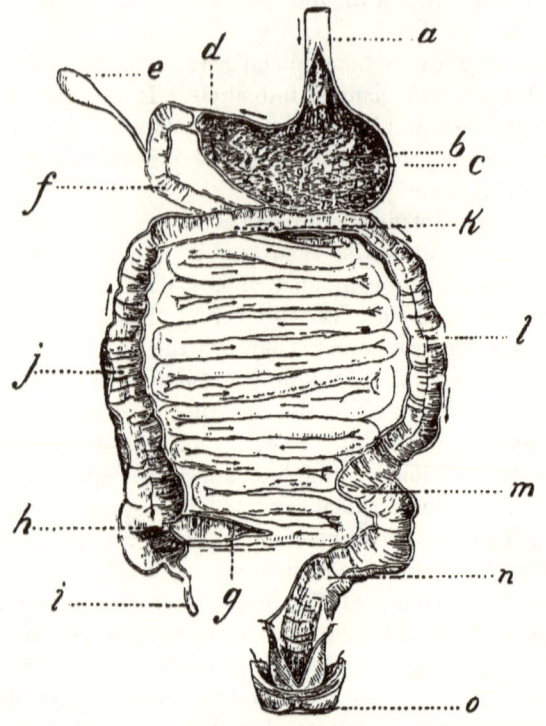

The digestive apparatus: A, œsophagus; b, stomach; c, cardiac extremity; d, pyloric extremity of the stomach; e, gall bladder; f, duodenum; g, lower end of small intestine; h, ileo-cæcal valve; i, vermiform appendix; j, ascending colon; k, transverse colon; l, descending colon; m, sigmoid flexure or S-shaped flexure of the colon; n, rectum; o, anus

II.—THE LARGE INTESTINE.

The large intestine begins at the termination of the ileum and extends to the anus. Its length is about five feet and its diameter is considerably larger than the small intestine.

The three names given to the different portions of it are the cæcum, colon and rectum. The cæcum is the beginning of the large intestine and is situated at the right and lower parts of the abdomen. Attached to it is the vermiform appendix, a small tube three or four inches in length and about a quarter of an inch in diameter. This is sometimes the seat of acute and chronic inflammatory action. It is a rudimentary sac and in man has no necessary use. (See appendicitis.)

From the cæcum the large intestine extends upward on the right side as far as the liver, then transversely across the abdomen then down on the left side. These portions are also known as the ascending the transverse and descending colon. The entrance of the ileum into the cæcum is known as the ileo-cæcal valve. The descending colon terminates in the portion known as the rectum, and owing to a curve at this point resembling the letter S, it is called the sigmoid flexure. The large intestine is retained in position by folds of the peritoneum. Its termination is the rectum which extends from the sigmoid flexure to the anus. As the rectum approaches the anus, it is more or less dilated in order to hold the accumulating contents of the bowel at this point. The large, like the small intestine, has four layers. The internal surface of the mucous layer is not covered with absorbent villi but merely lodges some simple follicles and glands. The rectal portion of the large intestine is subject to so many annoying affections as to deserve some special attention.

The outlet of the rectum is guarded by two circular or sphincter muscles under the control of the will; the internal sphincter being about an inch above the outlet while the external sphincter puckers the outlet like a purse string. Paralysis of the sphincter muscles though infrequent occasions much annoyance.

III.—DISEASES OF THE RECTUM.

Congenital Deformity.—There is sometimes the abscence of a rectal outlet or other congenital deformity. When a child is born with this defect death soon occurs unless relief is afforded by skillful surgery. Such deformities, if not too extensive, may often be completely relieved. The necessity for relief, however, should be recognized promptly, as delay might thwart the most skillful operation.

The number of children born with some deformity is large in the aggregate, those of the mouth and rectum being among the most frequent and important.

Injuries of the Rectum.—Injuries of the rectum may occur from falls or accidents, as in severe labor. From such injuries hemorrhage is usually profuse, but they generally heal kindly if the parts are thoroughly cleansed and properly treated. A good result is not likely to be obtained if constipation is permitted, as a difficult movement reopens the lacerated surfaces and prevents healing by first intention.

Fissure and Ulcer.—A fissure of the rectum is an irritable ulcer in which healing is hindered by its location and the spasmodic action of the external sphincter muscle. It is caused usually by a little rent or tear in the margin of the anus. The rectum is especially liable to irritation and injury from the passage of hard fæcal matter owing to the wide prevalence of constipation. It is chiefly owing to neglect that the rectum is so frequently affected by a large number of annoying diseases. A little rent or fissure if not properly treated, may exist for years and cause unlimited distress and suffering. It is attended by a disagreeable smarting sensation which is augmented by every movement of the bowels. The general health suffers, the patient is sallow and wears an expression indicative of prolonged suffering. This affection so trifling in itself is sometimes so painful as to be mistaken for a cancer.

TREATMENT.—The treatment, fortunately, is both simple and successful. At first laxatives should be administered as an ounce or two of castor oil or a generous dose of Epsom salts. The ulcer should next be washed over with a solution of nitrate of silver, ten grains to the ounce of water. This stimulates the ulcer and brings about a healthy condition of the surrounding tissue. It may then be dressed with benzoated oxide of zinc ointment or an ointment containing a dram of iodoform mixed with an ounce of vaseline. This method of treatment is suitable for any ulcer or fissure of the rectum about the margin of the anus.

When there is agonizing pain caused by the spasmodic action of the sphincter muscles, these measures alone will not be sufficient, but the patient should be put under an anæsthetic, and then the muscle should be partially or wholly cut through or stretched until its fibers are sufficiently lacerated to prevent future contraction or spasm, after which it can be healed as readily as if it existed in any other location.

Rectal Abscesses and Fistula.—The tissue about the anus is a frequent site for the development of an abscess which is frequently followed by a fistulous track leading from the rectum to the external surface in the neighboring vicinity.

The management of a rectal abscess differs only slightly from a similar affection elsewhere. A thorough incision is necessary to liberate the pus, and the after treatment consists in keeping the abscess cavity clean and healing it from the bottom. Rest in bed is recommended and soothing applications, as a warm poultice covered with laudanum.

A fistula usually has an external and an internal opening; the external is outside the anus and the internal is within the rectum, just above the sphincter muscle. The internal opening may be difficult to find. There are a few other causes beside the one already mentioned which may result in a fistula, as a fish bone, a pin or other foreign body which may become lodged above the sphincter muscle and ulcerate through to the external surface.

A fistula does not tend to heal of its own accord, but produces much uneasiness, disagreeable itching and pain. It is usually a source of no little annoyance.

TREATMENT.—The treatment is chiefly surgical, and usually requires a complete division of the tissue from the fistula into the rectum, cutting completely through the sphincter muscle. Recovery then takes place rapidly, and healing from the bottom of the wound goes on without interruption from spasm of the divided muscle. After the operation the wound should be cleansed each day and a little iodoform of aristol sprinkled between the surfaces. Other operations suggested for the treatment of a fistula have not yielded as satisfactory results as the one already detailed.

Itching of the Anus or Pruritus.—This is sometimes a disagreeable, obstinate and painful affection, which is usually worse at night.

There is often an excess of moisture about the rectal orifice, and unless removed by frequent bathing it is highly irritable, and the trouble is much increased if the inclination to rub or scratch is yielded to.

The causes are quite indefinite and perhaps numerous as high living, sedentary habits, overwork, irritating perspiration, eruptions, piles, eczema, seat worms and derangement of the nerve forces.

Why such causes should occasion pruritus in one and not in another is puzzling, and it may be doubted whether there is much connection between some of the causes recounted and the disease beyond the fact that some explanation must be offered for such a troublesome affection.

TREATMENT.—The treatment is simplified when the cause of the affection is known with certainty. Bathing the affected locality daily with warm or carbolized water is beneficial. The application of benzoated oxide of zinc ointment, to which a little chloroform may be added, is recommended by competent authorities. The application of alcohol when it can be borne is said to be of service. The following may be used each night at bed time, and if necessary in the morning.

  ℞ Carbolic acid   twenty grains
    Cocaine   ten grains
    Menthol   thirty grains
    Oxide of zinc ointment one or two ounces

Mix. Use externally.

If the patient is debilitated and suffering from nervous disorders the following in addition is suggested for internal treatment.

  ℞ Fowler's solution   one and a half drams
    Elix. calisayæ   four ounces

Mix. Dose one teaspoonful three times a day after meals.

Piles or Hemorrhoids.—Piles are a very common affection. In fact, there is no other disease of this region so frequent. There are two varieties, external and internal.

External piles are little tumors at or near the margin of the anus. Internal piles are little tumors within the orifice which are liable to become inflamed, bleed and protrude. The causes as commonly enumerated are constipation, long continued sedentary habits, irritating physic, high living, pregnancy or any obstruction of the pelvic circulation.

Piles are, in reality, little blood tumors or dilitations of pelvic blood-vessels and are chiefly caused by irritation of the anus and the obstruction of the venous circulation.

Internal piles are often painful, liable to bleed and to protrude as the result of straining at stool.

TREATMENT.—Rest, cold applications, astringent ointments or anodyne and astringent suppositories are appropriate. External piles can be permanently cured by making an incision into the little tumor and turning out its contents which is a clot of blood. Internal piles may be permanently cured by ligation.

Palliative treatment may afford relief for a long time. The diet should be regulated and constipation carefully avoided. The injection of a pint of warm water into the rectum before each stool affords considerable relief.

The following prescription is unrivaled.

℞	Pulv. opium	six grains
	Ext. hyoscyamus	six grains
	Ext. belladonna	three grains
	Tannin	twelve grains
	Cocaine	six grains
	Cacao butter q. s. to make	twelve suppositories

Insert one well into the rectum each night and morning.

Prolapse of the Rectum.—This is a protrusion of a ring of mucous membrane outside of the anus. It sometimes happens that several inches of the entire rectum is forced outside the external sphincter.

This affection in a mild form is common in young children in a debilitated condition. The immediate cause of this affection is relaxation of the sphincter muscle, irritation of the urinary organs, rectal irritation from worms, dysentery or constipation.

Prolapse of the rectum rarely happens in middle life except as the result of piles, but it frequently happens in very young children or very old people as the result of weakness and debility.

TREATMENT.—The protruding bowel should be returned. Place the patient in a recumbent position. Oil the fingers and gently push back the protrusion. The utmost gentleness should be used to avoid resistance which will increase the difficulty of reduction. Having replaced the prolapsed tissue a repetition of its descent may be prevented by a pad held in place with a bandage. The application of astringent washes may be necessary to prevent a return of the trouble. Constipation must be avoided and straining at stool.

Polypi.—A polypus within the rectum should be treated the same as in any other locality by removal.

IV.—OTHER RECTAL AFFECTIONS.

Stricture.—There are a number of other rare affections of the rectum. Stricture may result from some inflammatory process, as extensive ulcerations, syphilitic diseases and cancer. The diameter of the rectum is much reduced, and at length complete obstruction may result. The approach of this affection is often unrecognized.

The treatment consists in dilating the stricture by mechanical means, using a bougie or sponge tents. The latter method is considered the safer.

Cancer.—Cancer of the rectum is not a frequent disease. When it exists it is very painful and likely to terminate life. The causes are unknown. The prominent symptoms are pain, the dischage of blood and pus, constipation, sallow complexion, loss of strength, more or less obstruction, and finally exhaustion. When ulceration takes place with a breaking down of the tissues the discharge is very offensive.

TREATMENT.—When the disease is discovered early its entire removal may be accomplished and afford a good chance for a cure. When it has so progressed that removal is impossible palliative remedies are alone required. (See cancer.)

The old method of using paper with printer's ink upon it, or other harsh or unsuitable substances for toilet purposes was doubtless the cause of much irritation of the anus if not the actual cause of disease. The modern use of soft tissue is a much needed improvement and in the interest of better health.

V.—RECTAL ALIMENTATION.

The rectum has some ability to absorb, not only medicines which may be applied to it locally, but also nutrients. Life has been maintained for several consecutive weeks by the use of nutritive enemata. This fact is borne in mind by physicians who, not only relieve pain successfully by the use of suppositories, but when the stomach is disabled, resort to rectal feeding with satisfactory results.

VI.—INTESTINAL CATARRH.

Since the intestines are lined throughout with mucous membrane containing a vast number of mucous glands, any portion may become the site of a catarrhal inflammation. Different names are given to this disease, and different symptoms are manifested depending upon the portion of this canal which is involved. A catarrh of the duodenum is likely to obstruct the outlet of the bile duct and occasion jaundice, a condition liable to be mistaken for some disorder of the liver. The two most prominent causes of intestinal catarrh are changes of temperature and improper diet.

Among the various symptoms the following may be mentioned. Disordered digestion, nausea, vomiting, diarrhœa, pain and lastly jaundice if the site of the trouble is in the duodenum. Other symptoms may appear such as a coated tongue, fetid breath, headache, languor and a yellow condition noticed in the whites of the eyes.

TREATMENT.

This consists in regulating the diet, offending material may be removed by a dose of oil or other mild laxative. The following prescription may be used in these cases to advantage:

℞	Castor oil	one half ounce
	Paregoric	two drams
	Syr. acacia	one ounce
	Cinnamon water	one ounce

Mix. Dose one teaspoonful every four hours for a child one year old, adults in proportion.

Intestinal catarrh, especially of the ileum and colon, may terminate in cholera infantum when the patient is only several months old if the weather is hot. In such cases the stools are first slimy and often green in color and their passage attended with griping pain or colic. The patient gets thin rapidly, the heart is weak and the urine highly colored. This disease may become chronic and exist for a long time without the development of cholera infantum. Such cases usually recover after the heat of the summer is over.

In adults this persistent looseness of the bowels is known as chronic diarrhœa. It was a troublesome affection in the army.

For children chalk mixture and bismuth combined, are excellent remedies.

℞	Salicylate of bismuth	one dram
	Chalk mixture	two ounces
	Paregoric	two drams
	Syr. acacia q. s. to make	three ounces

Mix. Dose one teaspoonful every four hours for a child two years old.

For the chronic diarrhœa of adults the following is efficient:

℞	Tinct. opium deodorized	four drams
	Fowler's solution	one dram
	Wine of blackberry root q. s. to make	four ounces

Mix. Dose one teaspoonful every four hours.

VII.—DYSENTERY.

Dysentery is a disease of the mucous membrane which lines the large intestine. There is ulceration of this tissue attended by griping pain and the discharge of mucous, blood and pus. It may exist in any climate but is more prevalent in the hot season.

CAUSES.

Climate may be considered the most promiment cause. It prevails especially in July, August and September. Heat, moisture and atmospheric changes are a combination which favor its development and prevalence. The decomposition of animal and vegetable matter during hot weather are favorable to its appearance. Among other causes unsuitable articles of food, the fermentation of food and the impurities of drinking water deserve mention. It is common among prisoners of war, especially when they are confined to a coarse diet without vegetables or fruit. It is sometimes epidemic and some have favored the opinion that it was caused by a specific germ of which proof is wanting. If it can be proved that dysentery is contagious, then its germ origin becomes positively established.

SYMPTOMS.

These are intestinal catarrh, abdominal tenderness, peculiar twisting pains, colic and an urgent desire for the stool, straining, smarting and inability to leave the stool or a desire to return almost immediately. There may be from twenty to forty or more movements of the bowels in twenty-four hours. The discharges are scant containing strings of mucous tinged with blood. From this fact it is sometimes called bloody flux. Emaciation is rapid and the patient, if not relieved, soon enters upon a typhoid condition.

TREATMENT.

Rest in the reclining position is important and ought to be insisted upon. In a mild case a dose of castor oil may be given to relieve the bowels of offending matter before they are put to rest with anodynes. A pint of warm water or starch water containing twenty or thirty drops of laudanum and a pinch of pulverized alum may be thrown into the rectum with a syringe. Medicines introduced into the rectum have a local effect and are often much more efficient than when given by the mouth. A single astringent injection often completely changes the character of the disease. In severe cases a half dram of nitrate of silver dissolved in a pint of water and injected into the rectum with a syringe will produce surprising results. The syrup of acacia and a little laudanum may be added with advantage. The injection affords more relief if used cold, or nearly so, and may be repeated in two or four hours. Ipecac. is much lauded as a specific for dysentery.

Boiled milk is an excellent article of diet for these cases. Raw, chopped beef and soft boiled eggs may be used. In bad cases stimulants may be essential.

When for any reason the use of the injections are inconvenient suppositories may be used instead as the following:

R Ext. witch-hazel thirty grains
Cocaine three grains
Tannin twelve grains
Pulv. opium twelve grains
Cacao butter q. s. to make twelve suppositories

One of these may be pushed well into the rectum each night and morning. The cocaine in the above perscription causes the griping pain to disappear and the patient gets refreshing sleep, which is so much needed.

When the disease can be traced to a malarial origin, as is sometimes the case, the following is appropriate and will give satisfaction.

R Salol one-half dram
Quinine two scruples
Morphine three grains

Mix. Make into twenty pills, or put into capsules.

Dose one three or four times a day for an adult in addition to the other treatment recommended.

Ulceration of the bowels, it is to be remembered, is one of the conditions common to dysentery, and the above treatment is suitable for all such cases.

VIII.—CHOLERA MORBUS.

Cholera morbus is sometimes called sporadic cholera. It resembles true Asiatic cholera except that it is usually less severe and less liable to terminate fatally. It occurs in the hot weather of summer or in the autumn when hot days are followed by cool nights.

CAUSES.

It appears to result from a combination of causes, among which heat and indigestible food are prominent. Wilted vegetables, unripe fruits, articles of diet which favor fermentation and the excessive use of ice water seem favorable to its development. Sudden changes of temperature, and sudden checking of the perspiration are among the factors which may be mentioned as causative.

SYMPTOMS.

The attack usually comes on suddenly with nausea, vomiting, chilly sensations, colicky pain in the bowels and diarrhœa. Vomiting affords only temporary relief, and after the stomach is emptied of its contents, the vomiting continues at intervals with increasing distress. After the contents of the stomach are expelled, the vomited matter is yellow or greenish in color, leaves a bitter taste in the mouth and is mixed with a large amount of mucous. When vomiting continues long enough, these bilious secretions are succeeded by a thin fluid having the characteristic appearance of rice water. A similar fluid is passed by the bowels.

When the pain and diarrhœa are not promptly relieved, all the symptoms are aggravated; the patient becomes cold and clammy, cramps occur in the stomach and in the muscles of the arms and legs; there is great thirst, the heart's action wanes, the pulse becomes weak and thready, the sufferer appears exhausted, losing strength rapidly but cannot rest for a moment as the pain and suffering increase. A condition of pallor and prostration ensue which is known as collapse.

All cases are not thus severe because they are not permitted to reach the stage just mentioned. In mild cases as soon as the stomach and bowels are unloaded relief is sometimes experienced and recovery takes place rapidly.

TREATMENT.

A generous mustard poultice strong enough to redden the surface without blistering should be placed over the stomach and bowels.

When the thirst is excessive little fragments of ice may be used to allay it, or lemonade or bread coffee, well cooled, may be permitted for the same purpose. Small doses of aromatic sulphuric acid and tincture of opium may be given in camphor water to check the diarrhœa as follows:

℞ Aromatic sulphuric acid   one dram
  Tinct. of opium   one and a half drams
  Camphor water   four ounces

Mix. Dose a teaspoonful every hour as needed.

When marked prostration and continued vomiting take place iced brandy frequently repeated is beneficial. The following prescription will work well in mild cases if taken early.

℞ Aromatic spirits of ammonia   one dram
  Paregoric   four drams
  Magnesia   one dram
  Peppermint water q. s. to make four ounces

Mix. Dose one tablespoonful every hour or half hour.

No method of treatment affords so much satisfaction to the physician as the hypodermic injection of morphia combined with atropia. It quiets the vomiting, eases the pain and brings about hasty reaction which is soon observed. The pulse improves, the warmth of the body is restored, cramps subside, diarrhœa ceases, the patient rests and is better. When the patient is not relieved within an hour, the dose which is one quarter of a grain of morphia and $\frac{1}{120}$ of a grain of atropia may be repeated.

The diet should be simple for several days after recovery to prevent a relapse. In some cases complete recovery is retarded and such demand tonics or perhaps medicines to stimulate the action of the liver or the kidneys or both.

IX.—CHOLERA, ASIATIC.

This dreaded disease is not common in the United States, but is liable to be brought into our sea-ports and large cities. In 1832 the cholera visited New York City, and there were three thousand five hundred and thirteen fatal cases. It has raged in nearly all sections of the old world at various times, destroying multitudes of people or devastating large armies. It has existed in India from a very remote period, and from thence it has appeared to spread to other sections of the world.

CAUSES.

Cholera is caused by an extremely minute specific disease germ, which enters the human system in various ways. The spread of cholera is favored by over-crowding, poverty, intemperance, high temperature, unfavorable surroundings or vicious and unclean habits.

These do not originate cholera, but are favorable for its development. Water is, undoubtedly, the most effectual agent in spreading the disease when it contains the cholera germs.

SYMPTOMS.

In a very short time after the contagion is received into the system, profuse diarrhœa occurs with liquid stools, causing little or no pain, but followed by great prostration. This symptom intensifies, the stools take on the characteristic rice-water appearance, vomiting occurs, and if the attack is severe, cramps in the muscles of the legs, followed by pallor, chilliness, thirst, weakness and collapse. There is a marked decline in the bodily temperature, the patient sinks rapidly, the contenance appears pinched and shrunken with a leaden hue; the breathing becomes difficult, the pulse weak, the surface of the body cold and bathed with a damp perspiration; the fingers and face get blue and the voice weak and sepulchral. Reaction sometimes takes place even after the manifestation of all these symptoms, but death is more common and occurs in about twelve hours.

TREATMENT.

No treatment has ever been universally successful. About fifty per cent. of all cases die. When cholera is epidemic, no case of diarrhœa should be neglected or allowed to take its own course.

Nothing can render more prompt and certain relief, than the hypodermic injection of morphia with atropia. (Morphia one fourth grain atropia $\frac{1}{100}$ and repeat as circumstances require.)

Excellent results have been claimed from the use of the following:

℞ Aromat. sulph. acid   one ounce
    Tinct. opium   one ounce

Mix. Dose fifteen to thirty drops every hour.

Mustard poultices over the stomach favor reaction and often prevent vomiting. Pieces of ice may be given for the thirst or iced brandy may be used. The following is excellent:

℞	Carbolic acid	fifteen drops
	Tinct. of camphor	two drams
	Spirits of chloroform	four drams
	Peppermint water q. s. to make	two ounces

Mix. Dose one teaspoonful in water repeated every hour or half hour.

The diet must receive attention. Boiled milk, wheat gruel with milk boiled into it, mutton or beef broth and even raw or soft cooked eggs may be used.

Sometimes collapse and death occur so suddenly that very little can be done. Cholera is especially fatal to alcoholic drinkers.

X.—INFLAMMATION OF THE BOWELS, OBSTRUCTION AND APPENDICITIS.

Inflammation of the bowels may result from various causes. Any obstruction, if not soon relieved, develops inflammatory action, except the obstruction is partial, as from a growth or cancer. Inflammation may take place in any portion of the intestinal canal and the symptoms will vary somewhat with the portion affected.

Obstruction.—Obstruction of the bowels is sometimes caused by a strangulated hernia, by bands of fibrous tissue, or by the twisting of the bowel upon itself in such a way as to prevent the passage of its contents. At the junction of the ileum and colon the bowel may become obstructed by its fæcal contents. Habitual constipation may cause some of these difficulties, but on the whole fatal diseases of the bowels are less common than might be expected.

The symptoms are severe pain, similar to colic, impeded respiration, anxious expression, a cold sweat upon the brow, enlarged abdomen, vomiting of fæcal matter, and in desperate cases persistent hiccough.

Diseases of the intestines are so painful and dangerous that it is not customary to rely upon any course of domestic treatment for their alleviation. In some of these diseases the symptoms are too obscure to render their description intelligible or their treatment safe. The treatment in all these cases should be outlined in accord with the symptoms. Suitable directions for adequate treatment cannot be detailed in advance.

In a general way it may be said that diseases of the bowels require rest in bed. Constipation should be relieved either by laxatives or rectal injections. A hot poultice placed over the abdomen in some cases affords a measure of relief. Cold acid drinks, as lemonade and cream of tartar, are excellent to relieve the thirst.

Appendicitis.—This is a dangerous affection which may be caused by the lodgement of a foreign body as a grape seed, a prune stone, a cherry pit, a gall stone or hardened feces in the vermiform appendix. Many cases, however, cannot be traced to such a cause but appear to

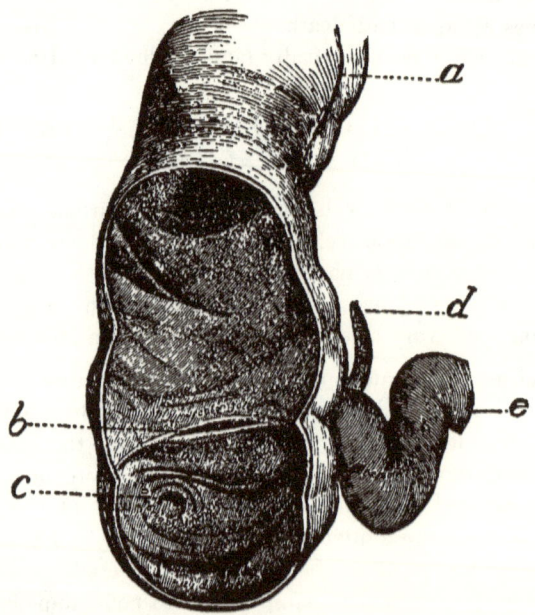

The cæcum and colon opened and front portion removed to show the ileo-cæcal valve: a, ascending colon; b, ileo-cæcal valve; c, opening into vermiform appendix; d, termination of appendix; e, small intestine.

be due to obstruction of the arterial circulation in the appendix or to local catarrhal or inflammatory action. If the blood supply is entirely obstructed or cut off, death of the part or gangrene results. When a foreign body becomes impacted, or local inflammation takes place in the appendix, suppuration and perforation are liable to occur.

When pus or fæcal matter pass through a perforation into the abdominal cavity, they cause fatal peritonitis. An abscess sometimes forms outside but in the vicinity of the appendix, which, if left to itself, will rupture into the abdomen, or in occasional cases it may work its way to the surface through the external abdominal walls.

SYMPTOMS.

The symptoms of appendicitis are similar to those of general inflammation of the bowels, for which in the past it appears to have been many times mistaken. The chief symptoms are tenderness upon pressure on the right side in front of the haunch bone accompanied with pain more or less severe. Sometimes the tenderness and pain are complained of as high up as the pit of the stomach and very commonly about the umbilicus or navel. Other symptoms are nausea, vomiting, loss of appetite, coated tongue, restlessness, fever and an anxious expression. Should pus be forming in or about the appendix, chills are likely to take place.

TREATMENT.

Before inflammation has developed, the sulphate of magnesia may be given in teaspoonful doses and repeated every hour or two. This remedy liquefies the contents of the bowels, relieves congestion and is not likely to be vomited or do harm. Warm water injections may be gently thrown into the rectum and colon by means of a syringe in the early stages of the affection.

More cases are relieved and cured by surgical interference than by any other method, and a disease of such grave import should have the benefit of early and skillful attendance.

Inflammation in the neighboring tissues of the appendix has been called typhlitis and perityphlitis. These terms are used much less than formerly, since appendicitis has come to be more fully recognized.

Hemorrhage of the bowels is a common occurrence in ulceration, dysentery and other acute affections, and is sufficiently noticed in connection with the acute diseases, which see.

XI.—HERNIA, BREECH OR RUPTURE.

Hernia is a protrusion of a loup of intestine or other tissue through the internal coverings of the abdominal wall. It is not commonly a rupture of these tissues, but the hernia follows some one of the natural openings which exist in the inguinal or femoral regions or at the umbilicus.

Inguinal hernia is the most frequent variety, it being eight times as common as femoral, and femoral being twice as frequent as umbilical. Other forms of hernia are too rare to receive attention except in an exhaustive treatise.

SYMPTOMS.

The symptoms of hernia are a peculiar fullness as of a bunch or tumor whose size is increased by standing or by the act of coughing. There may be considerable pain, nausea, vomiting and a feeling of weakness or prostration.

A hernia is reducible when it goes back of itself or with the assistance of manipulation. When it cannot be put back it is irreducible. When the circulation becomes much obstructed in a hernia it is known as strangulated.

TREATMENT.

The horizontal position should be assumed with the limbs drawn up and the head placed lower than the feet or body. This position is favorable to the reduction of the hernia, or it may go back itself without assistance. Chloroform or ether carefully inhaled at the hands of a competent medical attendant favors reduction. The same may be observed with respect to the hypodermic use of morphia.

For the treatment of congenital hernia, use a suitably adjusted truss which rarely fails to cure.

The manipulation used to replace a hernia is called taxis. It should not be continued too long, neither should too much force be employed. Taxis is an attempt to push the hernia back with the fingers, little by little, through the opening. A knowledge of the direction by which the hernia has advanced is very helpful and almost essential to its employment. In the hands of a competent surgeon taxis is much favored by the application of cold or a piece of cotton saturated with ether.

A strangulated hernia should receive attention without delay, as the condition is critical and constantly becomes more so. A hernia which cannot be reduced by simple means demands immediate and skillful attention, an operation being frequently required for its reduction.

XII.—PERITONITIS.

Acute peritonitis is an inflammatory disease of a serious character. It may be local and confined to a single part or general, extending throughout the abdominal cavity and the organs which are covered by the peritoneum.

CAUSES.

These are a cold or injuries sufficient to excite an inflammatory process. Peritonitis follows perforation of the stomach, perforation of the bowels, rupture of the liver, the rupture of an abscess or hemorrhage into the abdominal cavity. It is often the result of the extension of some inflammatory process, beginning in one of the pelvic organs. It may follow abortion or childbirth. It results sometimes from gonorrhœa in the female.

SYMPTOMS.

Sometimes it is ushered in by a chill followed by high fever and rapid pulse. If from perforation of the bowels, the onset is sudden and presents the symptoms of nervous shock, with faintness, clammy skin, perspiration and collapse.

The most prominent symptom is usually pain with great tenderness and distension of the abdomen. The pain is so peculiar and cutting that the patient is unable to bear the weight of the bedclothing or of the hand or finger. The patient lies upon the back and avoids moving, with the lower limbs drawn up to relieve the tension of the abdominal muscles. The breathing to avoid motion of the diaphragm, is short, shallow and rapid, also the countenance is anxious. The pulse is quick, reaching a hundred and forty or more. Nausea and vomiting may occur, and there may be diarrhoea or constipation.

Hiccough is often annoying, especially toward the close of the attack, and it is associated with other symptoms of prostration. When peritonitis is due to perforation of the bowels the mortality is great.

TREATMENT.

The responsibility of treating a case of peritonitis is so great and the issues are so uncertain that in every instance a trusted physician should be employed.

There has been much progress made in the treatment of this disease, for in former times nearly every case proved fatal. It was due to the efforts of Dr. Alonzo Clark that the disease became manageable and in a large per cent. of cases curable. The one remedy upon which he relied was opium in sufficient quantity to entirely relieve the pain. The preferable method of administration is morphia with atropia hypodermically in energetic doses. The amount required to allay pain is often astonishing.

A turpentine stupe over the abdomen or hot fomentations are often helpful. Carbonate of ammonia or other stimulants may be required. A mild injection may be administered to unload the bowels if necessary, but active cathartics ought not to be given. In recent practice Epsom salts in small and frequent doses is sometimes administered to liquefy the contents of the bowels and such practice has proved successful.

XIII.—COLIC.

This is a pain of the bowels without inflammation, and is caused by over-distension of the intestines with gas, indigestible substances as unripe fruits, and neuralgia of the bowels. It is sometimes due to malaria, to hot weather, impure water, or it may result from lead-poisoning. The pain occurs in paroxysms of a twisting, griping character.

SYMPTOMS.

These are pain in the center of the abdomen, more liable to occur at night. It differs somewhat from the pain in neuralgia of the stomach. It is abdominal. The pain may be very severe but there is little or no soreness or tenderness upon pressure. The attack may be brief or last several hours. A free evacuation of the bowels or discharge of gas may bring sudden relief. Infants often suffer much from this affection, as when they cry, draw up their limbs and show signs of intense distress. The pain from colic resembles that of gall stones, ulcer of the stomach, strangulation of the bowels and renal colic, but is easily distinguished from these by the observing nurse or practitioner.

TREATMENT.

Lead colic demands an evacuation of the bowels, as obstinate constipation has existed in these cases. The sulphate of magnesia is a safe physic to use in these cases. It is cooling in its nature and does not excite inflammation. When caused by distension of the bowels with indigestible substances, an emetic may be of service. Warm rectal injections help to unload the colon and rectum and can do no harm if carefully administered. Hot applications may be applied over the abdomen and hot herb tea administered, as catnip, spearmint, composition or Jamaica ginger. After unloading the bowels, a dose of paregoric may be administered.

Infants may be relieved of wind colic by a few drops of the essence of anise or an infusion of anise seed. When the pain is persistent and does not yield to warm external applications and hot internal remedies, the possibility of confounding colic with some more serious affection should be considered and timely assistance sought.

XIV.—CONSTIPATION.

Constipation is that condition in which the contents of the bowels are retained longer than is beneficial or proper, and when expelled the act is accomplished with difficulty, the fæcal matter having become dry, hard and scanty. It is conducive to health to have one full natural movement daily, and yet considerable departure from this rule often occurs without inconvenience or injury to health.

Nursing children, especially those artificially fed, are often troubled with constipation. Old people are liable to suffer from this common trouble, for their habits are less active, the bowels become torpid and there is much inaction of the whole system. The same is true of all persons whose habits are deficient in activities. Women are more liable to suffer from it than men owing to their habits of indoor life, insufficient exercise and other natural causes. Habit and occupation have their influence in causing this condition. Those who lead active and outdoor lives rarely suffer from it, while the sedentary rarely escape.

Constipation complicates certain diseases, especially those of the brain, also measles, small-pox and fevers, except typhoid. Persons suffering from dyspepsia, as a class, are troubled with constipation.

The taking of pills and harsh cathartics are prominent causes. Tea drinking, opium taking and lead absorbed into the system cause obstinate constipation. Certain articles of food are liable to cause this condition, as milk, cheese, crackers, wheat bread and many others.

SYMPTOMS.

These are generally well-known. Some of the more important are a sallow countenance, irritable disposition, headache, coated tongue, disagreeable or bitter taste in the mouth, distended abdomen, unrefreshing sleep, bad dreams and nervous disturbances as perhaps hysteria.

TREATMENT.

The treatment depends largely upon the age and occupation of the patient. Nursing infants may be relieved by regulating the diet and adapting the food to the especial condition of the little ones. These patients are benefited, when there is marked inaction of the rectal portion of the intestine, by warm water injections containing a little glycerine, or instead, a glycerine suppository may be used each morning until a regular habit is established.

Persons engaged in sedentary pursuits should give attention to exercise, as walking, riding, bathing and daily gymnastic practices. Such persons ought to form the habit of giving attention each day punctually to this important matter.

In most cases fruits are valuable, as an orange each morning before breakfast, grapes, peaches, figs, raisins, stewed prunes, apples, bananas and others in their season, including canned fruits at those seasons of the year when others cannot be obtained.

Fresh vegetables are of great service, as spinach, dandelions, lettuce, asparagus, peas, tomatoes, etc.

Fresh meats are preferable to those which have been salted or cured.

Graham bread, bread made from the entire wheat, rye bread, brown bread, cracked wheat, oatmeal, hominy well cooked, and corn bread, are all healthful and beneficial in relieving constipation.

Some persons are benefited by drinking a cup of cold water each morning on arising, or a cup of water to which a small teaspoonful of common salt has been added.

If, in addition to these simple and natural remedies, a laxative is occasionally required; the granular effervescent citrate of magnesia is recommended. In cases where more energetic remedies are demanded podophyllin, combined with nux vomica, will prove almost a certain cure for obstinate cases of chronic constipation.

These remedies may be rendered still more efficient by combination with cascara-sagrada and belladonna. The following formula may be used and will prove a positive cure for the most chronic cases:

R	Podophyllin	one grain
	Ext. nux vomica	three grains
	Ext. belladonna	four grains
	Ext. cascara-sagrada	twenty grains
	Oil peppermint	two grains

Mix and make twenty pills.

Dose one, two or three times a day, gradually leaving off the medicine as the natural habit becomes regularly established. This treatment may be continued, if necessary, for several weeks, or long enough to effect a cure.

Those cases complicated with dyspepsia are benefited by taking a two or three grain pepsin powder with each meal. Debilitated cases will need in addition to the foregoing remedies tonic doses of salicin or calisaya bark.

XV.—WORMS.

We understand by worms a variety of parasites which are found occasionally in the intestinal canal of the human body. These unwelcome guests occasion more or less inconvenience which is manifested in many ways.

Formerly they were regarded as of much more importance than at present. In fact, there are but few diseases and symptoms which have not been attributed to worms.

SYMPTOMS.

These are of two kinds, known as local and systemic. The former may be enumerated as uneven and fitful appetite, disordered digestion and abdominal pains; the latter are cough, chorea, convulsions and other nervous disturbances which may be either so slight as to escape notice or so grave as to occasion alarm. The most certain symptom, however, is the discovery of worms in the stools.

When these parasites exist in large numbers, they are undesirable mischief makers and their speedy expulsion is necessary.

The three most common varieties are the tape worm, the thread or seat worm and the round or stomach worm. There are several kinds of tape worm, but in this connection it is unnecessary to multiply descriptive details.

Tape Worm.—The mature tape worm is a long, flat white worm, deriving its name from a fancied resemblance to a piece of tape. The head is small, the neck slender and it gradually widens out toward the body. The tape worm fastens itself to the mucous lining of the intestines with a firm hold hanging on by means of hooklets. It maintains its position with such tenacity that its removal is difficult.

It is of interest to observe that the tape worm has no mouth, stomach or alimentary canal, but maintains its own life by absorbing the fluids with which it is surrounded.

As the lower segments mature and the eggs become thoroughly developed, they separate and are discharged with the stools. One of these segments or rings contains from thirty to forty thousand eggs, and since only one individual worm as a rule inhabits the human intestine, the query is of unusual interest, how does this parasite gain access to the human body in the first place?

ORIGIN.

A singular fact concerning this parasite is that it requires an abode in the bodies of two different animals in order to complete its development. Another singular fact is that this parasite reaches its habitat by means of the food supply. It has been explained how the lower segments containing a numerous supply of developed eggs are discharged with the fæcal matter. If the ripe eggs contained in one of these segments are in any way able to reach the stomach of the pig or ox they hatch out into larvæ and migrate into the muscles, where they exist one or two years enclosed in a small cyst. These encysted larvæ are so small as to escape detection in the flesh of beef. In pork they are slightly larger and can be detected by the naked eye.

We now see how easy it is, since these eggs retain vitality for an indefinite period, for them to be taken in with the food of animals, while feeding in the pastures and ranches far away from human habitations but under constant human oversight.

When the flesh of beef or pork containing one of these embryos or encysted larvæ is eaten without being sufficiently cooked, it is introduced into the human alimentary canal where the second or real development of the tape worm takes place.

The common source of tape worm is from beef, for although the larvæ are more numerous in pork, owing to the unclean habits of the pig, pork is seldom eaten rare or slightly cooked like beef, and thorough cooking destroys their vitality.

A full grown tape worm reaches its full second development after entering its human abode in the short space of three months, and in this brief time may reach a length of thirty feet.

A certain diagnosis of tape worm is easily made because the rings or terminal segments are discharged with the stools.

TREATMENT.

Preventive treatment consists in avoiding raw or very rare meat. Pork especially should always be adequately cooked before it is eaten. In order to commence medical treatment for the removal of a tape worm, a day or two of fasting and a mild cathartic to clear out the mucous and unload the bowels is essential. The preparatory cathartic should be taken at night and the expelling medicine given the next morning. It takes from three to four hours to remove the parasite after the expelling medicine has been taken. The prescription which will accomplish this result without danger and with absolute certainty is given and caution is emphasized to prevent an improper use of it.

℞	Ext. of male fern ethereal	three drams
	Chloroform pure	one dram
	Emulsion of castor oil	two ounces
	Croton oil	two drops
	Syr. of spearmint	one ounce

Mix. The preliminary directions having been followed, shake the bottle thoroughly and take one half of the above prescription on an empty stomach, and half an hour afterwards take the remainder. The patient should lie quietly on a lounge while under the influence of the medicine, as it makes one slightly drowsy, but no ill effects follow its use, and when the medicine acts the entire tape worm will be found in the stool.

Thread Worms.—These minute, but active parasites prevail the world over. They are sometimes called pin or seat worms. They are especially troublesome to children. They are remarkably prolific, a single female producing successively ten or twelve thousand eggs, which are deposited in the folds of the rectum, where they speedily develop. These worms inhabit both the small and large intestines.

SYMPTOMS.

Of the few unpleasant symptoms the most prominent is itching about the rectal orifice, which is always annoying. They cause children much restlessness at night, and sometimes convulsions or chorea.

TREATMENT.

A dose of Epsom salts and senna will remove them in large numbers. A dose of castor oil containing from three to five or ten drops of turpentine will also expel them. The following is an efficient and excellent prescription:

R	Santonine	twenty-four grains
	Podophyllin	six grains
	The mild chloride of mercury	twelve grains
	Pulv. sugar	forty-eight grains

Titurate these together thoroughly and divide into twenty-four powders, give one each night and morning for two or three days.

After the worms are expelled inject a mild decoction of aloes. Open and wash all the folds about the rectum with this bitter fluid, then apply a carbolized salve. This treatment persisted in faithfully a few times will destroy them utterly.

Round Worms.—These are also called stomach or lumbricoid worms. They are a common and well known parasite. They are supposed to reach the alimentary canal from unfiltered drinking water. Poverty and filth are conditions which favor their development, although they are found in all ranks of society. They are remarkably prolific, one female being adequate for the production of several million eggs, and these eggs retain their vitality for years.

SYMPTOMS.

These are foul breath, disordered appetite, flatulence, furred tongue, abdominal pains, dyspepsia, emaciation, grating of the teeth at night, picking the nose, pallor about the mouth and nose, bad dreams, muscular convulsions and fits. No one person is likely to present all these systoms, perhaps only one but more frequently several of them.

TREATMENT.

The fluid extract of pink root and senna is an old time remedy The dose is from one-half to two teaspoonfuls according to age. This is an efficient remedy but from its liability to produce temporary nervous symptoms it is not used as much as formerly.

The best because most satisfactory remedy and the one sanctioned everywhere by modern usage is santonine. It is given with sugar. The dose is two or three grains. Its efficiency is increased by combining with it the same amount of calomel. Should the latter remedy be considered objectionable, podophyllin in doses of from one-sixth to one-quarter of a grain can be combined with it with equal efficiency, although it is not as pleasant to take. The following prescription is admirable.

℞	Santonine	twenty grains
	Calomel	twenty grains
	Podophyllin	four grains
	Pulv. sugar	forty grains

Mix and make twenty powders. Give one each night and morning for two or three days at a time as occasion requires.

CHAPTER XXIII.

THE KIDNEYS AND THEIR DISEASES

I.—Description of the Kidneys. II.—The Secretion of the Kidneys. III.—Diseases of the Kidneys. 1. Gravel. 2. Renal Colic. 3. Pyelitis. 4. Abscess. 5. Cancer. 6. Hydatid Disease. IV.—Bright's Disease. V.—Diabetes. VI. How to Preserve the Health of the Kidneys. VII.—The Supra Renal Capsules.

I.—DESCRIPTION OF THE KIDNEYS.

THE kidneys are two small, but important, glandular organs, situated one on each side of the spine in the lumbar region. The right kidney is placed a little lower than the left to accommodate the liver, which occupies a large amount of space upon the right side.

The outer portion of the kidneys is known as the cortical substance. It is of a dark, red color, soft and easily torn. The inner portion is called the medullary substance. It is of a more dense structure than the outer portion and differs from it considerably in appearance.

The kidneys contain many little tubes which converge into pyramids, and the cones of these pyramids contain many hundreds of openings, minute outlets which empty into what is known as the pelvis of the kidney.

The pelvis is simply the upper and dilated portion of the ureter, a tube more than twelve inches long in the adult, and about the size of a goose quill. There are two ureters, one of which extends from each kidney and opens into the base of the bladder for the purpose of conveying the secretions of the kidneys into a common reservoir.

We will content ourselves with this brief description of the kidneys, since their anatomy is not of sufficient interest to be minutely detailed. The subject is complex and difficult to describe, and in fact but little was known of these organs till the power of the microscope rendered a study of their structure intelligible. There is no portion of the human body whose anatomical description is more technical and uninteresting to the general reader

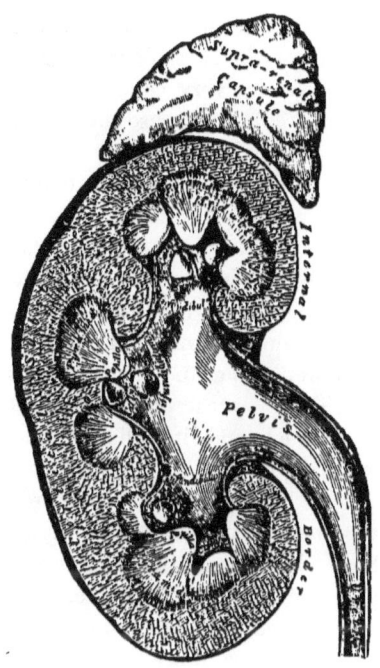

Vertical Section of Kidney.

The function of the kidneys, however, is very important. They are liberally supplied with blood from which they secrete a large amount of both solids and fluids, waste products which are held in solution until they can be eliminated from the system. If for any reason the work of the kidneys is impaired so that they fail to eliminate these poisonous products, serious or fatal consequences soon result. The health of these organs is of the utmost consequence to the well being of every one. The kidneys are subject to inflammations, degeneration and a variety of important diseases.

II.—THE SECRETIONS OF THE KIDNEYS.

The kidneys secrete from the blood an amber colored fluid of a peculiar odor. The color of the urine is derived from the coloring materials of the blood.

The amount secreted depends upon several things, as the amount of fluid taken into the system the nature of the food consumed and the temperature. In hot weather much moisture passes out of the body through the pores of the skin, decreasing the amount of urine secreted by the kidneys to a very considerable extent. Vegetable foods and fruits of many kinds increase the amount of urine, as does also the free use of water and liquids.

The specific gravity of the urine depends upon the amount of solids it contains and normal urine varies between 1015 and 1025.

In health the urine is acid in reaction and turns blue litmus paper red. After eating and during the process of digestion it may be slightly alkaline for a short time or turn red litmus paper blue. The urine contains in solution a number of solid products, as urea, urates, salts of sodium, potassium, lime and magnesium, the most abundant of which is urea. This is a waste product which results from the activities of the individual, and its elimination is as much a natural process as the taking of food. If for any reason the elimination of this waste product is hindered, the whole system is soon disturbed, and a complete stopping of the elimination of urea produces death in three or four days. In sickness the urine is often highly colored, showing that changes are rapidly taking place in the system. When the urine contains bile in considerable amount, it is of a dark brown color. The urine contains a large quantity of urates in many diseases which render it turbid on cooling.

It is to be remembered that certain medicines and food products affect perceptibly the color of the urine, and that upon standing, all urine deposits a sediment.

Such abnormal products as albumen and sugar in the urine are characteristic symptoms in certain diseases. From these facts and others of like import it is easy to understand that an analysis of the urine is frequently of the utmost importance in the diagnosis of disease.

Those deposits which are harmless and indicate no suspicion of organic disease are likely to excite great alarm, while those that indicate serious or incurable disease can only be discovered by the careful application of tests.

Albumen in the urine is easily discovered by means of boiling a small quantity of the suspected fluid in a test tube and then adding a drop or two of nitric acid. The acid dissolves any normal product as the phosphates, which the urine may contain but does not dissolve albumen.

Several chemical tests may be used for the detection of sugar. A very convenient and delicate one is made by boiling a small quantity of Fehling's test fluid in a glass tube, after which add a small quantity of the suspected urine and repeat the boiling. If the added urine contains sugar, the test fluid changes to an orange color and becomes turbid, otherwise it retains its natural color which is blue.

III.—DISEASES OF THE KIDNEYS.

Gravel.—There are a few diseases of the kidneys of sufficient importance to receive special notice. Among these may be mentioned gravel or calculi, which form in the pelvis of the kidney. Gravel exists in the form of sand or little stones formed from the crystallizable substances as uric acid, or oxalate of lime which is ordinarily held in solution in the urine. If these concretions are small, they are called gravel, but if large they are known as calculi. When a gravel forms in the pelvis of the kidney, one of two things may happen, it may pass down the ureter into the bladder, or it may remain in the pelvis of the kidney constantly increasing in size in which place sooner or later, it will excite inflammatory action.

Renal Colic.—When a gravel or a calculus passes from the pelvis of the kidney to the bladder, it occasions sudden and terrific pain of a cutting type. This pain is attended by a frequent and urgent desire to pass water which is voided in small quantities and usually contains some blood. In severe attacks there is nausea, vomiting, excruciating pain and coldness of the surface.

After the gravel or calculus has passed into the bladder, the patient experiences a glad sense of relief. An attack of renal colic may last a few hours or for several days.

If the calculus passes out of the bladder with the urine, it will occasion no further trouble, but should it remain it will become the nucleus of a stone in the bladder and occasion decided trouble later.

Treatment.—A warm bath may be employed and hot application over the seat of the pain, hot drinks may be taken and as suitable dose of some anodyne as morphine, administered. It may be necessary to give one-fourth of a grain to afford relief and to repeat such a dose in a short time, for renal colic does not yield to ordinary measures. The ease afforded by the morphine and the relaxation it causes favor the passage of the calculus into the bladder.

Pyelitis.—Inflammation of the pelvis of the kidney is known as pyelitis. When a calculus is too large to pass out of the pelvis of the kidney it is retained and is liable at any time to set up an inflammation, resulting in the formation of pus. The symptoms of this affection are difficult to detect. There may be pain in the loins, chills and fever, emaciation and exhaustion, accompanied by a frequent desire to pass water.

Abscess.—The formation of an abscess in the pelvis of the kidney is a rare and obscure affection. If it bursts and the pus passes into the bladder with the urine the result is favorable, but should the pus pass into the abdominal cavity it would most likely excite peritonitis, followed by death.

Sometimes, though rarely, a whole kidney becomes obliterated, having been converted into a mass of pus. Treatment for such an affection taxes the patience and skill of the surgeon. It is prolonged and must be adapted to the individual case.

Cancer.—Cancer of the kidney is a rare affection, but sometimes results from cancerous disease extending from some other organ or part of the body. The symptoms are obscure and often unrecognized. In general they are bloody urine, pain, emaciation, exhaustion and the development of a tumor in the lumbar region. The cure of such an affection is out of the question, and the best that can be done is to relieve the pain and make the patient comfortable.

Hydatid Disease.—Hydatid disease of the kidneys may occur. It is a parasitic affection, having the same origin as hydatid disease of the liver, which see.

IV.—BRIGHT'S DISEASE.

This name includes several organic diseases of the kidneys, in which albumen is found in the urine together with the epithelial casts which line the tubules. Richard Bright, a London physician, in the year 1827, was the first one to call attention to the symptoms and pathology of this disease, and hence its name.

Bright's disease may exist in either the acute or chronic form, and in either case it is an inflammation of the kidneys.

CAUSES.

The causes of this affection are acute diseases as scarlet fever, intemperance, mental anxiety, gout, lead-poisoning or taking cold. Pregnancy, in some instances, appears to favor its development.

SYMPTOMS.

The following symptoms may develop as the result of exposure, dull pain in the back, chills followed by fever, headache, pain in the limbs, nausea and vomiting, and a frequent desire to pass water.

Other less acute symptoms are the presence of albumen in the urine and the existence of dropsy. The face about the eyes is puffy and the limbs are swollen.

The dropsy may subside and the patient recover. This is quite likely to be the case when the disease follows scarlet fever. In other cases the severity of the symptoms may increase, dropsy becoming general and the termination of the case may be attended by a train of hopeless symptoms as convulsions, coma and death.

This disease may pass into a chronic state and continue for one, two or three years or any indefinite period. Recovery is said to have taken place even in the chronic stages, but more frequently the symptoms become severer until death ensues.

The detection of albumen in the urine constantly and the presence of tube casts are the two features which unite and confirm the diagnosis. The amount of albumen contained in the urine is in proportion to the extent and severity of the inflammation. The existence of albumen is easily detected. (See the secretions of the kidneys.) The existence of tube casts requires some experience and a good microscope. Tube casts are the lining of the uriniferous tubules and are composed of epithelial cells, and when they are found in the urine, they indicate that important and destructive changes are going on in the kidneys.

Dropsy is the escape of the watery portions of the blood into the various tissues of the body. It is often a troublesome symptom in Bright's disease. When the kidneys fail to eliminate the urea properly from the blood, uræmic symptoms develop such as a peculiar sweetish or sickish odor about the patient, headache, defects of sight and hearing, muscular convulsions, drowsiness and finally profound stupor from which the patient does not rally.

TREATMENT.

Since Bright's disease is a name which is applied indiscriminately to several forms of kidney disease, the difficulty in the way of domestic practice can be easily anticipated.

In addition to the acute and chronic inflammations are the changes which the kidneys themselves undergo during the progress of this disease. There is first the large white or waxy kidney, and later the granular or contracted kidney, also the fatty and amyloid degenerations which occur and are known under the general name of Bright's disease.

No uniform method of treatment can be recommended for a disease which presents so many different stages. There is no disease which requires more careful study to ascertain the condition of the patient, and no disease in which it is more important that the remedies selected should be skillfully chosen or employed. In a general way it may be said of all cases that hygienic measures are of importance Exposure to cold and other climatic changes should be avoided by wearing flannel next to the skin. Alcohol should be regarded as an injurious stimulant to the kidneys and avoided. In nearly all these cases milk, skim milk or butter milk, are excellent articles of diet. When the stomach is irritable milk may be combined with lime water. Meats should be used with caution, and if necessary, entirely excluded.

The activity of the skin should be encouraged, sweating is often beneficial and relieves the kidneys of considerable burden.

When uræmic symptoms appear much relief is often afforded by the free evacuation of the bowels. Cream of tartar water is excellent in these cases. It may be used freely and sometimes combined with digitalis to advantage. The prescription of digitalis and caffein, as found on another page, is excellent to remove dropsical effusions.

Complications of this disease are numerous and require appropriate treatment.

In every case it is better to regulate the diet and trust to nature rather than to adopt harsh remedies or excessive medication.

V.—DIABETES.

Diabetes is the name given to a set of symptoms associated with the derangement of various functions especially of the liver and kidneys and on account of which a large amount of sugar is passed into the blood and secreted by the kidneys.

Three things may be said to characterize this disease; they are a large increase in the amount of urine, the constant presence of sugar in it and a decided wasting of the bodily tissues.

CAUSES.

While the causes of this disease have not been satisfactorily determined, a hereditary tendency has been observed and has recently been coming more and more into prominence. Much attention has been given by way of study and research to the causes of diabetes, but they are still somewhat obscure.

These facts are established, namely, that males are more subject to it than females; that it is more prevalent between the ages of thirty and forty. Lean and fleshy persons alike are its subjects. Fleshy persons who indulge freely in the luxuries of the table, who live a sedentary life and are troubled with indigestion, are believed to be more liable to this disease than others who are abstemious, live an active life and have a good digestion. Lean persons who are the victims of business troubles, who are given to anxiety and mental worry sufficient to disturb the cerebral functions, are classed among those liable to the development of diabetes.

Among exciting causes may be mentioned nervous shock, mental distress or anxiety and profound emotion. Excesses of various kinds have been regarded as the starting point of this disease, as intemperance, high living and sexual indulgence. Some cases have been accounted for by injuries of the brain and nerve centers. It is also thought that some cases are caused by fevers, malaria, gout, rheumatism and exposure to cold.

SYMPTOMS.

It is probable that this disease may exist for some time without being recognized. The first thing noticed is usually the passing of a large amount of urine at frequent intervals, thirst and a peculiar dryness of the mouth and skin. Other symptoms which develop later are loss of weight, muscular weakness and diminution of sexual desire. There may be indigestion, vertigo, headache, double vision, wakefulness, neuralgia or an exhausting cough. Later symptoms are a flagging and irregular heart, peculiar fruity odor of the breath, and in extreme conditions coma. The thirst is excessive, there may be functional derangements of hearing or vision, and also impaired taste.

Boils and affections of the skin may occur. The amount of sugar contained in the urine varies greatly. Diabetic patients are sometimes the victims of consumption or jaundice.

TREATMENT.

The most important part of the treatment for diabetic patients has reference to the diet. From it must be eliminated all those articles which contain sugar and starch. The functions of the liver are so deranged that what are known as the carbo-hydrates cannot be handled, hence they increase the trouble and work mischief.

The most successful method of eliminating these objectionable articles of food is by an exclusive diet of milk. Skim milk is preferable. Its use often causes the disappearance of sugar from the urine and great amelioration of the condition. A tumbler full or more every two hours is necessary to maintain the bodily waste. Peptonized milk is excellent and the directions for preparing it are given elsewhere.

Other articles of food are admissible when the patient for any reason cannot subsist on milk exclusively, as beef, mutton, tripe, tongue, poultry, game, fish, lobsters, clams, oysters and soups, without rice or flour. The following vegetables are admissible: Cabbage, cauliflower, string beans, asparagus, spinach, dandelion, lettuce, radishes, onions, cucumbers and others of similar character. Among the fruits suitable to use are cranberries, plums, cherries, strawberries and apples, but without the addition of sugar. Saccharin may be used with entire satisfaction to take the place of sugar.

Bread made of gluten flour may be used, and from the above list a very agreeable and palatable bill of fare can be arranged.

Favorable hygienic surroundings and correct habits of living are essential. The functions of the skin and liver should be kept active. Mineral waters have been highly praised for this affection. Especially worthy of notice are Vichy and Carlsbad. The prepared effervescent salts may be used instead.

Codeia has obtained considerable repute for diminishing the amount of sugar, beginning with a fourth of a grain three times a day and gradually increasing the dose until characteristic effects are produced. Other remedies made use of in the treatment of this disease are ergot, iron, arsenic, strychnia, bromide of potash, the phosphates and the chloride of gold and soda. Claims have been made from time to time for many other remedies, but most of them have proved disappointing.

The best possible results are obtained by a carefully restricted diet, healthful surroundings and such medicines as are indicated by the symptoms and the idiosyncrasies of the patient. This disease is too formidable for domestic treatment, except from the hygienic and dietary standpoint.

VI.—THE SUPRA-RENAL CAPSULES.

Above and in front of the upper portion of each kidney is a small irregular shaped gland, known as the supra-renal capsule. These glands are not very liable to disease. Their function is unknown and their consideration is of minor importance.

The disease with which they appear to be most frequently associated is known as Addison's. This is characterized by excessive prostration, weakness of the heart and a peculiar bronze discoloration of the skin. The cause of this disease is unknown, but when it exists, it is found that the supra-renal capsules are in a condition of degeneration. It is not a common affection. No cure follows the administration of medicines and their use can only relieve the urgency of the symptoms.

Rest, pure air, a milk diet and tonics to prevent poverty of the blood are all of service in its treatment. The danger of exhaustion should be borne in mind and excessive mental or bodily exertion should be avoided.

VII.—HOW TO PRESERVE THE HEALTH OF THE KIDNEYS.

The health of the kidneys is best maintained by giving suitable attention to the diet. An excessive use of meat or nitrogenous food adds to their labor and may hasten a breaking down of their tissues when a tendency to disease exists.

Sudden changes of temperature often affect the kidneys unfavorably by checking the activity of the skin and increasing the eliminative work of these organs. Ice water, when over-heated, or other means of rapidly cooling off, getting drenched with rain and similar exposures may be the means of arousing to activity the slumbering tendencies to Bright's disease.

Exercise and life out of doors in an even climate and the practice of good habits, the use of pure water, the avoidance of alcoholic drinks are preventive measures worthy of earnest consideration by those who have reason to suspect any weakness or inherent tendency to disease in these important organs.

CHAPTER XXIV.

THE BLADDER AND THE URINARY APPENDAGES.

I.—Description of the Bladder and Neighboring Tissues. 1. The Ureters. 2. The Urethra. 3. The Prostate Gland. 4. Cowper's Gland. II.—Acute and Chronic Cystitis, or Catarrhal Inflammation of the Bladder. III.—Retention of Urine. IV.—Suppression of Urine. V.—Enuresis, or Incontinence of Urine. VI.—Stone in the Bladder, or Vesical Calculus. VII.—Enlarged Prostate. VIII.—Other Obscure Affections.

1.—DESCRIPTION OF THE BLADDER.

THE bladder is a membranous cone shaped sac or reservoir for the purpose of holding the urine until it is convenient to void it. It is situated in the front part of the pelvic basin, and when distended, ascends well up into the abdominal cavity. It is held in position by several ligamentous bands. Its average capacity is about one pint. It is made up of three layers or membranes, a serous, muscular and mucous. The muscular coat has two layers of tissue, the outer composed of longitudinal and the inner of circular unstriped muscular fibers. The mucous layer is a smooth surface covered by epithelium and forms the interior lining of the bladder. It is of especial interest on account of the several important diseases to which it is liable. It is supplied with vessels and nerves which are branches of those which supply the other parts of the pelvis.

The Ureters.—The ureters are canals leading from the kidneys and terminating in the lower portion of the bladder by means of small openings. Through these canals, about eighteen inches long, and the size of a goose quill, the urine passes from the kidneys where it is secreted, to the bladder.

The openings of the ureters are situated one on each side of the base of the bladder, about two inches apart and about an inch and a half from its neck.

The Urethra.—The canal which conveys the urine out of the bladder is larger than the caliber of the two ureters combined. It is sometimes the seat of annoying disease.

On the under side of the bladder in the male are small, irregularly shaped reservoirs, the vesiculæ seminales. These contain the seminal fluid and open by a duct into the urethra.

The Prostate Gland.—Just in front of the neck of the bladder, the male urethra is surrounded by a glandular body an inch or more in length, weighing nearly an ounce, and known as the prostate gland. It is about the shape and size of a horse chestnut. It secretes a milky fluid, which mingles with and dilutes the seminal fluid. When the condition of this gland is abnormal it occasions considerable annoyance.

A small amount of prostatic fluid appearing at the close of urination is often erroneously regarded as a symptom of some disease of the sexual organs. This is, however, of slight significance, having no connection with the seminal fluid, and should occasion no concern.

Cowper's Glands.—A short distance in front of the prostate gland are two other small glands about the size of a pea which open by means of ducts an inch and a half long into the urethra and known as Cowper's Glands. They secrete a thin fluid resembling mucous. The function of these glands has not been positively determined, and since they are not often subject to important diseases, their further consideration is considered unnecessary.

II.—ACUTE AND CHRONIC CYSTITIS OR CATARRHAL INFLAMMATION OF THE BLADDER.

Cystitis is the most frequent of all the diseases of the bladder. It may be acute or chronic. An acute attack usually precedes the chronic form of the disease. Mild forms of the disease may exist which are little more than an irritation and yield readily to treatment. In all cases the secretion of mucous is more or less augmented.

CAUSES.

It may result from a variety of causes, as stone in the bladder, an extension of gonorrhœal inflammation or stricture of the urethra. It may appear in dyspeptic subjects as the result of indigestion which causes the urine to be excessively acid. It may be caused by the excessive use of irritating drugs as the result of taking all sorts of patent medicines. The decomposition of retained urine is a frequent cause of cystitis in old people who are unable to completely empty the bladder. One or several of the foregoing causes may exist at the same time.

SYMPTOMS.

The symptoms are characteristic. There may be chills followed by fever, a frequent desire to void the urine and smarting or burning of the urinary organs. The act of urinating may be painful, attended by straining and afford no relief.

The symptoms become more intense in proportion to the extension of the inflammation. The urine presents an altered condition, containing a large amount of mucous and sometimes pus and blood. If the bladder is not thoroughly emptied, the retained urine becomes fœtid and ammoniacal, augmenting the difficulty.

TREATMENT.

In order to treat this disease successfully it is necessary, if possible, to ascertain its cause. When cystitis is caused by calculus or other foreign body in the bladder its removal should be accomplished. When caused by the drug-taking habit this foolish practice must be abandoned. If due to the retention of urine a catheter may be passed and the bladder completely emptied. This may afford relief. In an acute attack rest in bed is favorable to recovery. Alkaline drinks, as the effervescing bicarbonate of potash in teaspoonful doses, dissolved in water, afford a measure of relief. Flaxseed tea and milk may be freely used and are both soothing and nutritious. The following may be used with good results:

℞	Acetate of potash	one ounce
	Fl. ext. buchu	half an ounce
	Sweet spirits of nitre	one ounce
	Wintergreen water q. s. to make	four ounces.

Mix. Dose a dessert spoonful or more every four hours in a wine glass of water.

When there is much pain the following will be found efficient:

℞	Pulv. opium	six grains
	Cocaine	four grains
	Ext. hyoscyamus	six grains
	Cacao butter q. s. to make	twelve suppositories

Insert one into the rectum and repeat every four hours until the pain is controlled.

When acute cystitis has passed into the chronic form, it is often obstinate and hard to cure. Good results are obtained in such cases from washing out the bladder daily with a fountain syringe and the following:

℞	Pulv. borax	two drams
	Cocaine	four grains
	Hot water	one or two pints

A quart of water containing a little table salt is also excellent.

Stronger solutions containing more efficient remedies may be used by the physician.

Salol in doses of from two to five grains may be taken internally to prevent the decomposition of the urine. When much pain exists, phenacetine may be combined with it. Tablets containing two and a half grains of each remedy may be obtained and one taken an hour after each meal. The prescription of suppositories for acute cystitis will relieve the pain of the same affection somewhat when it has reached the chronic stage. Alkaline mineral waters are beneficial in the chronic form of cystitis.

III.—RETENTION OF URINE.

Retention of the urine is not a common affection, except it is caused by a calculus in the bladder, gonorrhœa, a stricture of the urethra, paralysis of the bladder, some injury, or the use of irritating drugs. It occurs sometimes in the case of very old people. Spasmodic retention may occur in acute diseases when nervous control is diminished or lost. In spasmodic retention hot applications, a hot hip bath, or hot water bags may afford relief. If such simple means do not avail the prompt use of a suitable catheter is demanded.

For the majority of cases the soft elastic is preferable to a hard or metallic catheter. When retention of urine is due to enlarged prostate that affection should receive attention. (See enlarged prostate.)

When it is due to a calculus or tumor it needs to be removed; when due to stricture or gonorrhœa these affections require appropriate treatment. When retention is due to paralysis of the bladder strychnia is the best known remedy. It may be given in doses of one-sixtieth of a grain two or three times daily after meals, and continued for a long time. Paralysis of the bladder often results from injuries or tedious labors, and requires the use of the catheter until this important viscus recovers its tone. Serious injury or disease of the spinal cord may cause paralysis of the bladder. A condition of paralysis resulting from labor usually recovers in a brief time without medicine.

The various remedies suggested for cystitis are appropriate to use in retention of the urine. In addition to alkaline drinks, mineral waters, washing out the bladder and diuretic mixtures, it may be necessary to dilate a stricture, pass a steel sound or resort to such other means as the individual requirements suggest.

IV.—SUPPRESSION OF THE URINE.

Suppression of the urine is a much more serious trouble than its retention. It may be due to inflammatory action or disability of the kidneys so that little or no urine is secreted

The poisonous products of the system which are constantly eliminated in health in this condition are retained, and unless relief is prompt, cause stupor, coma and death.

Suppression of urine may occur in Bright's disease or after scarlet fever and is a signal of imminent danger.

It is customary in these cases to administer remedies which act promptly upon the skin as jaborandi, and upon the bowels as the sulphate of magnesia and at the same time effort is made to induce the kidneys to act. Hot fomentations may be used externally. Cream of tartar lemonade, marshmallow tea, infusion of wintergreen and sweet spirits of nitre are among the best domestic remedies.

In the uræmic condition, after scarlet fever, one-twentieth of a grain of pilocarpin may be given to a child two years old once in four hours. This remedy causes profuse sweating. It may be obtained in the form of pills or tablets.

Suppression of the urine indicates an urgent condition, and when it exists for even a brief time, a competent medical attendant should be consulted, who can call to his aid a much wider range of efficient remedies than can be advised in this work.

V.—ENURESIS OR INCONTINENCE OF URINE.

This annoying affection may be due to a variety of causes, as congenital weakness, injury and paralysis of the nerves which control the bladder, or it may result from the infirmities of old age or from the pregnant condition. Thread worms, indigestion and an acid condition of the urine may cause irritation and incontinence. With children it may be the result of neglect and the formation of a bad habit. It is chiefly an affection of children who manifest some weakness of the pelvic organs or who have suffered from the want of proper care. When the habit of wetting the bed becomes fixed with such children, it is not only troublesome but difficult to overcome.

TREATMENT.

The cause, if possible, should be determined and remedied. Waking a child regularly after two or three hours of sleep helps to overcome the wrong and establish the right habit. Hearty suppers, especially of meat, should not be allowed and only a limited amount of fluid to drink as night approaches. It is useless to attempt to remedy this annoying habit by whipping. Judicious talk and moral impressions are preferable.

The operation of circumcision is recommended as it affords relief when the prepuce is long and has been the cause of the irritation.

For the weakness of small children there is no better remedy than atropia in doses of $\frac{1}{1000}$ of a grain two or three times a day. The last dose to be given at bedtime. Its preparation is easy. Dissolve a tablet containing $\frac{1}{100}$ of a grain in ten teaspoonfuls of water. One teaspoonful of this solution is the requisite dose.

For children over or under two years of age the dose may be increased or diminished proportionately. Other remedies which have proved useful are chloral, iron, phenacetine and ergot. The following prescription is excellent and can be used without danger, while such remedies as atropia and chloral must be used, if at all, with especial care. In preparing this the iron and acid should be combined first.

> ℞ Ext. of ergot fl.   three drams
> Muriate tinc. of iron   two drams
> Dil. phos. acid   three drams
> Syr. of orange peel   one ounce
> Water   one and one-half ounce

Mix. Dose a teaspoonful three times a day.

When worms cause the difficulty they can be removed by the treatment advised. (See worms.)

Enuresis of the aged, due to paralysis, may be benefited by the administration of strychnia in doses of $\frac{1}{100}$ of a grain three times a day. This remedy can be obtained in tablet form.

VI.—STONE IN THE BLADDER, OR VESICAL CALCULUS.

The origin of stone in the bladder is usually the descent into it of gravel or a small calculus from the pelvis of the kidney. It may be retained in the bladder and become the nucleus of a larger formation. Its increase is from the solid constituents of the urine which are attracted to it and deposited upon it, causing its constant growth. A stone is composed of the same material as gravel, the most common variety is made up of uric acid, and next in point of frequency is a stone composed of the oxalate of lime, and next to the latter is a stone composed of the phosphate of lime. There are several other rare varieties. In some sections stone in the bladder is a common difficulty.

The early symptoms may be slight and are often overlooked for several years. In general, the symptoms are similar to cystitis, a frequent desire to urinate, the act being attended by pain and a tendency to strain (tenesmus). During urination a sudden arrest of the stream is often observed, caused by the stone falling forward and obstructing the outlet of the bladder. The last drop of urine may be tinged with blood. In some cases there is more or less retention and incontinence of the urine. The pain may be slight or agonizing.

The chief danger of a vesical calculus is from its liability to produce organic changes in the kidneys and thus endanger life. The most characteristic symptom of this affection is the click which is heard by the ear and the impression conveyed to the hand of the surgeon after passing a steel sound into the bladder. Striking the stone with the sound renders the diagnosis certain.

TREATMENT.

The treatment is surgical and demands the removal of the calculus. Several methods are now employed as cutting into the bladder or crushing the stone with a powerful instrument which grasps it. This crushing instrument is called a lithotrite and the operation is called lithotrity.

Whether the cutting or crushing operation is selected depends upon the size and composition of the stone as well as the age and condition of the subject. The crushing operation is safe, if the kidneys are in a healthy condition, otherwise it is dangerous and liable to result fatally after a few days.

After the removal of a vesical calculus, the regulation of the diet and other habits are essential to prevent a recurrence of the trouble. Preventive measures may be employed with good hope of avoiding a similar trouble in the future. There are no drugs or remedies which will dissolve a calculus after it has once formed. The use of such mineral waters as Vichy and Bedford Springs are beneficial. Constipation should be avoided and the various eliminative organs encouraged to perform their functions in a normal manner.

VII.—ENLARGED PROSTATE.

A consideration of the prostate gland is important from the fact that it is liable to enlarge and occasion trouble after fifty or sixty years of age. When this occurs to any considerable extent, it interferes with the discharge of the urine, so that the bladder is never completely emptied; the retained portion called the residual urine may awaken inflammation accompanied by frequent and urgent desire to pass water.

It is believed that an enlarged prostate may not only awaken cystitis, but also an inflammatory condition which will extend to the kidneys and may result in the development of Bright's disease, hence the necessity of promptly recognizing and alleviating this affection.

SYMPTOMS.

These may be so obscure as to fail of recognition but ordinarily there is a frequent desire to urinate, the patient being obliged to arise several times each night for this purpose. The stream of urine is small and considerable effort is required for its expulsion. The irritation increases, being more urgent at night than by day. There may be uneasiness and throbbing pain with an involuntary escape of urine. An increasing portion of the urine may remain unpassed in the bladder where it decomposes and becomes ammoniacal, increasing the irritation until a chronic condition of cystitis is established. Enlarged prostate is recognized by means of a rectal examination, it being hard to the touch and greatly increased in size.

TREATMENT.

The treatment calls for a thorough evacuation of the bladder by means of the catheter, and washing it out daily with warm water, warm salt water or a solution of boric acid and water. The object of washing out the bladder is to get rid of the residual urine, the mucous and pus, and to leave the bladder in a cleansed condition, which tends to prevent an extension of the inflammatory action.

When much force is used in the evacuation of the bladder its walls become thickened or contracted, and piles or hemorrhoids may result from this daily and long continued effort to void the urine.

Mineral waters are beneficial and contribute to the patient's comfort. The citrate of potash makes a pleasant diuretic drink. The granular effervescent salt is very convenient and agreeable to take.

The bicarbonate of potash is prepared in the same manner and is also an efficient diuretic and antacid.

The following affords comfort:

℞   Pulv. opium   four grains
    Ext. belladonna   three grains
    Ext. hyoscyamus   six grains
    Iodoform   one grain
    Cacao butter q. s. to make   twelve suppositories

Use one placed well up in the rectum each night or each night and morning.

For internal treatment the syrup of hydriodic acid in teaspoonful doses three times a day is an excellent remedy. It should be diluted with water, and care taken that the syrup is not changed by age.

The fluid extract of saw-palmetto is a remedy much used in recent practice. One-half teaspoonful, in a little wine three times a day, is a suitable dose. Many cases have been benefited or cured by this remedy.

VIII.—OTHER OBSCURE AFFECTIONS.

There are a number of other rare affections of the bladder or its neighboring tissues, as ulceration, fistula, paralysis, tumors, tubercular disease, cancer, etc. These diseases are too infrequent to receive extended notice, too obscure to be diagnosed without professional skill and beyond the reach of domestic practice.

Benign tumors can be removed from the bladder by operative surgery but malignant growths can only receive palliative treatment.

Rare diseases of the bladder should be treated on general principles, the same as similar diseases of other organs.

Pain in the pelvic region can usually be relieved by the introduction of a suppository into the rectum. For formula see acute and chronic cystitis.

CHAPTER XXV.

THE MALE GENITAL ORGANS AND VENEREAL DISEASES.

I.—Description of the Male Genital Organs. II.—Affections of the Male Genital Organs. 1. Phimosis. 2. Para Phimosis. 3. Congenital Malformations. 4. Warts. 5. Cancer of the Penis. 6. The Testicles. 7. Varicocele. 8. Hydrocele. 9. Hæmatocele. 10. Orchitis. 11. Other Minor Affections. III.—Chancre and Chancroid, or Venereal Diseases. IV.—Acquired Syphilis. V.—Hereditary Syphilis. VI.—Gonorrhœa, Urethritis, or Clap, and its Complications. 1. Orchitis. 2. Bubo. 3. Chordee. 4. Gleet. 5. Stricture. 6. Gonorrhœal Rheumatism. 7. Purulent Ophthalmia.

I.—DESCRIPTION OF THE MALE GENITAL ORGANS.

THE male genital organs require but little anatomical description or explanation. The structure of the penis is somewhat peculiar. It is richly supplied with blood vessels and nerves. The substance of the organ contains a plexus of veins which when congested or filled with blood, much increases its size rendering it turgid, but ordinarily the organ remains in a flaccid condition. Irritated by disease as gonorrhœa, the erection of this organ may be both troublesome and painful; a condition known as chordee, which see. The penis suffers from venereal diseases, it being the usual location in the male of chancre and chancroids.

The penis being a part of the human body should not be regarded with such false modesty as to prevent it from receiving appropriate attention. It should not be permitted to suffer from untreated disease or from ignorance and neglect. Important reasons exist for the cleanliness of these parts which, if not observed, may lead to irritation, constant annoyance from itching, inflammation of the delicate mucous membrane and the contraction of habits which ought to be avoided. Young children should be taught the important lesson of cleanliness of these parts when taking a bath.

There is no reason why any mother should fail to attend to her duty in this respect, and her neglect may lead directly to those wrong habits whose formation she wishes her boys to avoid. It would be far better to remove the redundant integument as is customary with the Hebrews than to have it become the cause of disease or of evil habits.

II.—AFFECTIONS OF THE MALE GENITAL ORGANS.

Phimosis.—When the foreskin cannot be brought back over the head of the gland a condition exists known as phimosis. Children with phimosis are liable to be peevish, fretful and suffer from a train of reflex symptoms, such as too frequent urination, wetting the bed at night, irritation of the bladder and many nervous affections, including fits and paralysis. This condition is very common in male children. It prevents proper attention to cleansing and requires attention. It may lead in the growing boy to the vice of masturbation.

TREATMENT.—Stretching the orifice will sometimes avail. Circumcision is a certain cure. It is neither a difficult nor dangerous operation. Where the defect is slight, slitting up the foreskin may prove a satisfactory measure.

Para Phimosis.—When a narrow foreskin has been retracted over the gland and cannot be replaced readily the condition is known as para phimosis. Swelling takes place rapidly, the organ becomes distorted and strangulation occurs which, if unrelieved, may be followed by mortification.

TREATMENT.—Grasp the head of the penis, compressing it with one hand, and with the other pull forward the foreskin and at the same time push back the gland. If this method does not avail the fibrous band which encircles it like a rubber ring can be cut through with a surgeon's knife. Circumcision is recommended to prevent any further trouble.

Congenital Malformation.—Congenital malformation of these parts sometimes occurs, calling for the surgeon's art, and unless the deformity is great, he is successful in completing the work which nature has failed to perform.

Warts.—Warts about the foreskin and gland are usually of venereal origin. Proper treatment consists in their removal and the application of the nitrate of silver to the stump.

Cancer of the Penis.—This disease sometimes occurs after middle life. If left to its own course, its progress is onward and destructive. The treatment requires amputation of enough of the organ to completely remove the involved tissue. By the modern surgeon this operation is almost painless and entirely bloodless, it being performed with the platinum wire heated by a galvanic cautery battery.

The Testicles.—These are glandular organs averaging an inch and a half to two inches in length, an inch in thickness and weighing each about six drams. Their structure is somewhat complex. They are situated in the scrotum and suspended by the spermatic cords. During fœtal life the testicles are developed and remain in the abdomen until sometime prior to birth, when they descend through an opening in the inguinal canal into the scrotum which is simply a sac or pouch adapted to their protection. Their only function is the secretion of seminal fluid. They are richly supplied with arterial blood from the spermatic arteries which accompany the cord.

The seminal fluid is a thick, whitish substance containing spermatozoa in abundance. These are germs which manifest in various ways remarkable vitality. Their form and movement are observed by means of a microscope.

Their contact with the product of the female ovary causes conception, a process more fully described on a later page.

Varicocele.—Varicocele results from a varicose condition of the spermatic vessels. These knotted veins in the scrotum feel like a bunch of earth worms. This affection more often occurs upon the left side, owing to a peculiarity of the course and length of the left spermatic vein, and is sometimes supposed to be caused by masturbation or excesses. It is not a very important affection, and can usually be relieved by wearing a suspensory bandage to support the testicles and prevent their weight from dragging upon the cord.

When varicocele occasions serious symptoms or severe pain the surgical operation of passing a ligature around the vein affords relief. A surgical operation is never resorted to for this affection unless palliative measures have failed to afford relief.

Hydrocele.—Hydrocele is a collection of serous fluid or dropsy of the scrotum, which may distend it to an enormous size. This affection is usually more troublesome from the weight and size of the distended scrotum than from pain. Its discomforts are much relieved by wearing a suspensory bandage until other measures are instituted. In treating a hydrocele care must be exercised to ascertain that the enlargement is not due to hernia. The diagnosis is confirmed by means of a lamp in a darkened room, a hydrocele being translucent, while a hernia is opaque. A large hydrocele is treated by tapping with a trocar and canula. After the fluid is drawn off tincture of iodine may be injected into the sack, which will awaken sufficient inflammation to cause its obliteration. This method is known as the radical cure.

Hæmatocele.—Hæmatocele is a blood tumor of the scrotum. It may be caused by the rupture of a vessel, or from a blow or strain, or it may be the result of puncturing a vessel in tapping a hydrocele. It differs from a hydrocele in that the effusion is blood instead of serum, and it has a more rapid origin. This blood tumor is not transparent.

Its treatment demands rest and cold lotions or ice to check hemorrhage. If pus forms an opening must be made for its discharge. The formation of pus is a common result of a blood tumor, yet, if the amount of hemorrhage is small nature may be able to accomplish its absorption. If the blood remains in a fluid state it may be withdrawn by aspiration.

Orchitis—Orchitis, or swelled testicle, is a common complication of gonorrhœa. It may result from other causes, as an injury. It sometimes occurs during an attack of mumps, but the relation between an inflamed parotid gland and an inflamed testicle is not well understood. In this case recovery is generally satisfactory, but sometimes the testicles suffer permanent injury and atrophy. Inflammation of the testicles is generally very painful and attended by sickness of the stomach and disagreeable or protracted nausea. There may be chills followed by fever and a rise of temperature.

TREATMENT.—The treatment calls for rest in bed, support of the testicles and hot or cold applications as may be indicated. The lead and opium wash is soothing. It is known as Goulard's extract. A poultice made of flax-seed meal and fine cut tobacco affords relief.

When pus forms no external applications are available. It is then necessary to make an incision and allow the pus to be discharged.

Orchitis may have a syphilitic origin in which case the same treatment is required as for syphilitic affections in general.

Other Minor Affections.—There are other affections of the testicles such as tubercle, hernia, cystic and cancerous diseases, but these affections are so comparatively rare that the details of their symptoms and treatment is not considered essential.

Cystic and cancerous disease requires the early removal of the affected testicle, an operation of but little danger and usually successful if performed sufficiently early.

III.—CHANCRE AND CHANCROID, OR VENEREAL AFFECTIONS.

The effects of venereal diseases are similar on both of the sexes. A chancre is a venereal sore which is followed by syphilis. It is a hard lump appearing in from two to six weeks after exposure. Its presence is often unexpected and sometimes unperceived. It commonly exists by itself alone, and secretes a thin, scanty but contagious fluid. Occasionally, however, more than one chancre exists at the same time. In order to distinguish a chancre from the chancroid it is variously called hard, indurated, infecting or Hunterian chancre. It is fully described on a following page.

The term chancroid means like chancre. The chancroid is a contagious, venereal ulcer or sore, usually situated upon the private parts, although it may occur in almost any other situation. It secretes a thin pus, which if brought into contact with the mucous membrane or an abraded surface, propagates itself by the production of other similar ulcers.

The chancroid has received a variety of names to distinguish it from the true or infecting chancre. It is frequently called the soft, simple or noninfecting chancre. It has nothing to do with syphilis. It is simply a local, inflammatory sore with ragged edges, tending to spread rapidly and loath to heal. The soft chancre appears in from three to ten days after exposure. It is commonly spread by sexual contact, although it may be communicated by means of fingers, towels and in various ways. Usually a number of these sores exist at the same time.

It is not always easy to distinguish between the soft chancre which is simply a local sore, and the hard chancre which is the beginning of syphilis. The possibility exists of being inoculated with the virus of both, so that where several sores exist one of the number may be a genuine infecting chancre.

TREATMENT.

A soft chancre, or chancroid when left to itself, tends to spread in a destructive way, and a month or two elapses before it runs its course and begins to heal. Cleanliness and correct habits are important factors in the treatment of venereal sores. Alcoholic indulgence tends to increase their activities and prolongs the healing process. In the early stage, the chancroid should be thoroughly destroyed by the cautious and thorough application of strong nitric acid to the sore. This destroys the ulcerating surface and the infecting virus and changes an indolent and spreading ulcer into a healthy sore which readily heals. After thorough cauterization, the surface may be dusted with iodoform, aristol or iodol, and a cure usually follows rapidly.

IV.—ACQUIRED SYPHILIS.

Syphilis is a disease due to the action of a specific poison, propagated by local inoculation. The history of syphilis extends back many centuries, and its origin has never been traced. No portion of the world occupied by civilized man is exempt from its ravages. It is more common, however, in the great centers of population and in large cities. It may be acquired in several ways from those who are suffering from this loathsome affection, or its subtile poison may be inherited from one or both of the parents or other ancestors. It is a disease possessing great abilities to do damage and work destruction. Its evil progress is not confined to any single tissue of the body, but it may invade any or all of them.

Acquired syphilis is always announced by the appearance of a hard lump known as a chancre, usually upon the private parts.

Between the exposure and the appearance of the hard chancre there is usually a period called the incubation, which lasts from two to six weeks. Sometime during this period a hard reddish pimple is discovered which pursues an indolent course. It does not occasion pain usually, nor does it increase rapidly in size, neither does it occasion any special inconvenience. After awhile other symptoms appear. The glands in the groin enlarge and a peculiar copper colored eruption of the skin appears. These symptoms come on in from one to three months after the appearance of the chancre and are known as the secondary symptoms, and unless terminated by efficient treatment they last for a year or more.

In addition to the eruption upon the skin, eruptions are likely to appear upon the throat, tonsils, mouth, lips, nose and genital organs. The face and scalp are often the site of ulcers and sores which are exceedingly annoying to the patient and repulsive to those with whom he comes in contact. The mucous patches about the mouth and lips are liable to convey the syphilitic poison to others, and it is on account of the danger of spreading this contagion that public drinking utensils are to be avoided as much as possible. In using public drinking cups, rinse them thoroughly if possible, before placing them to your own mouth. The act of kissing is not without danger if one party is infected with syphilis.

During the latter portion of the second period the patient is likely to suffer from pain in the bones especially at night; thus sleep is seriously interfered with and the general health is deteriorated.

Syphilis is inclined to pursue a chronic course. It is one of the most persistent affections known, and after appearing to be cured for years, it may break out afresh on the slightest provocation. When the course of syphilis is not arrested by efficient treatment, it may harass the patient continually and prove a perpetual annoyance to the close of life.

Many physicians rightly believe that the efficient treatment of syphilis, prior to and during the secondary period will effectually cure it and prevent the approach of those more disgusting and persistent symptoms which characterize tertiary syphilis. When syphilis pursues an unmolested course, the tertiary symptoms appear in from one to two years. After tertiary syphilis has become permanently established, its cure is an utter impossibility.

The unaided system is not able to eliminate the poison of syphilis, and if the symptoms disappear for a time they are sure to reappear in some other form; for its power for harm appears never to be exhausted. The symptoms of tertiary syphilis are so varied, numerous and well known that few words are necessary to be said concerning them.

Tertiary syphilis attacks the deeper and more vital organs, as the liver, the kidneys and the brain. The bones are often attacked, the destructive process causes ulcerations that are difficult to heal and a great variety of abnormal growths and morbid conditions.

TREATMENT.

The remedies chiefly relied upon to cure syphilis are mercury in some form, and the iodide of potash. Mercury has a specific action in arresting the development of syphilis. It must be given in small doses as soon as the secondary symptoms appear, and continued for a long time; from one to two years or more. The proto-iodide of mercury may be given in doses of one-eighth of a grain in pill form, three times a day, or the biniodide in doses of one-sixteenth of a grain. A larger or smaller dose may be used if the condition of the patient requires. The treatment is tedious and must be continued long after the symptoms have disappeared.

The management of a case of syphilis ought to be intrusted to the judgment of a competent medical man, for a very serious affection is to be dealt with. In order to effect a permanent cure and forestall untoward results, the treatment must be faithfully carried out at least for two years, and then there is no question but what the suffering patient will be successfully and permanently cured.

Iodide of potash is made use of in tertiary syphilis to check the progress of the disease and assist the absorption of nodes and nodules. It is often combined with mercury, and after secondary symptoms have existed a year or so it is used with great benefit. The treatment of mercury and iodide of potash combined is known as the mixed treatment. The following is an excellent formula and specimen of the mixed treatment:

℞   Biniodide of mercury   two grains
    Iodide of potash   half an ounce
    Tinc. cinchona comp.   three ounces
    Peppermint water   one ounce

Mix. Dose one teaspoonful an hour after eating in a wine glass of water. This treatment is to be continued for a long time.

V.—HEREDITARY SYPHILIS.

Syphilis under certain conditions is wont to blight the progeny with fearful destruction descending as a curse from parent to child with the most disastrous effects. It is the most frequent known cause of miscarriage, stillborn children, and of infant mortality, a fact well known to all medical men.

Many believe also that scrofula is due to the remote effects of syphilis. The symptoms of hereditary syphilis are very similar to that of acquired with the exception that the hard chancre does not appear as the initial lesion. These symptoms are the characteristic affections of the skin, mucous membrane, bones and other tissues. Eruptions often appear, fissures about the mouth and nose, emaciation, swellings, tumors and chronic inflammations. The sight, the hearing, the teeth, the bones and any other part of the body may be involved to a greater or less extent.

Children inheriting syphilis are liable to eruptions, hydrocephalus tuberculosis, marasmus and many other diseases which it is needless to enumerate.

The treatment of hereditary syphilis is similar to that of acquired and is often attended with the most happy results. Nursing babies are benefited by the administration of remedies to the mother through the medium of the mother's milk.

A person who has had syphilis ought not to marry until a year after every trace has disappeared. Such a course would reduce to the minimum the risk of transmitting syphilis.

VI.—GONORRHŒA, URETHRITIS, OR CLAP AND ITS COMPLICATIONS.

Urethritis is either a simple or a specific inflammation of the urethra. The specific is otherwise known as gonorrhœa or clap.

Gonorrhœa is an acute, contagious inflammation of some portion of the mucous lining of the urethra in the male or the vagina and urethra in the female. The inflammation is accompanied by a fluid discharge of a whitish color, about the consistency of cream. This loathsome disease is produced by contagion and chiefly by impure contact of the sexes.

It is a local disease running a definite course, and tending toward recovery, though in some cases the recovery is retarded for several weeks or even months. The period which elapses from the time of the exposure to the outbreak of the disease is from three to five or more days. This period is designated as the incubation.

SYMPTOMS.

The first symptom is usually an itching about the urethral orifice. The passing of water, urination, is attended by a burning or smarting pain. After a short time the flow of a thick, whitish fluid is established. There is swelling, redness, soreness, and perhaps pain in the private organ or penis. These symptoms are more or less marked in different cases. In the female the seat of the inflammation is chiefly in the vagina, and occasions much less inconvenience and anxiety than in the male.

TREATMENT.

The treatment most highly and heartily recommended is preventive. There is nothing in a strictly continent course of life which is inconsistent with or antagonistic to good health. This fact needs to be widely known, thoroughly taught and persistently emphasized.

Having contracted this loathsome disease, rest in bed should be maintained during the severity of the inflammation, as going around aggravates the pain and retards recovery. Attention should be given to the diet. It should be light and unstimulating and consist of milk, broths, toast, stale bread, crackers and similar articles which characterize a mild regimen. Meat for the most part should be discarded. Tobacco should be restricted and alcoholic liquors ought not to be allowed.

Bathing the inflamed parts in hot water soothes the pain, relieves the soreness and reduces the swelling. This treatment may be used freely and always with comfort to the patient. Some benefit may be derived from drinking flax seed or slippery elm tea. When much discomfort attends and follows urination, the following affords relief.

℞ Bicarbonate of potash   four drams
    Tinc. hyoscyamus   four drams
    Syr. of orange peel   two ounces
    Wintergreen water   two ounces

Mix. Dose one teaspoonful every four hours in water.

After a few days the discharge becomes thicker, of a greenish color, and appears more purulent in character. There may be considerable elevation of temperature and other symptoms of general malaise. The acute stage of the disease lasts from one to two weeks, then a decline takes place. The discharge becomes thinner and finally disappears, except perhaps, that it is still noticed in the morning. This under proper treatment soon disappears and the disease is cured.

The following prescription may be successfully used for the acute stage of gonorrhœa:

℞	Carbonate of magnesia	two drams
	Oil of cubebs	one dram
	Balsam copaiba	one dram
	Oil sandal wood	one dram

Mix. Make sixty pills. Dose two every four hours.

Astringent injections have been much used and often abused in the treatment of gonorrhœa. In mild cases they are unnecessary, and in all cases unneeded till after the acute stage has passed.

The following is a good sample for injection:

℞	Sulphate of zinc	one grain
	Acetate of lead	one grain
	Ext. hydrastis (discolored)	one dram
	Water	seven drams

Mix. Inject a small syringe full two or three times a day.

The usual duration of an attack of gonorrhœa is about three weeks. It may continue much longer, and when improperly treated has been known to last for several months.

Orchitis.—There are numerous complications which may result from an attack of gonorrhœa. Orchitis, as a complication, does not differ from the same disease due to injuries or other causes.

In this case the inflammation extends from the urethra till it reaches the testicle, where it may cause an inflammation of the duct, epididymitis, or an inflammation of the testicle itself, orchitis. For treatment see affections of the male genital organs. In addition two drops of tincture of pulsatilla may be given every hour.

Bubo.—Bubo is an inflammation of the glands in the groin. These swellings sometimes suppurate. When pus has formed, the abscess should be opened and the cavity washed out with an antiseptic fluid, after which it should be dusted with aristol or iodoform and a pad of iodoform gauze placed over it and held in position as a dressing. In the early stage before the formation of pus spirits of camphor are an excellent external application to abort it. Bubo not only complicates gonorrhœa but is a frequent complication of chancroids. Venereal diseases, although loathsome and disgusting at the best, are quite amenable to proper treatment.

Chordee.—Chordee is sometimes a very painful and persistent affection due to the irritation awakened by an attack of gonorrhœa. It can be relieved by the following prescription.

℞	Pulv. camphor	twenty grains
	Ext. hyoscyamus	ten grains
	Ext. opium	ten grains

Mix. Make into twenty pills.

Dose one at night on retiring and repeat toward morning if needed. This complication is also relieved by suppositories. For formula see treatment of acute and chronic cystitis.

Gleet.—When an attack of gonorrhœa is neglected or for any reason is long continued, the discharge becomes thin and colorless resembling glycerine and is known as gleet. When gleet persists, it usually indicates stricture of the urethra. The following prescription is appropriate for chronic gleet:

℞	Tinct. cantharides	one half dram
	Muriate tinct. of iron	one ounce

Mix. Dose one-fourth of a teaspoonful three times a day in water.

Stricture.—In severe or protracted cases of gonorrhœa the mucous lining of the urethra becomes contracted in the process of healing and cicatricial tissue is formed, which obstructs to a greater or less degree the caliber of the canal. In some cases the urethra is almost completely obstructed, so that the urine passes in a dribbling stream or drop by drop.

Usually a stricture can be treated successfully by dilatation of the canal with steel sounds of different sizes. An ingenious instrument has been invented to cut through or stretch a close stricture.

Such injuries may result to the organs of generation from an attack of gonorrhœa as to prevent procreation.

Gonorrhœal Rheumatism.—A peculiarly distressing kind of rheumatism is a frequent complication of an attack of gonorrhœa. Severe pains and tenderness of one or more joints come on during the late stages of the disease. The ankles and knees are the joints most frequently affected. This complication is sometimes so desperate as to endanger life and no more obstinate grade of rheumatism is ever encountered.

Purulent Ophthalmia.—Those afflicted with gonorrhœa should be careful not to inoculate the eyes with the poison virus as may be done by soiled towels or fingers. This affection is sometimes followed by blindness. It is mentioned elsewhere. See diseases of the eyes.

It is important to say that stricture and orchitis often result from the prescriptions of druggists and incompetent persons who attempt to prescribe for gonorrhœa.

CHAPTER XXVI.

THE FEMALE GENITAL ORGANS.

I.—DESCRIPTION OF THE FEMALE GENITAL ORGANS. 1. THE FEMALE PELVIS. 2. THE OVARIES AND THEIR FUNCTIONS. 3. THE FALLOPIAN TUBES. 4. THE UTERUS OR WOMB. II.—MENSTRUATION AND ITS DISORDERS. 1. MENSTRUATION. 2. DELAYED MENSTRUATION. 3. PROFUSE MENSTRUATION. 4. CESSATION OF MENSTRUATION. 5. CARE OF MENSTRUATION. III.—AFFECTIONS OF THE FEMALE GENITAL ORGANS. 1. PRURITUS, OR TROUBLESOME ITCHING. 2. LEUCORRHŒA, WHITES, FEMALE WEAKNESS. 3. GONORRHŒA IN THE FEMALE.

I.—DESCRIPTION OF THE FEMALE GENITAL ORGANS.

THE Female Pelvis.—The female pelvis differs somewhat from the male, the bones are lighter and more expanded, making the hips prominent. It is owing to this fact that the motion of the female in walking is quite characteristic.

While the female is not so well adapted to walking or running as the male, the shape of her pelvis and the organs contained therein, especially fit her for the performance of those peculiar functions of reproduction which are essential to the perpetuity of the race.

The Ovaries and their Functions—There are two ovaries, one on each side of the womb, situated in the folds of the broad ligaments. They are about an inch and a half long and less than an inch in diameter. They resemble the testicles of the male in size, shape, and somewhat in their development and functions. They contain numerous little bodies known as Graafian follicles, in which an ovum, or egg, is ripened at regular intervals.

Each ovary contains several thousand immature ova, many of which never reach maturity, but some are in different stages of development preparatory to their expulsion. The human ovum is very small. It does not measure over $\frac{1}{120}$ of an inch in diameter. At each menstrual period a single ovum is usually matured, the ovaries alternating. When each ovary matures an ovum at the same time should pregnancy follow, the result would most likely be double pregnancy or twins.

Each month attending ovulation is a sensitive condition of the internal surface of the womb, and should impregnation take place the womb is thus prepared for undertaking the nutrition and development of a fœtus. Blood flows from the internal surface of the womb during ovulation for several days. This process is known by various terms as the courses, menses, or in medical language as menstruation or the catamenia.

The Fallopian Tubes.—The Fallopian tubes are the permeable ducts which convey the ovum to the uterus. They are about four inches long. Their distal ends are little cups surrounded by a fringed border called the fimbriated extremity which possesses the peculiar faculty of attaching itself to that portion of the ovary where the ovum is about to be expelled. This little cup shaped extremity catches the matured ovum from whence it is conveyed to the uterus where, if previously impregnated, it finds a permanent home and all necessary conditions for its development.

Impregnation is believed to take place most frequently somewhere on the journey of the ovum through the Fallopian tube. Sometimes though rarely the ovum fails to be grasped by the fimbriated extremity and is dropped into the abdominal cavity. This accident is the cause of what is known as extra uterine or abdominal pregnancy in case impregnation has taken place.

The Uterus or Womb.—The uterus is a hollow, muscular, pear-shaped organ situated in front of the rectum and behind the bladder. Above it rests the intestines while its lower portion rests upon and is supported by the walls of the vagina. The vagina is a distensible canal of from three to five inches long. The womb is held somewhat loosely in position by the broad and round ligaments. These ligaments are capable of permitting marked alteration in the position of the womb, as is required in pregnancy, and it is owing to this fact also, that displacements of the womb are more liable to occur than of any other organ.

The broad ligaments are composed of folds of the peritoneum. They extend outwards from the uterus on each side enclosing the Fallopian tubes and surrounding and holding the ovaries also in position. Folds of peritoneum attach the womb to the bladder in front and to the rectum behind. The round ligaments are two round cords four or five inches long which extend outward through the folds of the broad ligaments and downward until lost in the tissues of the labia.

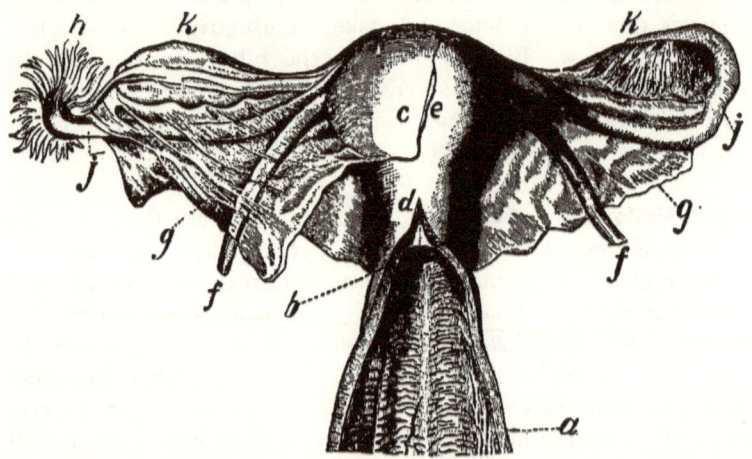

The uterus and adjacent tissues: a, the upper part of the vagina laid open to show internal appearance and mouth of the uterus; b, mouth of uterus at upper termination of vagina; c, the fundus or body of uterus; d, the cervix or neck of uterus; e, line showing the removal of the peritoneal covering from the right side of the figure; f, f, the round ligaments; g, g, the broad ligaments which give lateral support to the organ; h, the fringe-like extremity of the Fallopian tubes; j, j, the Fallopian tubes; k, k, the ovaries. On the right side of the figure the fringe-like extremity is closely applied to the ovary as when an ovum is ready to be discharged.

The upper portion or larger end of the uterus is called the fundus and the lower end is called the cervix while the canal which leads into it is the os uteri or mouth of the womb. The cavity of the uterus extends from the cervix to the fundus, and on each side of the fundus is the small opening of the Fallopian tube. The uterine cavity is capable of great distension and is thus admirably fitted for the process of reproduction. It enlarges during this process in order to accommodate the development of the product of conception to a couple of pounds or more in weight.

The nerve and blood supply of these organs are from several different sources and calculated to be as abundant as any occasion may require. It is owing to this fact largely that derangements of these organs are numerous and occasion a great variety of troublesome symptoms.

II.—MENSTRUATION AND ITS DISORDERS.

Menstruation.—Menstruation attends ovulation. It occurs in the mature female every lunar month, or once in about twenty-eight days, although slight variations are consistent with health and unimportant. Menstruation is commonly established between thirteen and fifteen years of age, but there are many exceptions. It may occur as early as eleven, or even earlier, and is frequently delayed till the eighteenth or nineteenth year, especially in cold climates. Warm climates and the excitements of fashionable life tend to hasten this well marked sign of maturity.

When menstruation occurs, many changes are observed in the habits, disposition, behavior and form of the young female. She ceases to be a romping girl, becomes modest, coy and ladylike, taking much care of her manners and personal appearance. It is noticed that her hips have become extended, that her form is more rounded and that her ways are more graceful and attractive, in other words, she has forever passed from girlhood to womanhood.

Normal menstruation is attended only by slight inconvenience, as perhaps headache, backache and some unimportant nervous symptoms caused by the congestion of the genital organs but these symptoms usually disappear when the flow becomes established.

Some females suffer from severe pain in the back or abdomen, heaviness and profound nervous symptoms previous to the establishment of the flow. When the pain is severe or the flow very scanty, absent or excessive, some disorder of the natural functions exists which should be ascertained and remedied. The amount of flow within the limits of health varies from two to ten ounces.

Delayed Menstruation.—Delayed menstruation in young females often indicates that the genital organs have not sufficiently matured for the performance of this function. It is poor policy to attempt to coerce nature. Such measures should be adopted as will improve the vigor of the feeble, anæmic, or those otherwise deficient in physical development. Better results are obtained from common sense measures than from the administration of forcing medicines. A nutritious diet, exercise in the country or at the seaside, gymnastic practices suited to the strength, and flannel or silk worn next to the skin are recommended as general measures calculated to improve the physical condition at this important period.

When the young female is pale and the condition of well-marked anæmia is present, suitable tonics to improve the appetite and iron in small doses to enrich the blood, are suggested as in the treatment of anæmia, which see.

Profuse Menstruation.—Profuse or too frequent menstruation indicates in some cases a lax and weak condition of the uterus, a condition which sometimes follows labor or abortion, or a succession of rapid pregnancies or abortions. Profuse menstruation occurs in certain abnormal conditions, as when a tumor or growth exists within the womb. The affection is rare in young females who have never borne children.

Excessive hemorrhage is debilitating from whatever cause, and when it exists for any length of time or is repeated at frequent intervals, it ought to receive careful attention. It should be borne in mind that what would be considered a scanty flow in one woman would rightly be considered excessive in another, each woman having individual peculiarities not to be overlooked. A full-blooded, plethoric woman would be benefited by a flow which would be too prostrating for a woman of the opposite type. When a uterine tonic like the fluid extract of ergot in half teaspoonful doses every two or three hours fails to relieve this condition, the pelvic organs should be explored to ascertain the cause.

Cessation of Menstruation.—Menstruation ceases temporarily during pregnancy and the whole or early part of lactation. The cessation of menstruation between the ages of forty-five and fifty is known as the change or turn of life and after this the power of reproduction is lost. This period in medical language is known as the climacteric or menopause.

Menstruation does not terminate abruptly but there is usually a long period in which the courses become scanty or excessive and irregular, a period in which are experienced many varied symptoms, as headache, backache, hot flashes, faint spells, nervous irritability and other derangements of the health. Pregnancy is quite rare after forty-five and occurs only in extreme cases after fifty.

After the change of life there are certain organic diseases, as cancer of the womb and breasts which are more liable to appear and a few previously existing diseases may become aggravated. When proper attention is given to this important period, the change of life is likely to be passed in safety and the subsequent health to be much improved.

Excitements are to be avoided during the change of life, and the sexual organs should enjoy perfect physiological rest. Digestion and nutrition should receive appropriate attention. Sleep should be abundant and exercise moderate, but persistent. The mind should be occupied with cheerful thoughts and not give way to melancholy.

It can hardly be expected that a complete line of treatment will be suggested for all the complex and varied disorders of the female genital organs. The most that can be attempted is to advise with respect to diet and nutrition, rest and freedom from excitements, and insist upon those general measures which will tend to prevent irregularities and preserve the genital organs in a normal and healthy condition.

From the anatomy and physiology of the pelvic organs the intelligent female ought to infer that lacing and tight clothing are injurious. They favor congestion and displacement of the womb, they obstruct the circulation, diminish the respiration, and are prominent factors in female weakness and debility, the effects of which are especially marked upon these organs.

Care During Menstruation.—Suitable attention should be given to the health during menstruation, for this function in the civilized world is especially liable to be disordered, and the prevention of such disease as may result therefrom is much more satisfactory than its cure. Many diseases of the female organs are the result of ignorance or neglect. During menstruation no carelessness should be permitted. Exposure, getting wet, getting the feet wet, or taking cold, may cause congestion of the genital organs and result in serious consequences.

Excitement, fatigue, drinking ice water, bathing in cold water or dancing may tend to increase or suppress the flow and result in inflammation of these organs. In many females of imperfect health rest for a day or so during menstruation is of great advantage and essential to the continuation of their well being. The amount of rest needed depends upon the condition of each individual case. The diet should be rather lighter than usual. A warm foot or hip bath is sometimes beneficial to assist in relieving the unpleasant early symptoms and aids in the establishment of the flow.

III.—AFFECTIONS OF THE FEMALE GENITAL ORGANS.

Pruritus or Troublesome Itching.—This is a troublesome affection of the external genital organs due to a disturbed condition of the nervous system. It may be slight or so troublesome and persistent as to occasion loss of sleep and endless annoyance.

It is often worse at night and the duration of the affection cannot be foretold. In some cases it is especially obstinate and lasts for years. The only symptom of importance is a troublesome itching and an almost uncontrollable desire to relieve it by rubbing or scratching. The remedy suggested by instinct affords only the most temporary relief and in the long run tends to aggravate the trouble. Scratching or rubbing draws an increased blood supply to the already sensitive parts, causes a thickening of the skin and favors the development of an eruption. It also adds to the trouble by further disturbing the sensitive cutaneous nerves and helps in various ways to aggravate a disagreeable condition.

Irritating discharges may be a factor in the development of pruritus and should receive appropriate attention. Cleanliness is within the reach of every one and ought not to require a physician's suggestion to render its employment popular. Vaginal injections of astringent lotions or of water alone may be frequently employed in addition to sponging the external surfaces with the same.

TREATMENT.—After thoroughly cleansing, the following ointment may be applied.

> ℞ Menthol half a dram
> Carbolic acid twenty grains
> Aqua rose ointment one ounce
> Vaseline one ounce

Mix. Apply as needed, especially at night.

The following is an excellent remedy.

> ℞ Acetate of lead one dram
> Carbolic acid one dram
> Tinct. opium one ounce
> Rose water two pints

Mix. This solution is to be applied by means of a piece of soft muslin. The following has succeeded in some obstinate cases:

℞ Bichloride of mercury .... half a dram
    Tinct. opium .... one ounce
    Water .... eight ounces

Mix and apply two or three times a day. Label poison.

When other remedies have failed, this may be tried with good hope of success.

℞ Chloroform .... two drams
    Oil bitter almonds .... two ounces

Mix and apply as needed.

In some of these cases the general health needs attention. Tonics containing iron and strychnia work well in a large majority of cases. When the trouble is due to a disturbed condition of the nervous system, the following will render invaluable service.

℞ Fowler's solution .... one and a half drams
    Elix. Calisaya .... four ounces

Mix. Dose one teaspoonful after meals. This prescription is for adults but may be used for young persons after suitable reduction.

Leucorrhœa, Whites or Female Weakness.—This is a common affection resulting frequently from some impairment of the general health. It is to be regarded as a symptom of some disease rather than a disease itself.

Leucorrhœa is a mucous discharge, more or less copious, from the glands of the vagina and cervix. It is often temporary from slight congestion of the mucous surfaces or a mild grade of inflammation. It often follows or precedes menstruation and occurs frequently during pregnancy. When persistent, it is a symptom of disease either of the vagina, womb or Fallopian tubes, and it is then necessary to investigate these organs in order to learn its origin or treat the affection intelligently.

It should be known that a thin, watery discharge, with offensive odor, takes place in cancer of the womb. When a tumor or polypus exists in the uterus hemorrhage, more or less profuse is a characteristic symptom, while pus, more or less tinged with blood, suggests discharge from an ulcer or abscess.

A slight discharge of mucous of temporary character, requires little notice except the suggestion of cleanliness. Assistance is not usually sought unless the discharge is profuse, persistent and annoying.

TREATMENT.—Persistent and severe cases are likely to resist the action of remedies. Ordinary cases of this affection are relieved by injections of tepid water, to which may be added such astringents as witch-hazel, alum, sulphate of zinc, or the glycerite of tannin, in suitable proportions. A heaping teaspoonful of pulverized alum to a pint of water makes a simple and convenient astringent wash. A tablespoonful of extract of witch-hazel or a teaspoonful of tannin previously dissolved by means of heat in half an ounce of glycerine and added to a pint of water, make applications equally beneficial. When a case of leucorrhœa does not yield to these simple remedies advice with regard to it should be sought.

When bloody pus is contained in the discharge, or an unpleasant odor is perceived, a wash containing a teaspoonful of carbolic acid to a pint or quart of water is appropriate. In using such a wash care should be taken to thoroughly mix the acid with the water.

A leucorrhœal discharge may be kept up by the irritation of a displaced womb, which will need to be rectified before a permanent cure will result. Constipation of the bowels is a frequent source of annoyance in nearly all pelvic troubles and should be remedied. The general condition may need attention. Many of these cases are in a run down condition and require tonics to improve the health.

It ought to be mentioned in this connection that leucorrhœa may prevent reproduction and be the sole cause of sterility. Directions for treating other diseases of the pelvic organs, such as tumors of the womb and ovaries, displacements, ulcerations and cancers, belong to the domain of surgery, and are intentionally omitted.

Gonorrhœa in the Female.—The general subject of gonorrhœa has been fully discussed. See previous chapter. The greater portion of what has been said applies to this loathsome disease in either sex. There are a few differences, however, which should receive mention.

There is always a possibility of contracting gonorrhœa innocently, and females are more often the victims of this unfortunate occurrence than males. An aggravated leucorrhœal discharge is sometimes mistaken for gonorrhœa, and may become the cause of unjust suspicion. Hence the wisdom always of a guarded professional opinion.

Peritonitis is an additional complication which may result from gonorrhœa in the female. The inflammation may travel up the Fallopian tubes to the peritoneum. When it occurs, it is to be treated the same as peritonitis from other causes, with rest and anodynes sufficient to allay pain. Pelvic abscess, or abscess of the labia may result from this affection.

Gonorrhœa may so injure the generative organs as to destroy their functions and prevent the possibility of maternity There is no more important requisite of treatment for gonorrhœa in the female than cleanliness, and this is readily accomplished owing to the access of the involved tissues. The irritating discharge should be washed away two or three times a day with tepid water and once a day the following astringent injection should be used.

℞ Pulv. alum   one dram
    Sulph. of zinc   half a dram
    Borax   ten grains

Mix. This makes one powder for a vaginal injection to be dissolved in a pint or more of warm water. In ordinary cases this treatment is sufficient, if used daily

CHAPTER XXVII.

CHILDREN'S DISEASES.

I.—CHICKEN POX OR VARICELLA. II.—CROUP, TRUE OR MEMBRANOUS. III.—CROUP, FALSE OR LARYNGISMUS. IV.—CHOLERA INFANTUM OR SUMMER COMPLAINT. V.—DIPHTHERIA. VI.—MEASLES OR RUBEOLA. MEASLES, GERMAN OR ROSEOLA. VIII.—MUMPS OR PAROTIDITIS. IX.—SCARLET FEVER OR SCARLATINA. X.—WHOOPING COUGH OR PERTUSSIS. XI.—DISINFECTION DURING AND AFTER DIPHTHERIA AND SCARLET FEVER.

I.—CHICKEN POX OR VARICELLA.

THIS is a mild contagious disease occurring chiefly among children under twelve years of age. It is accompanied by slight fever and an eruption which resembles that of small pox. It is caused by disease germs.

SYMPTOMS.

The first thing that attracts attention to the disease is the breaking out of an eruption which may be scanty, or extend over the whole body.

Vesicles soon form, containing a thin, watery fluid. In a day or two they dry in the center and a brown, umbilicated scab or crust is formed, which falls off in the course of two or three days, leaving underneath a reddened surface and a superficial scar which usually disappears after a few days, except in severe cases, when it may last longer. These vesicles are not in the same condition, but are in every stage of development, and this fact distinguishes the eruption from small pox or varioloid. Some are a red spot, still unformed; others have reached a more advanced stage and contain fluid, while others are drying up, revealing a scab. In small pox all the vesicles are in the same stage of development.

The vesicles in chicken pox are superficial, while in small pox or varioloid they reach down into the connective tissue under the skin. The disease is not dangerous and in many cases there is absence of all symptoms of sickness except the eruption. Recovery is usually rapid and perfect.

TREATMENT.

Domestic remedies are sufficient for this mild and harmless disease. Warm drinks may be administered to promote sweating, when the skin is dry, and the patient feverish. It is unnecessary to separate the patient from other children or to disinfect the apartments beyond the admission of sunlight and fresh air. It is important that care be exercised to prevent taking cold. A cold contracted might render a very mild disease severe or dangerous.

II.—CROUP, TRUE OR MEMBRANOUS.

Croup is an acute inflammation of the windpipe, involving also some of the neighboring tissues. With young children it is a frequent and sometimes a fatal disease. It rarely occurs after the tenth year of age. The climate is the chief factor in its causation, it being more prevalent in some sections than in others, and in cold, damp and changeable weather. Certain families and localities appear to be especially subject to it.

SYMPTOMS.

The disease comes on stealthily. The symptoms are fever, thirst, hoarseness and altered voice. Sometimes the child is able to speak only in a whisper. There is a peculiar paroxysmal, sharp, ringing, brassy, and frequent cough, which having been once heard is rarely forgotten, and the disease may be recognized by hearing it from an adjoining room without seeing the patient. The tongue is coated, the skin is hot and the secretions are checked. Respiration is obstructed, which at length becomes the most prominent symptom; the child makes a peculiar noise and suffocation threatens, rendering the situation dangerous and exciting. If the obstruction is great the child clutches at his throat with his hands, is thirsty and drinks freely, experiencing no difficulty in doing so. The symptoms are worse at night, but seem somewhat relieved in the morning, which inspires hope. On the whole, however, they intensify, the cough and thirst are constant; a little tough phlegm may be expectorated, yet the difficulty of breathing increases. In favorable cases the cough becomes softer, the false membrane may be coughed up entire or in shreds, and improvement rapidly follows.

In unfavorable cases the symptoms become alarming, the mouth is open, the head is thrown back to favor breathing, the lips and ends of the fingers get blue, the pulse become rapid and thready; air enters the lungs with increasing difficulty, and unless relief comes from opening the windpipe, tracheotomy, the case becomes hopeless. The mortality of this disease, especially among children under two years old is considerable.

TREATMENT.

It is necessary to recognize the danger early and combat the disease before the condition of the patient gets desperate. Prompt treatment is successful in a great majority of cases.

Emetics, in the early stage relax the spasmodic condition and may thwart the formation of the false membrane. The syrup of squills comp. in small doses of four or five drops, and repeated every half hour until nausea and vomiting occur is an efficient household remedy. The syrup of ipecac. is a safe remedy to use but is less energetic. Powdered alum answers well for an emetic. The vomiting ought to be followed by a dose of castor oil sufficient to move the bowels thoroughly. Hot cloths wrung out of mustard water and laid upon the neck and covered with flannel to keep in the heat are beneficial. The temperature of the room should be about seventy degrees and ought to contain moisture from steam produced by boiling water or slacking lime.

If the disease is taken in hand early and managed energetically, it can be overcome before the appearance of any distressing symptoms, but if neglected, less favorable results will be obtained even with the aid of all the efficient remedies known to the physician.

When the disease persists, the possibility of its being laryngeal diphtheria should be considered, for many cases of acute inflammation of the larynx and trachea formerly believed to be membranous croup are now believed to be diphtheria. There is no more dangerous form of diphtheria than this, owing to the difficulty in making local applications. Such cases should be recognized early, treated energetically and antiseptically with the same remedies as recommended for diphtheria, which see.

III.—CROUP, FALSE OR LARYNGISMUS.

This disease is due to a spasm of the glottis and neighboring muscles caused by some irritation acting upon the nerves of the larynx.

SYMPTOMS.

The early symptoms are those of having taken cold as in acute catarrh. The throat may be red and inflamed, the eyes heavy and the conjunctiva congested. There is some cough and slight hoarseness of the voice with more or less running from the nose. Toward evening the cold tightens, the running catarrh ceases, the voice gets hoarser and the cough has a croupy sound. In the night the child awakens suddenly and makes a loud crowing sound, as if partially choked, the air enters the windpipe with considerable difficulty, owing to the spasmodic condition of the muscles. In some instances it is thought to be due not so much to a sudden cold, as to irritation produced by a hearty supper and undigested food in the stomach. Under suitable treatment the child gets relief in the course of an hour or so and falls asleep, but the barking cough may continue at intervals till morning. The children of some families seem to be liable to such attacks and it is probable that they have an especially sensitive nervous organism. It rarely occurs in adult life. When spasm of the glottis occurs in diphtheria, it is of more serious import, and has been known to cause death.

TREATMENT.

The syrup of ipecac. administered often till nausea and vomiting are produced usually relieves. Another handy remedy is Hives' syrup, five to ten drops every half hour till relieved. Five grains of bromide of potash and one or two grains of chloral dissolved in water usually afford relief.

The following prescription is appropriate:

℞	Bromide of potash	four scruples
	Chloral	sixteen grains
	Paregoric	two drams
	Syr. tolu.	one ounce
	Anise water q. s. to make	two ounces.

Mix. Dose one teaspoonful every hour as needed.

Children who are accustomed to repeated attacks of false croup should be clothed warmly with woolen next the skin in winter, and accustomed to exercise in the open air. Tonic remedies are often necessary to improve the general condition of such children as follows:

℞ Iodide of iron pills, each pill containing one grain

Dose one pill three times a day, or the following:

℞	Syr. of hypophosphites comp.	three ounces

Dose half a teaspoonful in water, three times a day, after meals.

IV.—CHOLERA INFANTUM OR SUMMER COMPLAINT.

This is an acute and often fatal disease which occurs among infants and children in the hot weather usually from June to September. The higher the temperature, the greater the mortality which this disease reaches. Teething and nursing children are especially liable to attacks. The chief seat of the disturbance is the stomach, bowels and finally the brain.

CAUSES.

The two most important factors in the development of this disease are impure air and unfavorable hygienic surroundings. In cities where population is crowded, ventilation imperfect and the odor of cesspools or sewers contaminates the air, the mortality from this disease is alarming. Teething in summer disturbs the nervous system, impairs the digestion and renders these little patients liable to attacks of diarrhœal diseases.

Heat debilitates the stomach and disturbs the digestion. It favors the fermentation of milk and other food products, and hence it is an important factor in causing summer complaint. Children brought up by hand are in much greater danger from this disease than those supplied naturally with the mother's milk.

Children often thrive on cow's milk and other foods in cool weather, but they may be utterly unable to digest them when the stomach and bowels are weakened by the debilitating effects of heat.

SYMPTOMS.

The onset of this disease may be sudden, or it may be preceded by a persistent looseness of the bowels for several days. Nausea and vomiting are frequent symptoms. The bowels are tender, loose and move frequently. The stools are at first slimy and emit a peculiarly disagreeable odor. There is marked thirst, and so great is the desire for fluid that the danger of over-feeding is much increased. The child, after nursing, immediately vomits while at the same time movements of the bowels are numerous and attended by severe pain.

Emaciation progresses rapidly, the countenance has a pallid, pinched appearance, the eyes are full and bright and the tissues about them sunken. This rapid emaciation is due to the escape of the fluids of the body.

The stools become colorless and sink into the napkin, leaving only a slight stain. They are known as "rice water" stools. The urine is scanty. Unless the disease is promptly arrested the progress of emaciation is rapid, great weakness is observed and collapse comes on and foretells the fatal termination.

In some cases while the degree of emaciation and weakness is extreme, the child lingers, looking like a living skeleton, and these apparently hopeless cases sometimes recover; but whether this fortunate result is due to good nursing, skillful treatment or an unusual vitality, or all combined, it is difficult to determine.

The majority of these cases having once reached the desperate condition of emaciation outlined above terminate fatally.

TREATMENT.

It is important to give attention to preventive treatment. Particular attention ought to be given in hot weather to nursing and teething children. Their food ought to receive constant attention and not be left to the discretion of hired girls or unskillful nurses. The quantity and the quality of food and the intervals of feeding, must be well regulated, and when milk is used great pains must be taken to preserve it from fermentation. A child should not be weaned just before nor during the heated term. All mothers who can should nurse their babies till they are ten or twelve months old.

Removal of a child to the pure air of the country will often prevent sickness in hot weather. Children who are already puny and suffering from indigestion, begin to improve almost immediately on removal from the stifling atmosphere of the crowded town, and this improvement is sometimes so well marked as to be noticed on the journey away. The requisites for the health of the little one are pure air, pure water and healthy food. It is sometimes advisable to undertake the removal of a sick child, the effort being attended with surprising benefit.

Thirst renders the sick child liable to take too much liquid food, instead of quenching the thirst with the nursing bottle, a teaspoonful of cold water, to which a drop or two of brandy has been added, may be frequently given.

There is no better artificial food than peptonized milk for those deprived of the natural breast supply. The process of making is simple and as follows: Into a clean quart bottle put a powder containing five grains of extract of pancreatin and ten grains of bicarbonate of soda; add first one teacupful of water and after shaking, add one pint of fresh milk and again shake the mixture. Then place the bottle in water as warm as the hand can bear for twenty minutes, then remove and place on ice till needed for use. Powders for peptonizing milk can be prepared by any druggist, or they can be bought by the dozen in peptonizing glass tubes.

An easier way is, to prepare the milk for the nursing bottle and add the powder to the warm food every time before the child nurses. The process of digestion will thus go on in the child's stomach, but greatly facilitated by the digestive ferment. The simple directions for this method are as follows: Put into the nursing bottle one gill of fresh cow's milk, one or two tablespoonfuls of rich cream and one gill of warm water. Add a little milk sugar and a powder containing one and one-half grains extract of pancreatin, with four grains of bicarbonate of soda. This is to be prepared freshly for the child at each nursing.

Some children improve on barley gruel, to which a small amount of fresh milk is added, both being boiled together for a minute or so.

In making barley gruel, it is necessary to boil the grain for a long time. In some cases it is advisable to remove the milk altogether for a few days and substitute peptonized beef, or some other nutritious food. Sick children should wear thin flannel next to the skin in summer, and this precaution will prevent injury from changes of temperature, such as are experienced in removal to the country. When a child is taken away from the city, it ought to stay away until cool weather.

It is almost impossible to outline a treatment for cholera infantum, so much depends upon the necessities of each case. In the beginning, it is often beneficial to administer a mild cathartic, to clean out all irritating substances from the bowels. The following will serve an admirable purpose.

℞ Castor oil   two drams
    Paregoric   two drams
    Syr. acacia   one ounce
    Cinnamon water   one ounce

Mix. Dose one teaspoonful every two hours to a child two years old, others in proportion.

When vomiting is persistent give the following:

℞ Carbolic acid   two drops
    Water   ten teaspoonfuls

Mix. Dose a teaspoonful as often as vomiting occurs.

The following may be used to allay irritation and ease pain:

℞ Ext. opium   one-half grain
    Ext. belladonna   one-half grain
    Cacao butter q. s. to make   twelve suppositories

Introduce one into the rectum every four hours.

Bismuth is a valuable remedy and may be given in five or ten grain doses. In place of the suppositories, warm starch water, to which has been added from four to ten drops of laudanum, according to age, may be used as an injection with satisfactory results. Many other remedies have been suggested, but those most suitable for domestic use have been mentioned. Hot poultices or liniment applied externally over the abdomen afford some relief.

℞ Camphor liniment   three ounces
    Oil mustard   one-half dram

Mix. Apply externally, on a piece of flannel, as needed.

Lime water, added to milk in the nursing bottle, corrects the acidity of the stomach and is a good preventive measure. Vegetable astringents, such as infusion of red raspberry leaves may be added to the milk in suitable proportions.

In a condition of collapse, hot water bags should be placed to the feet and brandy frequently given, or other suitable stimulants.

V.—DIPHTHERIA.

Diphtheria is a disease which, although it attacks adults, is more common among young persons and children, and for the sake of convenience is here classified with children's diseases.

It is rightly regarded under the best management, as a very serious and fatal disease. Many cases are mild and tend to recovery. Sometimes an epidemic is mild, nearly all cases recovering while another epidemic is severe and many cases are fatal. Occasionally, a single case only occurs in a family or community, but more often it spreads from one to another and from family to family throughout whole sections.

The cause of this disease is believed to be a specific disease germ which enters the system in one of two ways, either through contaminated food or infected air. The germs cause fermentation in the blood with rise of temperature and lowered vitality. A poison is generated in the body which acts upon the nerve forces in a very depressing manner, while the site of the local manifestation of the disease is usually in the throat, upon the tonsils, or upon the mucous membrane in the vicinity.

Severe cases of diphtheria resemble the condition of blood poisoning more closely than anything else. Upon the throat are discovered distinct patches of an ashy colored membrane. These patches are adherent, and each one tends to enlarge and unite with others. In severe cases, their hold is so firm and deep, as to cut off the capillary circulation beneath and produce sloughing of the tissues. It is this sloughing process which sometimes produces the fearful odor.

The glands, in the neighborhood on the sides of the neck and under the jaw, swell up and are hard like tumors. These glands sometimes turn purple, which is an unfavorable symptom and indicates a changed condition of the blood.

Diphtheria is a contagious disease, and a child sick with it should be isolated from others to prevent its spread. See disinfection during and after diphtheria.

Some authorities describe two varieties of the disease, one called false diphtheria. There is but little fever and the child is but mildly sick. Health returns after a few days, and there are no unpleasant after symptoms, the system being but slightly affected. The other variety is more severe in every way. The whole system seems to be powerfully impressed. There are both local and systemic symptoms. Cases of recovery are attended with paralysis and other signs of debility, the whole system seeming to be overwhelmed with poison of a malignant type.

TREATMENT.

This disease should receive early, energetic and skillful treatment. In order to soften the indurated glands of the neck, applications of camphor liniment on a woolen cloth may be made to them. The following may be used as a gargle and taken internally.

℞	Chlorate of potash	one-half dram
	Muriatic acid, (strong)	twenty drops
	Water	two ounces
	Simple syrup	two ounces

Mix. Gargle a teaspoonful every hour and take a teaspoonful internally every two hours. This prescription is known as the chlorine mixture. It must be made carefully in order to prevent the escape of the chlorine gas, which is antiseptic.

Formerly the tincture of iron was much used for diphtheria. It is not so much used at the present time. It is a good heart tonic and in mild cases answers well.

Chloral hydrate may be used to produce rest. It is mildly antiseptic, but in severe cases cannot be relied upon as a germicide.

℞	Chloral hydrate	half a dram
	Glycerine	one ounce
	Anise water q. s. to make	two ounces

Mix. Dose one teaspoonful every two hours for a child three years old.

Powdered sulphur has been used extensively with good results. Some make use of equal parts of sulphur and quinine. Burning small pieces of sulphur or roll brimstone on a shovel, by means of a hot coal from the fire, carrying it around the sick room, is thought by some to be beneficial. Care must be taken not to inhale it too freely, or to make the fumes too strong for the comfort of the patient. Many other remedies have been suggested and tried for this disease, but the best ones are those most destructive to germ life. The most powerful antiseptic remedy for diphtheria is the bichloride of mercury or corrosive sublimate. It is destructive to all forms of parasitic or germ existence. It must be used cautiously. It is not a dangerous poison in small doses well diluted, as in the following:

℞ Corrosive sublimate   one grain
    Water   three ounces

Mix. Dose a teaspoonful every two hours or in very bad cases every hour. It may be alternated hourly with the chlorine mixture previously mentioned. It is claimed for this treatment, that recovery takes place without the unpleasant complication of paralysis in any of its forms. The use of this remedy is not recommended for domestic practice.

When paralysis occurs during the process of recovery either of the vocal cords or other parts, strychnia in doses of one $\frac{1}{100}$ of a grain is a remedy of recognized efficiency. It can be obtained in the correct adult dose in tablet form, and the dose for children can be regulated by dissolving one tablet in from five to ten teaspoonfuls of water, giving one teaspoonful of the solution every four hours.

Many physicians make a free use of stimulants, in all cases where the poison of the disease shows a tendency to depress and lower the vitality of the system. It is claimed that stimulants are unnecessary when the bichloride treatment is carried out.

*The antitoxine serum has been used with marked success by many eminent physicians, who believe that it reduces the death rate very perceptibly. The author has tested the antitoxine treatment and believes it to be the greatest advance ever made in the treatment of diphtheria, having lost no case since commencing its use. The internal remedies are given with the same persistency, where the injection of antitoxine is used, thereby increasing their efficiency. Its use demands professional skill.

Previous to the use of antitoxine no remedies availed in certain

---

*Antitoxine is prepared by treating a young and healthy horse for several months with injections of diphtheria cultures, beginning with small doses and increasing them as the animal's resistance increases, until the injections cease to produce effect. The horse is then said to be immune, and his blood serum is then known as antitoxine.

putrid or malignant cases. Antitoxine, when injected early enough and in sufficient quantity, appears to antidote the septic character of the disease, modifying its course. To many, the claim that it is a specific, does not seem extravagant. History is likely to rank its discovery with that of vaccination for the prevention of small pox.

VI.—MEASLES OR RUBEOLA.

This is a contagious disease caused by exposure to disease germs. See bacteria or germs in disease. For two weeks after the exposure no symptoms appear and the exposed person feels as well as ever. This is the period of incubation.

SYMPTOMS.

After the incubative period which may vary a little, symptoms of the disease begin to appear and the system is under the influence of an advancing sickness. The temperature rises, there is shivering, thirst, fever, a coated tongue, watery eyes, running at the nose, marked catarrhal affection, dry, hoarse cough, coarse and obstructed breathing, headache and loss of appetite. The patient presents every appearance of having taken a severe and sudden cold. These symptoms occupy three or four days and this period is known as the stage of invasion.

The stage of eruption which now follows is peculiar and characteristic. It appears first in the mouth and throat, next upon the forehead, and soon spreads over the entire body. It consists of dark red or purplish spots, slightly elevated, feeling somewhat dry, hot and rough to the hand. The rash is coarser and darker colored than that of scarlet fever, and unlike it, does not cover the whole body. This distinction is usually clear and well marked. The stage of eruption lasts four or five days. Before the rash appears, there may be vomiting; the patient appears drowsy and is inclined to sleep. Convulsions sometimes occur, especially in children.

The fever does not immediately and wholly decline upon the appearance of the rash, but the temperature is likely to remain high for two or three days. The urine is scanty and highly colored. The whole duration of the disease from the time of the invasion is about two weeks. With the fading of the eruption, the severity of the symptoms decline, the cough loosens, expectoration becomes more abundant and the tongue cleans off.

The final stage is that of desquamation or peeling. The fever declines, the rash gradually fades away and the surface of the skin peels in little fine dust like scales.

Army measles, owing to exposure and other causes, have been of a very severe and fatal type. Measles without an eruption is a dangerous disease.

The common complications of measles are bronchitis, pneumonia, tonsilitis and affections of the eye. Diphtheria, when it occurs as such, is a grave complication.

Ordinary cases tend to recovery, but complication with pneumonia is serious and may require earnest attention to save life.

TREATMENT.

This, for the most part, is simple and palliative. There is no preventive remedy after exposure. It is very difficult to quarantine the disease, because it is largely spread before characteristic symptoms have developed.

Cleanliness and disinfection of the room occupied by the patient are important. The temperature of the sick room should be uniform and not above seventy-two degrees. Free ventilation is essential, but draughts of air should be avoided, as a cold contracted by the patient may be a very serious matter. If the eyes are sensitive to light, the room should be darkened. The bedding should be comfortable but not too heavy, as it is unnecessary to keep the patient in a profuse sweat.

If the temperature is high, the tincture of aconite may be given in drop doses till the skin becomes moist. Cold drinks may be allowed in moderation. Cream of tartar lemonade is often very agreeable to the patient.

The diet should be nutritious, but not hearty. Milk, gruel, tapioca and similiar foods may be used as required. Complications should be met with appropriate remedies. The recovery of those who are much debilitated, or who are naturally troubled with scrofula and other constitutional diseases may be prolonged. The patient must remain in the house till recovery is fully established and avoid exposure to cold. Neglect in the after care of measles is the reason why so many cases develop lung and other diseases. If the cough is troublesome, the following may be used:

℞	Muriate of ammonia	one dram
	Syr. wild cherry	one-half ounce
	Syr. ipecac.	half an ounce
	Paregoric	one-half ounce
	Anise water q. s. to make	four ounces

Mix. Dose one teaspoonful every four hours. Stimulants are rarely needed. The application of carbolized oil or vaseline to the skin is agreeable. Five or ten drops of the acid to the ounce of oil may be used. Should bleeding at the nose occur, a cloth wet with vinegar and water and laid on the back of the neck will generally relieve it. Vaseline may be used on the margins of the eyelids if they stick together or are inflamed. Cold compresses of water and extract of witch-hazel, equal parts, may be used on the eyes. If there is much bronchial trouble, cover the chest with camphorated oil and place a flannel outside. If convulsions occur before the eruption, a bath in hot mustard water is advised. After removing the patient from the bath, wrap in warm blankets and administer bromide of potash. Put one teaspoonful of bromide of potash into half a tumbler of water; dissolve and give a teaspoonful every half hour until relieved. Every fourth dose may have combined with it a grain of chloral. When the temperature is high, quinine combined with phenacetine will lower it.

℞	Quinine	thirty grains
	Phenacetine	thirty grains

Mix. Make twenty-four powders or tablets.
Dose one three times a day.

VII.—MEASLES, GERMAN OR ROSEOLA.

This is a mild, infectious disease, known also as false measles or roseola. It is characterized by an eruption upon the skin, resembling measles, associated with a slight catarrh and other mild disturbances. It occurs but once. It is largely a disease of childhood, for the simple reason that adults having had it previously are exempt. It has been regarded by some, as a combination of measles and scarlet fever. This, however, is a mistake, for it has no relation to either. It resembles measles simply in its spread and mode of contagion. The course of the disease is so mild, and its character so simple, that it has received far less attention than other contagious diseases.

SYMPTOMS.

About two weeks after exposure, an eruption appears upon the surface of the body, without much of any fever or other indications of sickness. The eruption lasts but a short time, varying from a few hours to a few days. The rash is less purple than that of measles, and less bright than that of scarlet fever. Other mild symptoms, may be slight nausea and soreness of tne throat. The sore throat resembles that of scarlet fever, but is much less severe. The tongue is somewhat coated, and there may be sneezing and other catarrhal symptoms affecting the eyes, causing dread of light, there is also a mild cough. The temperature is but slightly elevated, and all of the disturbances are much milder in type than a case of ordinary measles.

It is rare for the patient to be confined in bed. Little or no treatment is required, a mild laxative may be administered and simple herb teas, taking care to prevent catching cold.

VIII.—MUMPS OR PAROTIDITIS.

This is an acute, contagious disease, characterized by an inflammation of the parotid gland, which lies just below and in front of the external ear. It is a disease common to children and young persons between the ages of two and fifteen years. Infants and old people are more or less exempt. The infecting agent or germ, has not yet been recognized. Epidemics of this disease are common in the spring and fall of the year, proving that cold and dampness have some influence in its production. Mumps ordinarily are mild, lasting only a few days and tending to recovery. Three stages are noticed. The first is the stage of incubation, and lasts from the exposure till the occurrence of sickness, a period of about fourteen days. The second is the stage of invasion, and lasts from twelve to twenty-four hours. The third is the active duration of the disease and occupies a period of three or four days. Recovery requires four or five days more.

SYMPTOMS.

The early symptoms are chills of a mild type; the patient appears pale and languid, complains of pain in the head and breast, with loss of appetite. Other symptoms of a marked character soon follow. There is rise of temperature; pain on moving the jaw; and the taking of acids into the mouth produces a peculiar pain. Vomiting or diarrhœa, restlessness or convulsions may occur. The pain increases if the patient moves the jaw, for the glands swell rapidly and form large lumps below the ear, pushing the lower lobe outward while the neck and cheeks are involved.

The swelling may begin first on one side, but during the attack both sides are usually affected. If both sides are much swollen, the patient holds the head stiffly and is unable to turn one way or the other without severe pain. The swollen neck, eyes and cheeks, alter the usual expression very much, and the patient, being destitute of the usual play of the expression, with the mouth open from which the saliva drains away, presents a stupid and almost idiotic appearance. Sometimes the amount of swelling is quite extensive. The patient is unable to eat, preferring to endure hunger and thirst, rather than experience the pain caused by taking nourishment. The tongue is coated; there is an increased flow of saliva; the pulse is more rapid than normal and the temperature is somewhat elevated.

If the tonsils are also swollen and enlarged, the patient breathes heavily and snores when he sleeps. After four or five days these symptoms subside, improvement follows rapidly and in four or five days more the patient is well.

Sometimes an abscess forms which opens on the inside of the cheek, but this result is rare. The disease is sometimes followed by a secondary inflammation in some remote part, as the breasts and ovaries in the female and the testicles in the male.

TREATMENT.

The treatment for mumps is simple. Patients should avoid taking cold. The diet should consist of beef tea, milk, gruel, broths and other suitable liquid food. The bowels should be kept open, using the citrate or sulphate of magnesia. Water, ice, lemonade and cream of tartar water may be allowed as needed to allay thirst. For the fever, tincture of aconite may be given, as in other febrile conditions, till sweating or moisture of the skin is produced.

Apply the following to the swelling:

℞ Tinct. opium   one dram
    Olive oil   one ounce

Mix. Use three or four times a day externally. Hot water dressings and hot poultices do good. Should the swelling become chronic, paint it each night and morning with the tincture of iodine. Hot foot baths containing mustard are good in the early stages of the disease. In scrofulous subjects, when recovery is prolonged, a one-grain pill of the iodide of iron may be used three times a day. If much debility follows an attack, cod liver oil is a good remedy to build up the system. To the tonsils, if much inflamed, may be applied a healing and astringent lotion as follows:

℞ Carbolic acid   ten grains
    Glycerine   one ounce
    Syr. acacia   half an ounce
    Chlorate of potash (saturated solution)   two and one-half ounces
    Tinct. of myrrh   one dram

Mix. Gargle the throat every two hours.

IX.—SCARLET FEVER OR SCARLATINA.

Scarlet fever and scarlatina are terms applied to the same disease. It receives its name from the scarlet color which it imparts to the patient. The disease is caused by contagious germs which gain admission in some way to the system. It never occurs apart from this specific principle. It is difficult often to trace it, when it appears to break out anew in some community where it has not existed for years, but in these cases it has come silently and unbidden, adhering to some book, piece of cloth, article of food, clothing or merchandise that has come to the family from some infected point.

This disease has been carried a long distance in a letter through the mails and been transported by means of milk from the family of the milkman. It may be carried in the hair, the whiskers, the clothing or the leaves of a book. The contagious germs may exist indefinitely in the meshes of a carpet or adhere to the paper on the walls of a room. They may be stored away in the attic with some doll or plaything and be brought forth at some future day, as vigorous as ever, to attack another victim after months or years. This disease has a short period of incubation, during which the patient feels as well as ever and has no reason to fear approaching sickness. This period varies from one to four days. The period of invasion lasts about one day.

SYMPTOMS.

The first symptom is usually a chill or chilly sensation, quickly followed by fever, with high temperature and rapid pulse; the skin is hot; the eyes are bright; the pupils enlarged and face flushed. Vomiting is rarely absent; there is usually great thirst, and sometimes stupor and delirium. The mouth and throat become rapidly inflamed and the papillæ of the tongue are enlarged. After these symptoms have lasted a few hours the eruption appears. The body looks as though it had been reddened with a strong mustard plaster, or like a boiled lobster. It is covered with a fine scarlet-colored rash, which disappears in a line when you draw your finger over the surface, but at once reappears. The rash causes a burning or itching sensation, very annoying to the patient. The stage of eruption lasts from three to six days, but reaches its height on about the third day. The temperature goes up to one hundred and one degrees, or perhaps as high as one hundred and four in very severe cases. The skin is hot; the lips are dry; and the patient is restless. The inflammation in the mouth and throat continue and the patient calls urgently and repeatedly for drink. The urine is highly colored. In favorable cases, the temperature declines after the eruption is fully established, and marked improvement is manifest. At the end of this eruptive stage the rash has faded away; the redness of the mouth and swelling of the throat subside; the appetite begins to return; the countenance brightens and the child takes an interest in objects that he has previously refused to notice. Next follows the stage of desquamation or peeling. This lasts five or six days, sometimes much longer. The skin peels off from the hands and feet in scales. If the rash has been slight, the peeling process will also be slight, but when the rash has been severe, peeling of the entire body occurs. There are other types of the disease, more prolonged and severe than that described. This disease has every type of manifestation, from very mild, to the most malignant sickness.

It is hardly to be expected that a severe type of scarlet fever with complications can be treated with household remedies. The onset of this disease is sometimes violent. There is great restlessness, twitching of the tendons, sometimes delirium and convulsions. In some cases there is irritability of the stomach, and the food and medicine necessary to sustain the strength and make an impression upon the disease are at once rejected. Sometimes the whole force of the disease, seems to attack the nervous system and acts with frightful energy, prostrating the vital forces with great rapidity, like a case of severe blood poisoning. Large swellings may appear on each side of the neck. The ear is sometimes involved, and discharges pus, with destruction of the tissues and loss of hearing. Diphtheria sometimes complicates scarlet fever.

Sometimes the kidneys become more or less disabled and dropsy manifests itself. This condition may arise from too early exposure, the patient being permitted to leave his room too soon. Albumen may appear in the urine and urea accumulate in the blood, presenting grave symptoms. Cases otherwise mild, that have progressed favorably and that have promised speedy recovery, may be complicated and the recovery prolonged. The patient should be kept in doors and exposure avoided, until full recovery has taken place and the stage of desquamation is complete.

TREATMENT.

Belladonna has been recommended to prevent scarlet fever, but it appears to have no power whatever to do so. The following treatment is adapted only to ordinary and uncomplicated cases.

The room occupied by a scarlet fever patient should be well ventilated without subjecting the patient to the danger of catching cold. The temperature should be kept at about seventy-two degrees. For the throat inflammation the chlorine mixture may be used. See treatment of diphtheria. This mixture is to be gargled every hour and a teaspoonful taken internally every two hours. Camphorated oil may be applied to the swollen glands in the neck. Quinine and phenacetine may be given to reduce the temperature. See treatment of measles for formula. The body may be sponged over with warm water and alcohol, after which the itching and burning of the skin may be relieved by the use of carbolized vaseline as follows:

℞ Carbolic acid   one-half dram
    Vaseline   four ounces

Mix. Apply over the entire surface of the body as needed to relieve the skin of itching.

The diet should consist of milk, gruel and light articles of food. An excellent drink in fevers is made by dissolving a teaspoonful of cream of tartar in a pint bowl of hot water, adding lemon juice and sugar to taste. Stimulants may be required. Sweet spirits of nitre may be used as a diuretic. In cases of threatened dropsy, one-twentieth of a grain of pilocarpin may be given three or four times a day. This remedy causes profuse perspiration and aids the kidneys in the work of eliminating the poison.

In the treatment of scarlet fever the septic character of the disease should be borne in mind, and in all severe cases the bichloride treatment as recommended for diphtheria, alternated with the chlorine mixture is appropriate.

X.—WHOOPING COUGH OR PERTUSSIS.

This is an acute contagious disease of uncertain duration, often lasting six weeks or more, depending somewhat upon the season of the year. Its course is more brief when contracted in the spring; warm weather and out-of-doors life being favorable to recovery. It occurs but once in a lifetime, usually in childhood, but it may be contracted by persons of any age.

SYMPTOMS.

These are a catarrhal condition of the air passages and a nervous paroxysmal cough which is easily recognized. The characteristic whoop occurs during the paroxysms of coughing. The cough is rapid, the breathing is obstructed by the spasmodic condition at the entrance of the windpipe, the child turns blue in the face, the eyes are congested and bulge from the head, and tears flow unbidden from the eyes. Previous to a paroxysm of coughing the child usually runs and seizes hold of some neighboring object for support. At the close of coughing the spasm relaxes and air is powerfully drawn into the lungs with a whooping sound. The characteristic whoop may occur several times during a fit of coughing. The cough reaches its height about the third or fourth week, after which, there is some decline in its frequency and severity.

When there are but two or three paroxysms of coughing during the day, the case is mild and the health suffers but little. When they run up to thirty or forty during the twenty-four hours, the case is severe and demands earnest attention. Vomiting is common during the spasms of coughing, and ruptures have been known to result from the severe strain upon the abdominal walls.

Whooping cough is often a severe ordeal for young persons of slender build, or weakly and poorly nourished children. Death rarely results from whooping cough, except when there are complications, which affect the lungs or brain. Pneumonia is the most unfavorable and frequent complication with young children.

Whooping cough is conveyed from one to another, by contact sufficiently close to inhale the breath. The time of incubation between the exposure and the appearance of the first symptom is from one to three weeks. It comes on like a cold or some catarrhal affection. This condition lasts several days, sometimes two weeks, during which time the eyes are heavy and the conjunctiva congested, there is more or less cough and expectoration, with loss of appetite and slight fever, as in a case of acute bronchitis. These symptoms occur before the character of the disease can be determined; for the paroxysmal cough and whoop are the only symptoms which render the diagnosis certain.

TREATMENT.

During the catarrhal stage the same remedies may be used as for an ordinary cold. Avoid exposure, as colds increase the severity of the attack. Should the lungs be loaded with mucous which the child is unable to raise, an emetic may be necessary to loosen it. Half teaspoonful doses of the syrup of ipecac. will accomplish this result without depressing the system. If there is some fever the following prescription is suitable to use:

℞ Syr. squill comp.   two drams
  Tinct. aconite   sixteen drops
  Paregoric   two drams
  Syr. tolu.   half an ounce
  Anise water q. s. to make   two ounces

Mix. Dose: half a teaspoonful for a child a year old, increasing or diminishing it as age or circumstances require.

Lobelia has been highly recommended in whooping cough and from its antispasmodic action, excellent results may be expected from its use, after the disease is recognized. Thirty drops of the tincture may be added to half a glass of water. Dose: one teaspoonful every hour or two. It is claimed by some, that quinine in full doses will arrest this disease.

Atropia often acts beneficially. Dissolve one tablet containing one $\frac{1}{100}$ of a grain in ten teaspoonfuls of water. Give one teaspoonful of this to a child a year old three or four times a day.

After the catarrhal stage has subsided, the child should be allowed to go out of doors in good weather. One of the best remedies in the spasmodic stage is chloral, in small and repeated doses, combined with bromide of potash as follows:

℞ Chloral	one-half dram
Bromide of potash	two drams
Syr. tolu.	one ounce
Anise water	two ounces

Mix. Dose half a teaspoonful to a child one year old, and a full teaspoonful for a child two years old, and repeat every two or three hours as needed. These remedies allay the spasm, relieve the cough and favor sleep, and when administered properly, the result is surprising. In all cases the coming of spring, a change of air or the sea air when available, act beneficially. The ammoniacal odors of gas works are said to be curative. A spray of carbolic acid solution is worth trying. Ten drops of carbolic acid should be added to an ounce of rose water and an ounce of glycerine. Spray this frequently into the mouth from an atomizer or load the air of the apartment with it for inhalation. Cod liver oil in the form of a palatable emulsion is good in cases of prolonged recovery.

Whooping cough is not only tedious and debilitating, but frequently fatal to children under two years of age, from some complication, hence it is wise to avoid the exposure of such children to it. Vaccination, as ordinarily performed, appears to modify the severity of the disease and is worthy of trial. This is probably owing to the fact that different disease germs sometimes antagonize each other.

XI.—DISINFECTION DURING AND AFTER DIPHTHERIA AND SCARLET FEVER.

After diphtheria or scarlet fever has invaded a household, it is important to know just what ought to be done to prevent its spread.

The patient should be quarantined in an upper room. The lower rooms will then be comparatively safe. Well children, if possible, should be sent away before they have been exposed to the contagion. If this is impossible they should be kept down stairs and away from the sick room.

They must not be allowed to attend school. The nurse ought not to mingle with the other members of the family. As little furniture should be allowed in the room occupied by the patient as possible, and that of the plainest kind. Carpets and stuffed furniture are to be excluded, as they furnish a lodging place for disease germs. The sick room should have some arrangement for ventilation, as a board placed under the bottom of the window to admit air between the sashes in cold weather. In warm weather, freer ventilation may be allowed by opening doors and windows, remembering always to keep the patient out of the way of a draught.

Disinfectant solutions should be used freely in and about the sick chamber. Cloths wet in these solutions and hung about the room are helpful. The patient can be sponged over with alcohol and rubbed with carbolized vaseline. This prevents the scales of the body from flying about, and is soothing to the patient when there is an eruption, as in scarlet fever.

The bedding, pillow cases, sheets, night dresses and other articles worn by and used about the patient should be changed frequently. The soiled clothing ought to be put into boiling water immediately and boiled for ten minutes. The bed clothing used by the nurse should be treated in the same manner. Everything that can be submitted to boiling water is rendered safe to use without the addition of chemicals, as boiling water destroys disease germs. For the discharges of the patient, dissolve two drams of corrosive sublimate and two drams of permanganate of potash in one gallon of soft water and use as follows.

Keep a little in the chamber, and when the patient has a movement, add to it a pint or more of this disinfectant solution. Let it stand for a short time and disinfection will have taken place. A carbolic acid or copperas solution should be used in the closet and urinals.

When the patient has sufficiently recovered, still more thorough methods of disinfection should be instituted. Playthings and valueless articles or articles of slight value should be burned and never thrown into the rubbish or into a running brook. Other articles should be subjected to the fumes of burning sulphur in a thorough manner.

Place a tub in the infected room with three inches of water in it. Put three or four bricks in the bottom of the tub, and on the bricks place an iron kettle. Into this kettle put two or three pounds of roll brimstone broken into fragments. Set it on fire by means of coals from the stove or a little alcohol and a match. Close the room tightly and fumigate it thoroughly for thirty-six hours, then throw open the room and ventilate it thoroughly. Afterwards wash the floors with hot soap suds. Repaper or repaint the walls and woodwork. Repaper or whitewash the ceiling. This work should be thoroughly done in order to destroy the innumerable and invisible germs which cause these infectious diseases. In addition to the fumigation of the room occupied by the patient, the whole house should be looked over, and attention paid to its sanitary condition. Everything in and about the house should be cleansed, as furniture, clothing, carpets and curtains. The cellar should receive most careful attention. Foul air, mould and dust should be cast out. Every room and its contents, from attic to cellar, should be cleansed and no dark corner or neglected spot be allowed to escape. The whole house should be cleansed, aired and ventilated.

Different disease germs require somewhat different methods for their extermination, but the same general principles apply to all.

After small pox it is better to destroy all the infected clothing and bedding by fire, as they are not worth the effort which would be necessary for their complete disinfection.

It is believed that under each disease sufficient directions are given for proper disinfection in every instance, but diphtheria and scarlet fever are diseases of such importance, that a special article on the necessary precautions will no doubt be appreciated. See bacteria or germs in disease.

CHAPTER XXVIII.

FEVERS.

I.—Bilious or Remittent Fever. II.—Malarial or Intermittent Fever. III.—Catarrhal Fever, Influenza or La Grippe. IV.—Neuralgic Fever or Dengue. V.—Typhoid Fever. VI.—Typhus Fever. VII.—Yellow Fever. VIII.—Puerperal Fever.

I.—BILIOUS OR REMITTENT FEVER.

THIS is a continued malarial fever, due to malarial poisoning, but is very severe. The symptoms are influenced by a disordered state of the liver, there being an excess of bile which occasions persistent vomiting, and for this reason it is called bilious fever. It prevails in malarial regions in the summer and fall, and manifests every type of severity. It is sometimes called typho-malarial fever.

SYMPTOMS.

These are fever, hot, dry skin, high temperature, offensive breath, a yellow coated tongue, nausea with vomiting, headache and chills. The vomited matter is composed chiefly of mucous and bile. On alternate days the symptoms usually abate somewhat, the skin becomes moist and the temperature declines. On the following day another chill occurs, succeeded by a rise of temperature. The patient is uneasy and restless at night, tossing and moaning. If the case is a grave one, the fever pursues a more persistent course and delirium is common. There is often hemorrhage from the nose; the tongue is dry; there is tenderness over the liver and spleen; the skin has a yellow hue, a condition which suggests jaundice, especially noticeable in the whites of the eyes. The urine is scanty and very highly colored. This condition may persist for a couple of weeks, when the symptoms abate in favorable cases, and the patient recovers. After recovery sores often break out about the mouth and lips. In malarial districts this disease is often severe, and takes on a form resembling yellow fever, which may terminate fatally.

TREATMENT.

A generous dose of quinine taken every morning before going out of doors is said to prevent attacks of bilious fever. In regions where this fever prevails in the fall, and quinine is usually relied upon to prevent it, the dose must be generous, five or ten grains each morning. When the fever is established it requires the same treatment as malarial fever or fevers in general. Remedies which act upon the liver are beneficial. The following is serviceable:

℞ Quinine   one dram
    Salol   one scruple
    Podophyllin   two grains
    Oleo-resin of ginger   ten drops

Mix. Make into twenty pills or capsules.

Dose one each night and morning. Acid drinks are often relished by the patient, as lemon juice, jelly water, cream of tartar water, and other similar and cooling drinks.

The mineral acids, well diluted, are often made use of in the treatment of this fever. Fowler's solution, in three drop doses, is a good tonic during recovery, and may be used in connection with quinine to prevent its recurrence.

II.—MALARIAL OR INTERMITTENT FEVER.

This disease is caused by a specific poison or germ which may enter the system in several ways, but chiefly by an infected malarial atmosphere. It may gain admittance to the system by means of the food and water supply, especially water and milk which are contaminated with malarial poison. After a period of exposure of longer or shorter duration, averaging about thirty days, the affection begins to manifest itself.

SYMPTOMS.

The symptoms are many and various, but the following are those more common and more readily recognized. The appetite is fitful, food producing sometimes a sudden nausea, followed by vomiting before the meal is finished. Digestion is deranged; headache is common, and pain in the back, back of the neck and limbs or elsewhere about the body. The tongue is pale and perhaps coated; the bowels are usually constipated, but sometimes the opposite condition is observed. Dizziness may occur; the countenance has a sallow look; the urine is highly colored, almost as if mixed with blood. Chilly sensations are experienced over the surface of the body, or creeping down the spine; the skin is pallid and little elevations known as goose flesh may be seen. Yawning may occur and decided shivering. The teeth chatter; the patient feels cold and shakes with chills, even though warm drinks are taken, hot applications applied externally, and blankets multiplied over him. Nausea and vomiting may continue, and the pain in the head and limbs increase. This is a description of the cold stage. The symptoms narrated may be more or less marked. Other symptoms may be noticed or some of those enumerated may be wanting. This stage lasts only a short time, varying from half an hour to two hours, during which, the circulation of the blood is much disturbed. It is driven inward, and with every chill there is more or less congestion of the internal organs, while the external surface is well nigh bloodless.

Soon reaction takes place and the patient begins to get warm. The blood returns to the surface and the equilibrium is somewhat restored. The face, so recently pale, begins to be flushed, the eyes blood shot, the veins fill up and appear turgid, the patient complains of headache, heat and thirst. The temperature rises rapidly, and the skin is hot and dry. Should the temperature run very high, there is usually marked restlessness and delirium. The patient seems burning with fever and calls for cold water, and the bedclothes are thrown off. This describes the hot or fever stage, and the two together are known as chills and fever, fever and ague or the shakes. The hot stage lasts from two to four hours, when profuse sweating followed by a decline of the temperature takes place. The delirium disappears and the patient feels much relieved, the attack being ended for the present, only to return with greater vigor in a couple of days unless prevented by treatment. This state of affairs might go on almost indefinitely at fixed intervals, but most commonly every other day.

TREATMENT.

When the chill follows a hearty meal, if vomiting does not occur spontaneously, it is a good idea to unload the stomach with an emetic, as digestion is impossible. Warm water, warm mustard water, or the syrup of ipecac, are suitable to accomplish this purpose. Blankets should be allowed as desired, and warm infusions may be given. Hot cloths wrung from mustard water may be applied over the stomach or elsewhere as needed. Bottles filled with hot water may be placed at the feet or along the spine, to assist in restoring the circulation and give comfort to the patient. Alcoholic stimulants seldom do good, and may do harm. They should not be administered unless, for some reason, their use is necessary.

The best remedy, because the most prompt to relieve the severe pain and distress in these cases, is from one-sixth to one-fourth of a grain of morphine combined with atropia and given hypodermically. This soon relieves the pain in all parts of the body. In family practice, it may be given by the mouth if the stomach will tolerate it, or in place of it a five or ten grain dose of Dover's or Tully's powder could be administered with similar results. To children suffering from violent pain, a one or two grain dose of Tully's powder may be given; or a cup of herb or ginger tea with a few drops of paregoric may be administered. Cream of tartar lemonade, hot or cold, may be freely used. It favors sweating and increases the eliminative action of the kidneys and bowels.

As soon as the hot stage subsides, a generous dose of quinine, five to twenty grains, may be given to prevent the return of a similar or more severe attack. One or two grains three times a day is sufficient for a child a year old. To such patients it may be given with the cream of tartar lemonade or in liquid form as follows:

℞ Quinine   half a dram
   Syr. of liquorice   two ounces

Mix. Dose a teaspoonful three times a day. This makes a palatable prescription out of a bitter drug.

After an attack of malarial fever and chills, the patient is usually more or less debilitated, and requires the administration of medicine to eliminate the remaining poison and restore health. The following prescription is an excellent one, and has cured many cases debilitated by malarial poison.

℞ Quinine   one dram
   Reduced iron   ten grains
   Ext. nux vomica   four grains
   Podophyllin   one grain
   Oleo-resin of ginger   ten grains

Mix. Make into twenty pills. Dose one pill three times a day after meals.

The following prescription may be used for children one year old and upward, who need building up after attacks of chills and fever.

℞	Quinia muriate	twenty-four grains
	Fowler's solution	half a dram
	Elix. calisaya	one ounce
	Syr. liquorice	two ounces

Mix. Dose one teaspoonful three times a day after meals.

III.—CATARRHAL FEVER, INFLUENZA OR LA GRIPPE.

This is an acute, epidemic, catarrhal fever which at times has prevailed over wide sections of the globe, attacking a large number of persons almost simultaneously. Its history shows that it is no new disease. In the fifth century it prevailed in Europe, and since that time its history has been frequently recorded. It has always approached our own country, advancing from the East. In 1890 it swept around the world with great rapidity and again appeared in the years 1891 and 1892, rendering its history and course to us of universal interest. It prostrated thousands, increased the death rate enormously, and left its depressing effects behind it for a long time. It paralyzed business to a great extent, and checked the progress of many enterprises. Its character at first was but little known. It was more carefully studied after its arrival, and proved to be a more debilitating and fatal disease than had been supposed. Many people in the decline of life succumbed to its ravages.

SYMPTOMS.

The symptoms are numerous. The onset is usually sudden, the patient being seized with chilly sensations and nervous chills, alternating with hot flashes and a marked tendency to internal congestion. These nervous chills are followed by high temperature, and pains of an intense character, as headache, lumbago, pain in the limbs and elsewhere throughout the body. The patient is uneasy and complains of aching in every bone. The flesh is sore as if it had been mauled. Even the eyeballs and the scalp are sensitive to pressure and there is often tenderness over the spine.

The sense of taste and smell may be disturbed. In severe cases delirium is common, and in a few instances meningitis or insanity have been known to result. The disease sometimes begins with sneezing, a hoarse cough and other symptoms of a sudden cold. There is a catarrhal condition of the mucous membranes and well-marked bronchitis, as in measles. At first the pulse and temperature may be but little altered; the patient complains of feeling chilly, even when in a warm room or seated near the fire. The inflammation of the mucous membranes is well marked. There is redness of the throat and bronchial breathing. Acute bronchitis or pneumonia are some of the diseases to be most dreaded as complications. Sometimes there is constant nausea and vomiting, and a tongue resembling typhoid fever. The liver is torpid and the bowels constipated. The skin may be sallow, the eyes yellow, and the urine scanty and highly colored.

In all cases marked nervous symptoms may be observed. There is loss of strength, an unexpected and unaccountable debility, the lower limbs being scarcely able to sustain the weight of the body. There is pain at the pit of the stomach, severe neuralgic pains, with well marked prostration and a peculiar tendency to heart failure in severe cases.

TREATMENT.

This disease is modified when treated early and efficiently, and its entire character changed. When neglected mild cases may develop into severe ones, and grave complications are liable to occur, entailing fatal results.

Rest should be enforced. This is imperative. The pain must receive attention. This sometimes yields to the administration of phenacetine or acetanilid in five grain doses, and repeated every two or four hours. When the pain is severe and the prostration well marked there is no better remedy than morphia. One-eighth of a grain may be given by the mouth, or if there is nausea hypodermically. In many cases double the amount is required to relieve the pain.

Morphia is a powerful nerve stimulant and strengthens the heart's action, hence it is the remedy above all others for pain in cases of depressed vitality. Quinine administered early in full dose may practically abort the disease. It may be combined with other helpful remedies as phenacetine or morphia, thus:

R   Quinine   thirty grains
     Phenacetine   thirty grains
     Morphine   one or two grains

Mix. Make twelve pills or capsules. Dose one every four hours in the acute stage.

The liver should be gently moved to action by a safe cathartic.

Expectorants may be needed as in bronchitis. Stimulants may be required in cases of excessive prostration, or when the patient is old or especially debilitated, or suffering from some other disease, so that recovery is retarded.

Camphor is well spoken of as a stimulant in this disease, and opium is a remarkably reliable stimulant to the cerebro spinal nerves. Digitalis is a valuable heart stimulant.

Acetanilid, antipyrine and phenacetine are capable of working mischief in unskillful hands, but are safe and reliable agents to relieve pain and reduce fever if used in the first stages, before the system is depressed by the disease. Their effects must be closely watched. After effects of the grip require tonics, such as quinine, iron and nux vomica, malt and a judicious diet.

Complications must be met as they arise and a relapse avoided. The disease possesses the most danger for old persons of feeble circulation and delicate health, and such patients require faithful care and attention. Recovery is sometimes retarded by a chronic discharge of pus from the middle ear, otitis media.

For an attack in a person of robust constitution the following prescription is recommended as combining suitable remedies.

R   Quinine sulph.   one dram
    Phenacetine   two and one-half scruples
    Tully powder   two scruples

Mix. Make into twenty pills or capsules. Dose one every four hours.

A mustard plaster applied over the chest when there is pain or hoarseness in that region, or symptoms which indicate bronchitis or pneumonia will afford no little relief. The diet should be simple and nutritious.

IV.—NEURALGIC FEVER OR DENGUE.

This is an acute febrile disease of malarial origin which occurs in the southern states. It reached as far north as Philadelphia in 1780. It resembles "La Grippe" in some respects. It is sometimes called breakbone fever.

SYMPTOMS.

These are chills and fever, flushed face, coated tongue with bitter taste in the mouth. Vomiting, diarrhœa and cramps may occur. Severe pain is experienced in the knees, ankles, wrists, fingers, toes, head and back, with marked soreness of the muscles and joints. Whole households are often down with it at the same time. In a couple of days the severity of the fever and the intensity of the pain subside. After about a week, a rash resembling scarlet fever appears, though somewhat darker in color and more in patches. Just before the outbreak of the rash the fever returns, but disappears again after the eruption is established. The disease lasts a little over a week, and leaves the patient prostrated, with marked symptoms of debility. In young children it may cause convulsions.

TREATMENT.

The pain may be relieved by morphia hypodermically or a five or ten grain dose of Dover's powder, or for a child, a two to five grain dose of Tully's powder, according to the age. A cathartic to move the bowels and arouse the liver is essential. Quinine should be given freely to allay the fever and antidote the septic nature of the disease.

For itching of the skin, carbolized water or vaseline, ten or twenty grains to the ounce, affords relief. For subsequent debility, use the medicines recommended for debility following La Grippe. In the fever stage the prescriptions given for the treatment of malarial and catarrhal fever are appropriate, and need not be repeated.

V.—TYPHOID FEVER.

This is an acute, infectious disease, which lasts from three to four weeks. It does not come on suddenly like scarlet fever or La Grippe, but gradually. It is a week after the first feeling of illness before the disease is fully developed. It is caused by disease germs and never occurs spontaneously. The germs multiply in the bowels and perhaps in the urine of the person suffering from the disease, causing fever of a high grade, and marked prostration of the vital forces. The germs of typhoid attack the glands of the bowels and cause them to inflame and sometimes to ulcerate. It is not contagious form person to person, and typhoid patients are admitted to hospitals without fear of spreading the disease. The period from exposure, to the onset of the disease, averages about three weeks. Young people are more likely to contract it than mature persons. It is more prevalent in the fall than at other seasons, and on this account is sometimes called autumn fever. Hot dry seasons, when the water supplies run low, increase the number of cases. See bacteria or germs in disease, drainage and sewerage, and the other sanitary subjects, for origin of typhoid fever.

SYMPTOMS.

For several days the patient feels ill with vague symptoms, as headache, aching pains in the body, especially the back and limbs, with nausea, vomiting and sometimes profuse diarrhœa. The stools are thin, watery, and of a light ochre color. The pulse is quick, the skin hot and dry, the tongue coated, and sooner or later marked tenderness from pressure upon the abdomen, especially upon the right side is observed. These symptoms continue to increase, until the patient gives up and takes his bed. The patient is restless and wakeful, grows weaker constantly, and in severe cases may appear dull and slightly deaf.

The diarrhœa increases in severity, the abdomen seems full and bloated. Gurgling sounds are heard in the bowels, and bleeding from the nose is common during the first week. By the close of the first week the temperature may reach a hundred and two, or a hundred and four degrees. The fever thermometer is an excellent guide to the severity of the attack. See temperature in disease. The urine is scanty, thick and highly colored. The eye is bright, the temperature is high, the skin dry and the cheeks red and burning.

In most cases a rose-colored rash appears about the twelfth day over the abdomen and chest. These spots disappear under pressure from the hand.

In severe cases there is an intensity of the symptoms, the tongue gets brown and dry, and perhaps so fissured as to bleed; the pulse is rapid and feeble from exhaustion. The temperature is more elevated and the diarrhœa becomes persistent. The nervous system manifests symptoms of marked disturbance. There may be mutterings or acute delirium. In these severe cases where the nervous symptoms are aggravated, the limbs tremble and the protrusion of the tongue is difficult and trembling.

Unfavorable cases are liable to terminate in hemorrhage or perforation of the bowels. There is liable to be great variation of the symptoms in different cases.

Mild cases occur in which the patient feels ill, has headache, but keeps about. These are known as walking cases of typhoid The most common symptom in nearly all cases is persistent diarrhœa.

The history of the temperature ordinarily is as follows :

It rises gradually for about seven days, remains nearly stationary for ten or twelve days more, when the fever declines and the temperature falls. There is a marked difference between the morning and evening temperature.

This disease is remarkably liable to complications, owing to which it may last from forty to sixty days. When it lasts over four weeks complications of some kind exist. Pneumonia is sometimes an unpleasant complication. There may be a relapse from injudicious food or exercise, taken before recovery. Hemorrhage of the bowels is sometimes a troublesome complication. Great care is required in the nursing of typhoid patients up to the time of complete recovery.

TREATMENT.

It ought to be known that typhoid fever runs a distinct course and cannot be broken up. A fever that yields quickly and readily to treatment is not typhoid. Caution is necessary for the patient not to use cathartics, as the mildest laxative acts with great energy, owing to the disturbed condition of the bowels. The patient should stay in bed, for to attempt to drag around as long as possible is not without danger. Some patients appear to have a dread of taking the bed, and think if they do so they are more likely to be seriously ill or to die. This is wholly a false notion.

If the bowels move more than three or four times a day they should be checked by a pill containing one grain each of opium and camphor, repeated as needed.

The diet should be liquid, and consist of milk, gruel or beef tea. Milk at the present time is considered the most appropriate article of food for fever patients. It may be combined with bread coffee, or lime water, when too hearty.

In ordinary cases very little medication is necessary, good nursing being more essential than medicine. When the temperature is high and the skin dry, the following prescription is appropriate:

℞	Quinine	two scruples
	Phenacetine	two scruples
	Salol	one scruple

Mix. Make into twenty powders or capsules.

Dose one every four hours. When there is troublesome nausea, six drops of carbolic acid in half a tumbler of water given in teaspoonful doses every hour, usually affords relief.

The patient must be restrained from going about too soon before recovery. It is wise to intrust the responsibility of a fever patient to some one, who is competent to watch developments and safely guide the patient past the signals of danger.

In order to prevent the spread of typhoid fever, it is necessary to know something of the source of infection. The stools from a sick person, without proper disinfection, should never be thrown out upon the soil, a compost heap, or near some stream of water. This disease could be banished as effectually as small pox by making a little effort. The infectious principle usually enters the system in the drinking water. This may be bright, sparkling, tasteless and free from odor, and yet contain disease germs in countless numbers. The germs leach through the soil and reach the water supply. They maintain their vitality for a long time. The stools of a tyhoid patient ought to be thoroughly disinfected, by which means, the danger will be averted.

VI.—TYPHUS FEVER.

This is a contagious fever of severe type, occurring rarely in this country. Up to the present century typhus fever was not distinguished from typhoid, both being regarded as the same and due to the same cause. In 1846 William Jenner made an investigation and arrived at the conclusion that they are two distinct and different diseases. The same view is held by all physicians at the present time. It has been known in the past by several names, as spotted, ship, famine, camp and jail fever. Severe epidemics of typhus fever have raged in the old world, where people have been crowded together and suffered for lack of food and the want of cleanliness. In 1846 it prevailed in Ireland, and was known as famine fever. This disease destroyed more soldiers in the army of Napoleon than the sword. It caused a frightful loss of life in the French and Russian armies in the Crimea. It breaks out among those who suffer from exposure and want, and in the poor quarters of the great cities where filth and misery abound.

The incubation of this disease requires about twelve days and it lasts from two to three weeks. Its onset is more sudden than that of typhoid.

SYMPTOMS.

The early symptoms are loss of appetite, headache, restlessness and chills. The symptoms increase rapidly, the patient soon takes his bed, has a peculiar expression, seems weary and dull, lies on the back, and is indifferent to his surroundings. The pulse is rapid, the skin dusky, the eyes dull and leaden, there is languor, moaning, and marked prostration. The tongue becomes brown, or even black, cracked and fissured. The temperature rises rapidly, reaching one hundred and three, four or more degrees. There is great thirst. The heart is weak; trembling and prostration are noticed. The body is covered with fine pink spots, which become brown, and have given to it the name of spotted fever. The body emits a very peculiar and unpleasant odor. The odor of the breath is offensive; the hearing is dull. The nervous system is profoundly impressed. In severe cases the patient cannot be aroused, and soon dies from exhaustion. In favorable cases the tongue moistens, the fever declines, sweating is noticed and the patient recovers rapidly.

TREATMENT.

This disease is feared by the nurse and physician, owing to its contagiousness. It cannot be shortened by treatment or broken up. The treatment consists in combating the severity of the symptoms. Appropriate nourishment is essential. After a time the patient cares for nothing but cold water. Then nourishment must be given like medicine, in small and repeated amounts, such as beef tea, broth, milk, custard, barley water, lemonade, carbolic acid water and stimulants. There is no specific line of treatment for this disease. It requires skill and treatment on general principles. Do not visit a person suffering from typhus fever, unless it is a necessity, and you are willing to contract the disease. The germs of contagion may be transmitted a short distance through the air. They are destroyed by the fumes of burning sulphur. Without a knowledge of sanitary science, a single case of typhus fever brought into a great city like New York, would be the beginning of a disease conflagration, which might sweep over the whole country.

VII.—YELLOW FEVER.

Formerly the port of Havana was never without yellow fever, and nearly every outbreak of this terrible disease has been traced from this starting point. It is entirely unlike typhoid, running its course in four days. It does not resemble malarial fever, which runs an indefinite course. It is a fever of hot countries, caused by disease germs. Certain conditions are essential to its development. Cold prevents it and checks its progress. It requires heat and moisture to assist in its propagation. It is rarely contracted the second time. The colored races are less susceptible to it than the whites, and with them it is less likely to prove fatal.

SYMPTOMS.

The attack comes on suddenly, three or four days after exposure, ushered in by a chill, pain in the back, nausea, vomiting and great thirst. After the chill the temperature rises to about one hundred and three degrees. The skin becomes dry, the face flushed, eyes congested, and pain is experienced in the limbs. The tongue is heavily coated, except about the edges. The fever rages for about three days, when a decline in the temperature takes place, and the patient feels so much relieved as to express a desire to have something to eat.

The mortality in this disease is great, but when the patient lives beyond the third or fourth day, the chances of recovery are improved. In severe cases the skin and whites of the eyes are yellow, and the vomited matter looks like coffee grounds, owing to hemorrhage from the mucous lining of the stomach.

TREATMENT.

The treatment needs only to be briefly outlined. It consists in combating the severity of the symptoms. The feet may be soaked in hot mustard water, a mustard poultice applied over the stomach, and sweating induced, in order to favor the elimination of the poison from the system. Mild cathartics and diuretics may be given with the same object in view. Soothing lotions may be applied to the head, ice allowed to allay thirst, and lime water and milk as the most suitable nourishment.

Nearly a fourth of those attacked by yellow fever die; hence, an outbreak is dreaded by any community. The germs of yellow fever attach themselves to woolen clothing, leather, sawdust, rotting wood, straw and the filth of dirty streets. The progress and spread of this disease resembles grease upon a piece of paper. Beginning in the filthy quarter of the city it extends in every direction, the infected circle becoming larger and wider each day. A tight board fence or brick wall arrests its progress. The danger of transporting yellow fever is very great, as will be seen from the following.

A young woman requested to have sent to her, a lock of her dead father's hair. It was placed in an envelope and folded in, and sent as requested. After a few weeks she examined it and showed it to another young lady, both of whom contracted the disease and died within six days.

VIII.—PUERPERAL OR CHILD BED FEVER.

Puerperal fever is an acute inflammatory disease, following child birth. It is due to the absorption of septic material, or the entrance of bacteria into the blood; hence, it is similar in its origin to surgical fever, and in its results, resembles blood poisoning.

The investigations of recent years have thrown much light upon the origin and nature of this disease. Formerly, it was very prevalent and fatal in the hospitals, before the importance of antiseptic treatment was understood. It was once the dread of the prospective mother and her medical attendant, but antiseptic measures have relegated this disease to oblivion, and at the present time its occurrence should be regarded in the majority of cases, as positive proof of incompetence on the part of the medical attendant. It can nearly always be prevented, and when it occurs; generally, some one has blundered in the simple performance of duty.

SYMPTOMS.

About three days after labor a chill occurs, ushering in a fever of high grade, accompanied by headache, restlessness and inability to sleep. There is usually some pain and swelling of the lower portion of the abdomen and sensitiveness upon pressure. The tongue is coated. There is nausea and vomiting, loss of appetite, and usually constipation, but sometimes looseness of the bowels. The secretion of milk is usually arrested and other secretions diminished.

TREATMENT.

Puerperal fever ought in every instance to be prevented, but when the septic germs which cause it have once entered the circulation, they are largely beyond reach, and the disease must be treated as the symptoms demand.

A measure so simple as the vaginal injection of a carbolic acid solution each day will prevent the development of septic poison. The directions are as follows: Mix half a dram of carbolic acid thoroughly with a pint of hot water. This solution is strong enough to prevent septic trouble. For cleansing purposes a solution of half the strength is sufficient. Its use should be continued for at least a week after confinement or until all discharges have ceased.

When the disease cannot be prevented, rest should be secured by a combination of morphia and chloral. The temperature should be reduced by the use of quinine and acetanilid. The patient's strength should be maintained by milk, animal broth and stimulants if needed. A flaxseed poultice or a turpentine stupe may be applied over the abdomen. Other measures should be made use of as needed.

CHAPTER XXIX.

NERVOUS DISEASES.

I.—EPILEPSY. II.—HYSTERIA. III.—CATALEPSY. IV.—ECSTACY. V.—CHOREA OR ST. VITUS DANCE. VI.—CONVULSIONS, FITS OR SPASMS.

I.—EPILEPSY.

EPILEPSY is a nervous disorder, closely allied to hysteria, and frequently associated with it. In attacks of epilepsy the patient usually falls and is unconscious, while in hysteria the patient is usually more or less conscious. In connection with falling, convulsions occur. The fit may last only a few minutes, and months may elapse before its recurrence. About fifty per cent. of all cases can be traced to a hereditary origin. Syphilis is thought to be an agent of some prominence in causing epilepsy. Some cases may be traced to falls and injuries, either recent or remote. Fright or the use of alcoholic liquors, may account for some cases. It has been known to follow meningitis, measles and scarlet fever. A disturbed condition of the sexual organs is generally mentioned among the causes. Diseases of the internal ear, and a large variety of other conditions, could be mentioned which are supposed to have some relation to this affection.

SYMPTOMS.

Before a seizure of epilepsy, some premonitory symptoms are usually experienced, as dizziness, headache, certain vague and confused feelings, drowsiness, irritability, a peculiar restlessness, a feeling of fear, and threatened danger, and a feeling of depression or exhilaration. Disorders of vision are common. The epileptic subject may see floods of light, balls of fire, or other brilliant displays. The attack may be preceded by a sense of suffocation, palpitation, roaring in the ears, and other vague disorders. Children sometimes manifest a disposition to fright. In mild cases there may be a simple change in the expression, a rolling upward of the eyes, a sudden cessation of the conversation, while the head may be thrown upward for a brief space, the lips momentarily convulse, and consciousness is briefly lost. The person thus affected may resume work, conversation, eating, or whatever he was doing at the time of the seizure, as if nothing had happened. In more severe cases the victim utters a scream and falls to the ground. Convulsions occur with frothing at the mouth, grinding of the teeth, biting of the tongue, and similar symptoms. The respiration is labored. The face, at first flushed, becomes pale. The attack may last a few minutes or half an hour, after which the patient is usually inclined to sleep. There is less danger from epilepsy even when of long duration, than from falling. Full recovery from genuine epilepsy rarely takes place. The most that can be done is to extend the intervals between the attacks.

TREATMENT.

During an attack, first, place the patient in a position of safety. See that respiration is unimpeded and that the patient is supplied with fresh air. Then place a few drops of nitrite of amyl upon a handkerchief and apply to the nose. This repeated a few times usually brings the patient quickly to consciousness. If the patient can be supplied with this remedy and use it during the premonitory symptoms, it will ward off an attack. The following prescription is a good one for epilepsy:

R   Bromide of soda   one ounce
    Fl. ext. ergot   two ounces
    Anise water   two ounces

Mix. Dose teaspoonful three or four times a day in water.

Medicines should be used to improve the general condition. A nutritious diet, good habits and regular methods of life, are important.

A ten-grain dose of chloral is sometimes necessary to produce sleep. The use of alcoholic liquors should be abandoned, moderation and self-government should be maintained.

II.—HYSTERIA.

This is an affection which, though difficult to define, is known to be a functional disease of the brain and spinal cord. The methods of manifestation are numerous and varied. The causes of this affection are often vague and obscure. It may occur at any age, but is more common between fifteen and thirty. It occurs among the rich and poor and in every condition of life. Females are much more liable to hysteria than males. The ratio is estimated as fifty to one. Among the causes, heredity has been considered important. Occupations which are uncongenial, may so irritate the nervous system, and studies at school so overtax and harass a sensitive brain, as to predispose to hysteria.

Educators, rarely consider sufficiently the wide difference in the intellectual capacity of those entrusted to their care. Some have little or no taste for mathematics or are terrified by a problem in geometry. Others have no ability to remember dates or abstract facts; yet they must all pursue the same course as those who have a liking and faculty for such things. The slow scholar is urged on to keep pace with the more active, and those physically weak must be prodded, shamed or ridiculed, to make them keep up with the strong.

With the dreaded examinations always approaching, is it any wonder that many suffer from overwork and become the victims of nervous disorders? The brain is a complex organ, and especially liable to suffer from modern methods of educational work. Anæmia, chlorosis, and disorders of menstruation are some of the causes of hysteria in young women.

The pregnant condition may so disturb the nervous system as to develop it. Any irritation in any part of the body, any special strain or exhaustion of the nervous system, especially on the part of those who are previously disposed, may be the means of causing hysteria.

SYMPTOMS.

These have no order in their manifestation. They present an unusual variety, including thousands of strange actions and proceedings. Among the common symptoms are the sensation of a ball or lump rising up in the throat, and impeding the respiration, crying, moaning, laughing, shrieking, spasms and insensibility to pain. Sometimes appearances are feigned, in order to excite sympathy. It is common for a physician to be awakened at night by some excited messenger, who reports that somebody is dying, and he is urged to make all possible haste. Upon his arrival he may find a case of hysteria without the least suggestion of danger to him.

TREATMENT.

The ignorance or foolishness of the patient's friends is often the most annoying thing encountered by the physician in these nervous cases. They are sure that some grave or fatal inflammation or some dreadful malady exists, and that the doctor fails utterly to comprehend the situation.

Hygienic measures are essential. The will power must be strengthened, and moral influences made use of, by parents and educators. Children should be taught to control their nervous emotions by the will. Morbid fancies, false ideas and notions should be scouted and the follies of fashion and society sensibly prohibited. Emotional excitements as developed by novel reading should be guarded against. Food, sleep, exercise and recreation should receive special attention. Fatigue, anxiety, overstudy and all depressing and exhausting influences should be avoided. In a few cases, harsh measures have proved beneficial, but they should be employed, if at all, with great caution and good judgment. If the condition of anæmia exists, it ought to be remedied by increased nutrition, physical exercise and iron tonics.

In the convulsions of hysteria, three or four drops of nitrite of amyl, inhaled upon the handkerchief, often affords speedy relief, and it may be repeated as occasion requires. A pill of assafœtida is a remedy of considerable value in hysterical cases, and may be given three or four times a day. Massage and electricity may do good.

The patient should be encouraged to expect a speedy cure, for hope and faith are essential in the treatment of these cases. The patient should be encouraged to exercise and cultivate the will power. These patients are much benefited by relying upon those persons who are strong in character, who can influence them to disregard trifles and exercise strength and determination.

Tablets of sodium and gold chloride, in doses of one-twentieth of a grain, are beneficial. The bromide of soda may be given in doses of from three to thirty grains. The following is often beneficial:

    ℞   Elix. valerianate of ammonia   four ounces

Dose one teaspoonful three or four times a day.

III.—CATALEPSY.

This is a rare nervous affection, quite similar to hysteria, but differing in some particulars. It is usually a disease of females between the ages of fifteen and thirty, and due to nearly the same causes as hysteria.

SYMPTOMS.

The seizure comes on suddenly, perhaps with some premonitory symptoms as hiccough, the victim becomes rigid and as immovable as if petrified. The temperature, respiration and pulse are diminished. The patient looks pallid and composed. If changed from one position to another she remains in the new position, no matter how uncomfortable, just as if moulded there. This is the most characteristic symptom. In some cases the patient is unable to move or speak, but is conscious of everything that is going on about her. There may be no sensibility to pain. This condition may continue for a few minutes, several hours or days. When returning to the normal condition, the patient arouses, yawns and appears as if waking from a long sleep. This condition is sometimes feigned.

TREATMENT.

The treatment is similar to that of hysteria. When the disease is continued for several days, artificial or forced feeding becomes necessary. Antispasmodics, as valerian, camphor and assafœtida render good service. The patient usually requires medicine to improve the nervous system, as the compound syrup of the hypophosphites, or the following:

    ℞   Tinct. chloride of iron   half an ounce
         Dil. phosphoric acid   half an ounce
         Syr. of orange peel   two ounces
         Water   two ounces
Mix. Dose teaspoonful three times a day after meals.

IV.—ECSTACY.

This is a state of exalted feeling which indicates derangement of the nervous system and is usually due to some excitement long continued. It is usually caused by a high pitch of religious excitement, and may be regarded as a sort of temporary religious insanity. The patient is in a peculiar state, and gives way to visions and fancies of the mind. This condition has been epidemic in some places. During the seizure the expression is radiant, and the patient appears to behold and enjoy beauties and glories not permitted to ordinary mortals. The fancies which take place in this visionary state are afterwards remembered and recounted.

TREATMENT.

This consists in those moral measures which influence the mind. Such persons are benefited by contact with those who possess a strong will power, and are able to control and influence minds of less strength. When medical treatment is necessary, benefit will be derived from the remedies recommended in hysteria. The elix. of the phosphate of iron and strychnia is appropriate for such cases, in teaspoonful dose three times a day.

V.—CHOREA OR ST. VITUS DANCE.

Chorea is a spasmodic affection of the nervous system, manifesting itself in the irregular jerking of certain muscles or groups of muscles. These movements are involuntary, but usually cease during sleep. The children of parents, who suffer from derangement of the nervous system, show a strong tendency to nervous diseases. Heredity, therefore, occupies a prominent place in causing chorea. A large share of the cases occur between six and fifteen years of age. Whatever tends to disturb the nervous system may appear to cause chorea, as overstudy in school, anxiety in regard to examinations, or other matters. These, even if they do not originate the trouble, seem frequently to aggravate it. A close relationship has been noticed between rheumatic affections and the development of chorea. Malaria should not be overlooked as a possible cause, and others worthy of mention are fright, blows, falls and various mental excitements. Some of the most unfortunate cases of chorea have occurred during pregnancy.

SYMPTOMS.

Some decline in the general health, and considerable disturbance of the nervous system is usually noticed previous to the onset of this disease. The appetite fails somewhat. The patient is restless, irritable and excitable. Slight irregular movements are noticed, the speech is affected, and there are contortions of the face, which suggest an idiotic appearance. The action of the heart may be disturbed. The intellect may appear to be weakened and the memory impaired. These symptoms are rarely mistaken for any other disease. Chorea is not often fatal, except in cases of unusual severity. After apparent recovery a relapse may take place.

TREATMENT.

Children suffering from this affection should be removed from school, have wholesome food, abundance of fresh air, and be prevented from playing games of an exciting nature. Baths and friction are beneficial. Change of air and residence may be required. The patient must be kept free from all annoyance, irritation and excitement. The peculiar movements ought not to be noticed, for remarks about them and scolding are injurious. Fowler's solution is a very reliable and efficient remedy, and may be given in the following manner:

Give a child six years old three drops in water after each meal, and add to the dose one drop a day until eight or ten are taken. If vomiting occurs, or puffiness is noticed about the eyes, stop the medicine for one or two days. Then begin again with three drops, and increase daily as before, until eight or ten drops are borne, or until all the symptoms entirely subside. At first no improvement should be expected, and the patient may seem worse, but in a week or so improvement begins and progresses rapidly. In obstinate cases the subcutaneous injection of the foregoing remedy has proved even more successful. If a remedy is required to produce sleep, the following may be used:

℞		
	Chloral hydrate	one-half dram
	Bromide of soda	one dram
	Syr. simple	one ounce
	Anise water	one ounce

Mix. Dose a teaspoonful before going to bed to a child six years old to secure sleep. To a child twelve or fifteen years old, double the amount may be given. In some cases iron is a valuable remedy. A one grain pill of the iodide of iron is suitable, or troches of the subcarbonate may be more convenient to administer to children. One three times a day is a suitable dose.

The following is a good preparation:

R̃ Tinct. of iron (muriate)   two drams
   Dil. phosphoric acid   three drams
   Syr. simple   one ounce
   Cinnamon water   one ounce

Mix. Dose one teaspoonful three times a day after meals.

Strychnia is a valuable tonic. It may be given in tablets, containing one $\frac{1}{100}$ of a grain two or three times a day. Scutellaria and black cohosh are vegetable remedies which have been used in this disease with more or less success. The adult dose of scutellaria is one dram, and of the fluid extract of black cohosh one-half that amount.

VI.—CONVULSIONS, FITS OR SPASMS.

Convulsions are common, and often alarming, with children whose nervous system is excitable. Prior to the fifth year children are subject to convulsions from the ordeal of teething. Many acute diseases, as diphtheria and scarlet fever, may have their onset in a convulsion.

They are more likely to occur in those of an excitable temperament and may be caused by anything which irritates or impresses the nervous system. The causes, which produce convulsions in children, would frequently have no perceptible effect upon a healthy adult. Among these causes may be enumerated fright, indigestible food, worms, constipation, and others of a similar nature. Teething is especially irritating to the nervous system, and is an ordeal of no little moment in the life of a child. See teething.

Desperate cases of convulsions may occur from eating unripe fruits or vegetables not thoroughly cooked. These cases sometimes prove fatal from inability to unload the alimentary canal promptly and completely. The occurrence of convulsions in the outset of any acute disease is not so unfavorable as their occurrence in the last stages.

SYMPTOMS.

The symptoms, although well known, may be briefly stated. They are restlessness, fretfulness, gritting of the teeth, trembling of the muscles, twitching about the mouth, rigid limbs, eyes rolled back in the head, hurried and labored breathing, muscular rigidity with jerking movements, and others of like character. A spasm may be of any grade of severity, from mild to violent. It may be of brief duration or last for hours. One convulsion may subside and be immediately followed by another. Death sometimes occurs without return to consciousness.

TREATMENT.

Preventive treatment is especially important with respect to children. Their diet demands healthy and nutritious food with light suppers, consisting of food easily digested.

Great caution is necessary to prevent nervous children from fright. Nurses and others should not be permitted to rehearse exciting stories about ghosts or make untruthful representations respecting the dark, or anything whatever which is calculated to shock the delicate nervous organism of a child.

In an actual case of convulsions it is necessary, for intelligent treatment, to ascertain the cause, and this may prove a puzzle. When the child is teething with the gums inflamed and swollen, lancing them may be attended by the most happy results.

If indigestible food has been eaten the stomach may be safely unloaded by giving the syrup of ipecac. in teaspoonful doses. A rectal injection consisting of warm water, castile soap and castor oil, will assist in unloading the lower portion of the alimentary canal. Cold compresses of vinegar and water may be applied to the head if indicated.

In the beginning of a convulsion it is appropriate to place the child quickly in a warm bath, containing a little mustard just enough to stimulate the cutaneous nerves. Rub the surface of the body briskly and thoroughly. After the bath apply friction by means of rubbing with a towel until the skin is dry, then roll up the child in a flannel blanket. Two or three drops of nitrite of amyl inhaled from a handkerchief will prove to be a timely and efficient remedy in all but the most desperate cases. The following prescription secures rest and prevents the return of the convulsion:

℞ Chloral   sixteen grains
   Bromide of soda   half a dram
   Syr. orange peel   one ounce
   Wintergreen water   one ounce

Mix. Dose one teaspoonful to a child one year old, and repeat every hour as needed.

The inhalation of ether and chloroform is sometimes cautiously used, but cannot be recommended as suitable for private practice.

CHAPTER XXX.

GENERAL OR UNCLASSIFIED DISEASES.

I.—Rickets or Rachitis. II.—Erysipelas. III.—Rheumatism. IV.—Gout. V.—Obesity. VI.—Small Pox or Variola. VII.—Varioloid. VIII.—The Prevention of Small Pox or Vaccination.

I.—RICKETS OR RACHITIS.

RICKETS is a disease of childhood in which the nutrition is so disordered that the bones are affected by irregular growth and deformities. This disease is very common among the over-populated and large cities of Europe, especially among the poverty-stricken laboring classes, whose food is deficient in nutrition, and whose habitations are unhealthful. In this country it is comparatively unfrequent, but it sometimes occurs among the well-to-do classes.

CAUSES.

The causes which contribute to the development of rickets are commonly regarded as lack of nutrition from poverty or dark and damp habitations. Children resulting from the marriage of relatives and from those who are physically incompatible, are thought to be more liable to this disease.

A mother's health may have much to do with the development of her offspring. If she is feeble and lacking in vigor, it is hardly to be expected that she can impart health and vigor to her children. Hence, whatever tends to enfeeble and deteriorate the original stock may be a factor in the development of this unfortunate condition.

SYMPTOMS.

These should be detected early, since deformities once established are prone to continue through life.

The first symptoms are usually associated with the digestion, as poor appetite and wasting. The child does not thrive, and a lack of nourishment is detected. The stools are clay-colored, and the formation of bile is thereby shown to be scanty. The pulse is quick and the child is peevish and fretful. There appears to be tenderness over the body and pain in the joints and lower limbs. The child has a peculiarly wasted and aged appearance, a wizen and pinched look, and the limbs seem unable to support the weight of the body. The fontanelle, or soft spot in the head, is large and continues open longer than is natural. When the child attempts to walk the head sinks between the shoulders, the face inclines upward and the head appears to be drawn backward toward the spine.

The head appears to be too large for the body to support and carry. The abdomen is full and swollen. The bones are soft and deformities of the chest and spine begin to be noticed more and more. When the disease begins early, the deformities are more extensive, the bones are more yielding and hence more marked curvature in the spine takes place. The tendency of the disease is chronic in character. Later in life the bones become harder, but the deformities continue.

TREATMENT.

The most satisfactory treatment is preventive. The faults of diet should be corrected. Disorders of digestion should be remedied. If the child nurses, the mother's milk should be looked after, or if bottle fed, attention given to the quality of the milk used. Hygienic measures should be earnestly considered. Air, sunshine and proper clothing should come to the rescue of the child living in dampness and filth.

The sea air is beneficial. It aids the appetite and digestion. Rock salt added to the child's bath is beneficial. Foods rich in phosphates as oatmeal are essential. Among the remedies which aid in arresting this disease the best are phosphorus, iron and cod liver oil. The form of iron best adapted to this disease is the iodide. It may be given in pills or the syrup. The latter injures the teeth, but is not so objectionable prior to the appearance of the permanent set. A one grain pill or from ten to twenty drops of the syrup is a suitable dose for a child three times a day. Cod liver oil may be given in half teaspoonful doses or more twice a day. Phosphorus may be given as follows:

℞	Phosphorus	one-fourth a grain
	Cod liver oil	four ounces

Mix. Dose a teaspoonful twice a day after meals.

Massage should be practiced for a few minutes every day with the hand covered with olive oil.

When constipation exists, a drop of the tincture of nux vomica given in water two or three times daily will afford relief.

Supports and surgical procedures have their advantages in appropriate cases.

The plaster of Paris jacket when suitably used affords marked comfort and improvement. Slight deformities can often be corrected by surgical genius.

II.—ERYSIPELAS.

This is an acute febrile affection, characterized by a deep, red-spreading eruption upon the skin, which is sensitive, painful, and accompanied by a peculiar tingling and burning sensation.

The disease may occur on any part of the body, but is more usual about the face. In hospital practice, it is prone to attack wounds and causes much concern, for it is liable to spread from patient to patient, and its work is of a destructive character. It has been maintained, with good reason, that erysipelas is closely related to puerperal fever. It is due to a specific germ poison. The lymphatic vessels of the skin are inflamed by the growth of the germ, which causes a spreading eruption upon the surface. It is somewhat contagious, but not so much so, as many other contagious diseases.

SYMPTOMS.

The first stage or period of incubation is short, though its duration is not accurately known. The second stage or period of invasion lasts from half a day to three days. The stage of inflammation may last from six to ten days, the whole duration of the disease being from one to two weeks. The invasion is usually accompanied by a chill, followed by fever and the appearance of an eruption upon the skin of a local character. This is scarlet, hot and painful, and tends to spread on all sides. The site of the eruption is tender to the touch, and there is a peculiar creeping, burning and tingling sensation, which is characteristic. When erysipelas invades the tissues about the eyes, they are usually swollen, so that it is impossible for the patient to see or to open them.

When the scalp is invaded, delirium is common. There is usually some irritation of the stomach and disturbance of the digestive system.

The bright red and shiny appearance of the skin over the affected locality is so well marked, as to attract the eye of the physician and enable him to diagnose the trouble at sight. The sensitiveness, heat and burning of the skin, combined with its glossy appearance, render the diagnosis certain.

The disease tends to spread from the first center of infection for a few days in either a regular or irregular manner, after which the advance ceases and the inflamed surface quickly loses its scarlet color and appears darker. If the disease has been severe or has invaded the scalp, the hair is inclined to fall off more or less after recovery.

TREATMENT.

The application of carbolized vaseline to the surface affords great relief. It allays the tingling and burning sensation, and soothes the inflamed skin. Twenty grains of carbolic acid, mixed with one ounce of vaseline is the right proportion. Apply two or three times a day, avoiding the eyes. This keeps the air from the skin and checks the spread of the disease. The tincture of iodine, painted entirely around the eruption in a band one-half inch wide, seems also to check the spread of the disease.

Two grains of concentrated pepsin with every attempt to take food aids its digestion and assists in maintaining the strength. Tincture of the chloride of iron, in from ten to twenty drop doses taken in water, has been a standard remedy. Injury to the teeth should be guarded against, by taking the medicine through a glass tube, or rinsing the mouth afterwards with soda water. Quinine is a valuable remedy. Two or three grains should be given in a pill three times a day. The diet should consist of animal broths, eggs and milk.

III.—RHEUMATISM.

There are several varieties of this affection, as for instance, muscular, articular, acute, inflammatory and chronic. Then too, the prominent cause is often made use of to designate the character of the affection, and hence we hear of malarial, gonorrhœal and syphilitic rheumatism.

It is unnecessary to discuss each of these varieties separately. Technical differences and close distinctions are only of interest to the medical profession. Since this work is designed for the general reader, distinctions unless important are confusing and out of place.

Rheumatism, as known by the household, is a frequent and distressing disease. Its course is uncertain, and recovery may be tedious and delayed. Repeated attacks may occur to render the time of recovery indefinite.

Certain families inherit a tendency to the development of rheumatism, and generation after generation suffer from it. The cause of this disease is somewhat uncertain, as is seen from the differences of opinion which are held concerning it. The prevailing opinion, however, is that a residence in moist regions, in cold, damp dwellings, favors its development. Often an attack seems to be induced by some slight exposure, as taking cold. Whatever reduces the vitality may favor an attack, as fatigue, prolonged lactation, loss of blood, local injuries or any bodily exhaustion. The most prominent factors are diminished activity of the functions of the liver, skin and kidneys. It has been maintained that an excess of lactic acid is always found in the blood during an attack of rheumatism and hence must be the cause. Rheumatism attacks all ages and conditions. The young and the old, the rich and the poor, those scantily and especially those luxuriously fed. Acute attacks are more common in early life.

Muscular rheumatism is probably caused by exposure. It yields to applications of heat and anodyne lotions. The acute inflammatory form is of a more serious character. It attacks the joints, one after another, sometimes until nearly every joint in the body has been invaded, and in such cases may last from three to six weeks or longer. As improvement takes place in one joint the inflammation, pain and swelling attack some other.

SYMPTOMS.

These are fever, thirst, high temperature, coated tongue, impaired appetite, constipation, scanty and highly colored urine, associated with one or more swollen, sensitive and painful joints. Sleep and rest are much disturbed by pain, which in some cases is severe and exhausting. The breath is feverish and offensive, and the early symptoms are followed by perspiration, which has a peculiarly sour odor. The pain and inflammation subside in one place only to reappear in another. When the inflammation is of a severe type and the temperature reaches a high degree, the heart may be involved in the inflammation and its valves may be seriously impaired. The results of rheumatism upon the heart and its valves are often discovered by the physician years after an attack.

TREATMENT.

The treatment of this disease is sometimes very trying and unsatisfactory. For cases of moderate type the following line of treatment is effective. Hot applications and soothing lotions are used externally for the relief of pain.

Warm poultices with laudanum over the surface may be applied, and afford the needed relief. The swollen joint may be enveloped in cotton batting, and outside a flannel or piece of oiled silk may be placed. This is a helpful measure. It excludes the air and allays pain. Cloths wrung out of hot water or hot fomentations are excellent. The following liniment may be used:

℞	Camphorated oil	three ounces
	Chloroform	seven drams
	Oil of mustard	one dram

Mix. Apply as needed to the sensitive joint.

Recovery is favored by keeping the bowels and kidneys active. The cream of tartar lemonade is a useful and cooling drink. The granular effervescent bicarbonate of potash is an excellent alkaline drink. A dessert spoonful in a half glass of water may be taken every two or four hours. The granular effervescent salicylate of soda or salicylic acid are good remedies. A teaspoonful or more every four hours. Wine of colchicum seed is one of the old but efficient remedies. It may be given with the bicarbonate of potash, as in the following prescription:

℞	Bicarbonate of potash	two drams
	Salicylate of soda	four drams
	Sweet spts. of nitre	half an ounce
	Wine of colchicum seed	half an ounce
	Syr. of orange peel	one and a half ounces
	Water q. s. to make	four ounces

Mix. Dose one teaspoonful in water every four hours.

Salicin is a good remedy. It must be taken in large doses, as a heaping teaspoonful for an adult three times a day. When pain is severe a ten-grain dose of Dover's powder may be given at night to allay it. This remedy given to children must be in properly reduced doses.

While the fever lasts, the diet should consist of simple foods, as gruel, milk, animal broths, rice, cornstarch, tapioca and similar appropriate articles. When the disease has produced marked debility, tonics as quinine or iron aid recovery. The prescriptions for anæmia are suitable for these cases. (See page 182.)

Those who inherit rheumatic tendencies, or who have suffered from previous attacks, should seek to ward them off in the future by appropriate living and preventive medicines.

The functions of the liver and kidneys should receive attention. A sallow complexion and constipated bowels should be remedied, and care taken to see that the waste products of the system are promptly eliminated.

Those liable to rheumatism should protect themselves with suitable clothing from cold, dampness and other climatic changes. Getting wet or getting the feet wet and other exposures should be avoided, and persons subject to rheumatism will be benefited by wearing flannel or silk next to the skin the whole of the year. Silk may take the place of flannel during hot weather. Rheumatism is a disease closely allied to gout. Prevention, if possible, is desirable for when once rheumatic trouble has been neglected or has become the habit of the system, it has been known to last for months or even years and sometimes throughout life.

IV.—GOUT.

There is a marked resemblance between gout and rheumatism, as both are hereditary in character. Gout is associated more with the small joints than rheumatism, and is more chronic in its course. There are enlargements of the joints which become permanent, especially the toe and finger joints. It is usually attributed to high living, indolent habits, excess of animal food, together with the use of wines, liquors and lack of exercise.

The fever is not so well marked as in rheumatism. The attack comes on suddenly, often at night, awakening the victim by the severity of the pain. The affected joint, perhaps that of the great toe, is tender, hot and somewhat reddened. The pain is very excruciating and sleep is impossible. The urine is scanty, highly colored, and contains a large amount of uric acid and urates. The urate of soda is often deposited about the joints.

TREATMENT.

Regulation of the diet is the most important part of the treatment. The patient is usually more or less troubled with dyspepsia, as shown by fermentation of the food or acidity of the stomach, and is unable to digest starchy foods properly. The amount of sugar used should be restricted to the smallest quantity possible. Potatoes and corn meal if used at all should be in moderate quantity. The patient ought to abstain from wine, beer and liquors. Abernethy's pet rule for gouty patients was "Live on a shilling a day and earn the shilling."

Sedentary habits are not conducive to the well being of gout subjects. An increased amount of exercise is recommended. This disease is said to be much less prevalent in mild climates, where outdoor life is the rule. Bathing in hot water followed by friction to stimulate the pores of the skin is serviceable. Pepsin may be used to aid the digestion, or pepsin combined with pancreatin. If the liver is sluggish, podophyllin in doses of one-tenth of a grain frequently repeated is excellent to regulate its functions. This remedy may be obtained in parvules or tablets, and while the dose is small, if persisted in daily, it will do its work satisfactorily.

Colchicum is a remedy which has stood the test of time, and has the reputation of affording relief. Fifteen or twenty drops of the wine of colchicum seed three times a day is a proper dose. It is an efficient remedy and may be combined with liquid ferro-salicylata. It is also a powerful remedy and must be used with caution. See prescription below.

Lithia is a good remedy for gout. The granular effervescent lithiated potash, a heaping teaspoonful in half a glass of water three times a day is appropriate. The various remedies for rheumatism are appropriate for the gout. The chief difference in the two diseases being that gout is more chronic, more likely to recur and to continue on to the close of life. The following is an excellent prescription for chronic cases of gout:

    ℞ Liq. Ferro-salicylata   three ounces
        Wine of colchicum seed   one ounce

Mix. Dose for an adult one teaspoonful in water three times a day. If this prescription loosens the bowels unpleasantly the dose must be diminished or omitted for a day or two.

V.—OBESITY.

This is a subject of considerable interest to a large number of persons who constantly increase in weight and become more and more corpulent, contrary to their wishes and well being. A certain amount of fat may be regarded as natural, favorable to good appearance and to good health. It gives to the body a condition of plumpness, protects the joints and nerves from injury, and prevents too rapid radiation of the animal heat. When the accumulation is excessive it interferes with the movements of the body and its natural functions. It is then to be regarded with apprehension, and the means for holding it in check are to be considered.

In some instances this condition seems to be due to hereditary tendency, to inactivity, sedentary occupations, high living, or a diet composed of rich and fat producing foods. The means by which it is induced furnish us with important suggestions as to the best means of preventing it. If no attention is given to this matter the fat of the body may increase to an enormous extent. Most medicines which diminish the surplus fat are of doubtful utility, since they are liable to interfere with the process of digestion or prevent the assimilation of food.

TREATMENT.

The fluid extract of bladder wrack, a common sea weed, has some reputation as a remedy for obesity. Whatever efficiency it possesses is probably due to its cathartic properties and to the iodine which it contains. The dose of the fluid extract is one or two teaspoonfuls three times a day. It is a harmless drug, and must be continued for a long time.

The best plan for reducing surplus fat is to place restrictions upon the amount and kind of food taken. A habit should be established in reference to the diet and made permanent. The process of reduction should be gradual. Hasty reforms are less likely to be lasting. The temptations of the table should be removed. Pastry, fatty foods and rich gravies are to be avoided. Starchy foods, like potatoes, peas and rice, are objectionable. Sugar and other sweets must be used, if at all, sparingly. The amount of tea and coffee used should be reduced to the minimum. Butter, cheese, cream and similar articles are to be given up on general principles. Lean meat, eggs, fish and green vegetables, with a limited amount of bread, are the standard articles of diet. Plenty of exercise and the Turkish bath are beneficial.

Of late the fluid extract of pokeroot (Phytolacca) is attracting considerable attention as a remedy for obesity. It is used also for chronic rheumatism. The dose is from one-fourth to one-half of a teaspoonful three times a day. A thorough trial of this remedy in small doses, together with the other measures suggested, is recommended. Ten drops taken one-half hour before each meal, and again ten drops after each meal, will produce better results than larger doses.

VI.—SMALL POX OR VARIOLA.

This is an acute, contagious disease accompanied by a high fever, and a peculiar eruption on the skin. Ancient writings prove that it occurred very early in the history of the human family. At present it is much less common than formerly, owing to the discovery of Dr. Edward Jenner, and the general protection afforded by vaccination.

It is the most contagious disease known. It attacks all ages and conditions, male and female alike. It is due to a specific germ, which acts upon the system as blood poison. You can no more have small pox without the introduction into the system of the proper germ, than the housewife can have her bread rise and omit the germ of fermentation. This disease is more prevalent in cold than in warm weather. It is a loathsome, terrible and dreaded scourge which is attended by a large mortality. It reaches the unprotected usually through the air, entering the system by way of the lungs. The disease germ may come from the breath, skin and all parts of the body of an infected person.

It may be transported by means of clothing, paper money, rags and various articles of merchandise, as the germs retain their vitality for a long period. Vaccination is the only protection which the physician, nurse or other persons can have, unless they have previously had the disease itself.

The time between the exposure and the breaking out or incubation of this affection is on the average fourteen days.

SYMPTOMS.

These begin to appear after the stage of incubation or fourteen days after exposure. The stage of invasion lasts about two days. There is great thirst, chilly sensations, high temperature, bounding pulse, loss of appetite with a severe cutting pain in the back and head. The poison acting on the nerve centers produces an intense headache and an agonizing backache. During the incubation the patient enjoys perfect health, but with the period of invasion the symptoms are so conspicuous that the disease, when prevailing, may be correctly suspected before the eruption appears. The onset of the disease with children is sometimes attended with delirium and convulsions. After the above symptoms have lasted about two days, the characteristic eruption appears in minute points. With the breaking out of the eruption, the headache and backache disappear, the temperature declines and also the pulse.

The eruptions somewhat resemble measles at first, but rapidly increase in number and size. A hard feeling as if shot were imbedded in the skin may be detected by the hand. In about three days these indurated spots are transformed into vesicles and contain fluid. A depression forms in the center of the vesicle and to this depression the term umbilicated is applied. This umbilicated depression is characteristic of small pox. By the sixth day the pock reaches its maturity and is filled with pus. These pustules are in some cases very numerous, covering over the entire body. The whole appearance is now repulsive. The eyes are swollen and closed, and in severe cases the condition is fearful and deplorable. The mouth is sore, pustules form on the tongue, inside of the lips and sometimes in the throat and elsewhere. The patient's condition is one of extreme distress and suffering. After several days the pustules dry up, and scabs appear which finally peel off and leave a scar. If the patient has been previously vaccinated, the disease runs a milder course, and is called varioloid.

TREATMENT.

Having been exposed to small pox, vaccination should at once be performed. If a person is vaccinated six days after exposure to small pox it will modify the disease, but the sooner vaccination is performed after exposure the better.

There is no specific or satisfactory method of treatment for small pox, beyond meeting the symptoms and relieving the patient as much as possible from suffering. The itching is well nigh intolerable, and yet the patient has to be prevented from scratching off the scabs. Chloral may be used, if there are no signs of heart failure, in doses of from ten to twenty grains to promote sleep. The diet should consist of milk, beef broth, oysters, and similar foods. Ice may be allowed to relieve the burning heat from the pustules in the mouth. Water dressings have been successfully used on the face and hands. A soothing ointment may be applied to the face, composed of carbolic acid, ten grains and vaseline one ounce. Many other remedies have been recommended. Cream of tartar lemonade is a cooling drink, and helps to keep the kidneys active in this disease.

The stools of the patient should be disinfected by strong carbolic acid, copperas or corrosive sublimate solution.

After recovery the room should be treated with thorough fumigation, as for diphtheria, and the clothing and bedding used by the patient destroyed by fire. See disinfection after diphtheria.

VII.—VARIOLOID.

This is usually a mild form of small pox, the disease being favorably affected or modified by a previous vaccination. The symptoms of the disease are similar in every respect to small pox, except that they are very much less intense. The eruptive process is cut short at an early stage and fails to reach its full development. It seems probable that varioloid could be avoided if every one would pay attention to revaccination after the lapse of a few years.

There are many cases in which the primary vaccination works in an unsatisfactory manner, and the amount of protection it affords is not sufficient for the whole term of life. Revaccination would fortify the system in these cases and prevent the outbreak of varioloid.

TREATMENT.

The treatment of this mild form of small pox is the same as that of the genuine disease, and does not need to be repeated. Isolation of the patient, care respecting diet, and a few simple remedies adapted to the manifestations of the disease will be sufficient to carry the patient through it successfully. The same care is required to prevent the spread of the disease as in small pox and the same measures of disinfection should be carried out after the disease is over.

VIII.—THE PREVENTION OF SMALL POX OR VACCINATION.

It is now agreed with but little dissension that the best means of preventing small pox is vaccination. Before the process of vaccination was discovered, it was customary to inoculate with the genuine small pox. This process, it was found, modified the disease, rendered it comparatively mild, and in the great majority of cases was successful; yet it occasionally proved fatal, and great care had to be exercised as inoculated persons could communicate the genuine small pox. Long ago this method was abandoned, owing to the discovery of one, more simple and as effective.

It was observed that those who accidentally contracted cow pox, did not subsequently contract small pox, no matter how much they were exposed to the contagion. The credit of making known this discovery to the world is due to an English country physician by the name of Edward Jenner. By actual experience it is learned that out of a great number vaccinated in infancy, a few only ever contract small pox, and that they have the disease in a much milder form than those who have never been vaccinated. It has been ascertained that positive protection requires the repetition of vaccination, more especially when it was performed in infancy.

An outbreak of small pox in any community renders it advisable for all persons to be immediately revaccinated as a measure of prudence. The trouble is small compared with the benefit conferred, and though it is not likely to take, in many cases, with anything like the vigor of the first vaccination, it affords a sense of security which is valuable.

The idea that vaccination is injurious as at present conducted, ought not to be entertained for a single moment. The method now employed avoids every possibility of introducing syphilis, or anything harmful, and to oppose vaccination is proof that one has become the victim of a silly and needless prejudice.

Time tends to diminish the degree of protection which vaccination affords. On this account it is well to have the operation repeated every few years, especially if the original scar becomes indistinct.

Formerly the matter used for vaccination was the pus taken from the pustule of a healthy infant, or young person, but as infants may be supposed to be healthy who are not, it is admitted that in the old way there was a possibility of introducing some impurities into the system of the person thus vaccinated.

This objection does not hold under the present method of procedure, which is sufficiently perfect to satisfy the most fastidious. The present method is as follows: A clean ivory point is dipped into the pustule of a healthy calf previously vaccinated. When withdrawn it is covered with matter which is allowed to dry upon it. This dried matter, like a dry yeast cake, is full of germs, which will do effective work when placed in favoring conditions. This dried point is securely wrapped, kept in a cool place and used within two or three weeks.

Directions for the operation are as follows: Dip the ivory point into pure cold water to moisten the virus. The point thus moistened must not be placed in contact with any contaminating substance. From the arm or leg scrape off a portion of the scarf skin, about the size of a child's little finger nail. This should be done with a sharp, clean knife. It is unnecessary to draw blood, but only moisture or serum, and little red points are to be observed on the denuded surface. Then take the moist point by the dry end and rub the moistened end over the prepared spot repeatedly until you have wiped off all the virus upon it. Let it dry a few minutes and the operation is complete. It does not involve pain if properly done, but only a slight sensation, hardly noticeable.

Children ought not to travel on the cars or in public conveyances before vaccination, and this simple and certain protection should be afforded previous to attending school.

A child should be vaccinated at about three months of age. This will obviate the necessity of vaccination during dentition, when the child has enough to contend with. Vaccination should not take place in houses where diphtheria or erysipelas exists, as there would be some danger of inoculating these diseases. With the exercise of proper care vaccination may be considered to be without risk.

It often causes some temporary eruption, fever and swelling of the vaccinated arm, but these are of short duration and of trivial consequence.

CHAPTER XXXI.

VARIOUS INFLAMMATORY AFFECTIONS.

I.—INFLAMMATIONS. II.—ABSCESSES. III.—FELON OR WHITLOW. IV.—ONYCHIA OR SUPPURATION OF THE MATRIX. V.—INGROWING NAIL OR ONYXIS. VI.—CHILBLAINS. VII.—BOILS AND FURUNCLES. VIII.—CARBUNCLES. IX.—MALIGNANT PUSTULE OR ANTHRAX. X.—GLANDERS. XI.—HYDROPHOBIA OR RABIES. XII.—TUMORS.

I.—INFLAMMATIONS.

WASTE products, or poisonous bacteria, multiplying in the system depress its vitality, weaken the circulation, and may give rise to inflammation.

Malarial and other poisons enter the system in the act of respiration. Bacteria may reach the system by means of the drinking water or food products. Other septic material may find an entrance into the system through an abrasion upon the skin or some wound. Nature is not only obliged to carry on a constant warfare with poisonous substances elaborated in the tissues, but also those which may exist in the air and water supplies. The more vigor and vitality a person possesses the better nature is able to perform this constant and important work. When the vitality is weak or the amount of poison to be eliminated is excessive, nature may be overwhelmed and unable to perform successfully the task which she attempts. Such failure may result in prostration, sickness, and perhaps death. Inflammation is a common and frequent method of proof that nature has been unable to successfully eliminate various poisons from the system.

The symptoms of inflammation are redness, heat, pain and swelling. The redness is due to congestion, the result of obstructed circulation of the blood. This is the first stage in many acute diseases, as pneumonia, meningitis, etc.

Heat is an important factor. Its degree determines the character of the inflammation. Most acute sickness shows elevation of the temperature. Any decided variation from the normal temperature shows that a person is sick, for in health the bodily temperature manifests almost no variation. This increase of temperature accounts for many of the symptoms to which we have so frequently referred, as thirst, loss of appetite, quickened respiration, emaciation and arrested or altered secretions. When inflammation goes on to the formation of pus the temperature continues to be elevated, and this fact often aids in suspecting and locating the trouble. Diseases resulting from germs or bacteria cause an elevation in temperature. Their multiplication and growth produce fermentation in the blood, which, coupled with the efforts of nature to eliminate them, accounts for the rising temperature, the thirst, fever and other symptoms.

The pain of inflammation is due to irritation, swelling and pressure upon the nerves produced by the inflammatory process. The greater the swelling, usually the more intense is the pain, owing to increased pressure. Those parts which are most liberally supplied with blood and sensitive nerves, are more responsive to the action of inflammation and experience more pain than other parts less liberally supplied. The swelling of inflammation is due to several causes, as the extravasation of blood, lymph, and serum into the tissues. The white blood corpuscles possessing the ability to pass out of the blood vessels into the inflamed tissues, may also increase the swelling.

There are many causes of inflammation, as traumatic, or those due to injuries and accidents; toxic, or those due to the action of poison; infectious, or those due to the action of septic germs; constitutional, or those due to diseases of a hereditary type. Traumatic inflammations are produced in a great variety of ways, as cutting, tearing, crushing parts of the body, and injuries produced by blows, falls, or from machinery, or the application of heat and cold, or contact with caustic chemicals, acids and poisons.

The inflammation of rheumatism and gout are caused by a retention in the system of waste materials which nature has been unable to properly eliminate, and is toxic in character.

The inflammation of tubercular consumption is caused by septic disease germs, producing fermentation in the blood and the destruction of tissue in the lungs, where they congregate and multiply in immense numbers. Many other varieties of inflammation are produced by disease germs, as erysipelas, diphtheria, scarlet fever, typhoid fever, glanders and a great many others.

The treatment of any inflammation depends largely upon the cause which produces it. It is evident to every one that the cut of a sharp knife requires very different treatment from the bite of a rabid animal.

II.—ABSCESSES.

An abscess is a collection of pus or matter in some portion of the body. This pus is usually loaded with multitudes of bacteria or germs. When an abscess forms rapidly, it is known as an acute abscess, but when it is a long time developing, it is a cold or chronic abscess. Abscesses are frequent in the debilitated, and are supposed to have some relation to a depraved condition of the blood. They are liable to originate in the glands of those who are afflicted with scrofula or other constitutional diseases. They sometimes result from injuries.

Nature sometimes attempts to relieve the system of certain poisons by establishing an abscess. An acute abscess disturbs the normal condition and produces the symptoms of inflammation, as redness, heat, pain and swelling. As the abscess progresses, the symptoms become more marked, and the pain is of a throbbing type. A chill may take place followed by fever and profuse sweating.

The pus in an abscess tends to work its way in the line of the least resistance, either towards the surface of the body, or some of the great internal cavities and often doing much damage while seeking an outlet. If the pus is prevented from traveling in one direction by dense tissues as the periosteum, it burrows its way in another direction, often reaching a joint or some remote outlet far away from the site of the original abscess. A superficial collection of pus can generally be detected by the fingers.

TREATMENT.

An abscess may sometimes be left to nature when it will reach the surface, rupture, discharge and disappear, but such a result cannot always be expected. It is often necessary to stop the destructive process of an abscess by opening into it, and giving exit to the pent up pus. This operation should be performed with care, as large blood vessels might be wounded and other dangers encountered. Hot fomentations and warm poultices of flaxseed meal, slippery elm, or bread and milk, may soften the swelling and ease the pain, thus hastening the opening of the abscess and affording at the same time no little comfort. They should only be applied when an abscess is near the surface and to hasten its rupture. The pus of a deep seated abscess is often drawn off by an aspirator, but it is sometimes better to make a free opening into the abscess sac so as to thoroughly liberate the pus. When an abscess has been opened, it should be kept open by the application of a hot poultice for a short time or warm water dressings. If the abscess cavity is large, it should be thoroughly cleansed each day by a carbolic or other antiseptic wash. In debilitated cases tonics are necessary. The contents of an abscess is sometimes absorbed. The aspiration of the pleural cavity to remove purulent matter from the chest has often resulted favorably. Drawing off the pus is the most rational method of treatment in empyema, a condition which may follow a severe attack of pleurisy. This and other special conditions as quinsy and whitlow are mentioned elsewhere under their appropriate heads.

III.—FELON OR WHITLOW.

This is a very painful affection, well known and easily recognized by those who have suffered from it. A felon has its origin in an abscess which forms between the bone and the thick inelastic membrane which covers it, called the periosteum.

Owing to the density of this tissue the pus cannot work its way through it easily, and so it often works its way along, burrowing underneath this membrane seeking an outlet, doing a great amount of damage and causing great pain. Sometimes a portion of the bone is destroyed, and sometimes a joint of the finger is stiffened or destroyed altogether, when proper treatment is delayed. Fever sores are similar in some respects to a bone felon, for they are due in the first place to an abscess which causes the death of a portion of the bone, and so long as this dead bone remains the abscess will continue to discharge pus. Felons are caused usually by some slight injury, often unobserved at the time, or perhaps only faintly remembered. The inside of the hand or finger is hit against some object, which may cause a deep-seated abscess. In the palm of the hand they are often caused by pressure or friction. They may result from an axe or hoe handle, a scythe snath, plough handle or other implement used by one previously unaccustomed to labor. It is probable that heat, pressure and friction, combine to cause these inflammations.

The first thing noticed is a callous or blister, beneath which is experienced a sense of soreness, which the patient usually attempts to treat by pricking with a knife point or needle. Suppuration follows the inflammation. It is a painful process, owing to the situation of the affection, and also to the fact that the periosteum is unyielding.

TREATMENT.

Abortive treatment must be applied early in order to be availing. Put the finger or hand into a hot alkaline solution, as hot as can be borne. To make the solution, add to water either wood ashes, soft soap, baking soda, or a small amount of liquid ammonia or potash. The solution must be kept as hot as can be borne by the painful finger or hand, which must be held in it a long time, and then paint the finger over with the following mixture:

℞	Nitrate of silver	twenty grains
	Spirits of nitrous ether	one half ounce

This will abort a felon if applied soon enough. The tincture of iodine, if painted on early, will also abort a felon.

The following is said to work well: Moisten common salt with turpentine and keep it applied, renewing it twice daily.

The surgeon rarely sees a felon before suppuration is well advanced, and then the only treatment is to cut with a sharp knife or bistoury down to the bone. This opens through the periosteum and allows the pus to escape. If too long delay occurs before the felon is opened there is liable to be not only the destruction of bone, but a tedious process of healing. After a felon is opened it should be dressed with soft poultices for a day or two to relieve pain and favor the exit of pus.

IV.—ONYCHIA OR SUPPURATION OF THE MATRIX.

Onychia is the suppuration of the root of the nail or matrix. It is a disease common to unhealthy children, and usually originates from some slight injury. It commences with the symptoms of inflammation, redness, pain and swelling about the root of the nail, followed by the development of pus or matter. Sometimes the nail loosens and falls out. This disease is sometimes associated with a syphilitic taint.

TREATMENT.

Apply stimulating remedies as the tincture of iodine. When pus forms, remove it, and apply cleansing lotions as carbolized water, ten grains of the acid to the ounce of water. This cleanses and improves the condition of the sore. After thorough cleansing, apply aristol powder or iodoform, dusting it well into the diseased parts.

Tonics and constitutional treatment are in order to improve the general condition. Such well known tonics as the syrup of the iodide of iron, ten or twenty drops, three times a day, or iron and calisaya, or the compound syrup of hypophosphites is beneficial to improve the general condition.

V.—INGROWING NAIL OR ONYXIS.

This is sometimes a troublesome and painful affection. It may result from pressure of the shoe or boot on the outside of the great toe, pressing it so that its inner corner overrides the second toe. When long continued, this crowds the soft flesh against the edges of the nail, and bends the nail into the flesh, causing irritation and soreness. Sometimes ulceration takes place as the result of the continued irritation, generally on the inside of the great toe, and while the cause exists, the ulcer refuses to heal.

TREATMENT.

The first indication is to remove the pressure by wearing broad or box-toed shoes. Relief is afforded in less severe cases by soaking the feet often and removing the callous and dead skin along with any fungous portion of the edge of the nail.

Removing the soft portion of the toe which bulges over the margin of the nail has sometimes afforded relief. After such removal the wounded surface may be painted over with collodion or treated as any slight wound. Caustic potash can be applied to a portion of the nail; this will soften it, when it may be pared away with a sharp knife. If at any time proud flesh or unhealthy granulations are observed, they should be touched with a pencil of nitrate of silver.

The following recommendation for the treatment of ingrowing toe nail has recently appeared and may be tried: Remove all pressure by wearing a loose shoe or slipper, for this is imperative. Have a pledget of cotton crowded under the nail so as to somewhat elevate the point which occasions the trouble, then allow a few drops of the muriate tincture of iron to fall upon the cotton. The iron deadens the sensibility so that the next day the cotton can be worked down further under the nail. This course must be continued until the point of the nail is lifted away from the flesh, when it can be snipped off. The author of this method of treatment assures us that patience, cotton, iron and the endurance of a little pain will work a cure in every case.

A sure cure may be obtained by having the whole or a portion of the nail removed. This operation will be successful if thoroughly done. The root portion of the nail must be drawn out and removed at the same time to prevent a recurrence of the trouble. This operation effects a certain cure, and is the best when one has neither time nor patience to submit to a less rapid method. It may be done with the patient under the influence of an anæsthetic, and is then rapid and painless.

VI.—CHILBLAINS.

These are superficial inflammations of the skin of a local character. The common sites of chilblains are the heels, toes, and sometimes the ears and nose. They are frequent with those whose circulation is lacking in vigor, and who are especially sensitive to changes in the temperature. The cause of chilblains is principally sudden changes of temperature, or chilling or slightly frosting the skin.

They are characterized by excessive tenderness and troublesome itching. These symptoms are aggravated by the approach of evening or the approach of changes in the weather and the application of external warmth. It is on this account that they are often troublesome at night and prevent sleep.

TREATMENT.

Avoid tight-fitting shoes and wear warm stockings to improve the circulation in the feet, and to prevent the chilling of the skin. This is preventive treatment, but when blisters have formed the following should be applied:

℞ Vaseline two ounces
Carbolic acid ten to twenty grains
Ext. of opium one dram

This is to be mixed into an ointment and applied two or three times a day.

If the skin is unbroken the tincture of iodine or camphor liniment will afford relief. If the chilblains are painful add one dram of laudanum to each ounce of camphor liniment for this disagreeable affection or use the following:

℞	Menthol	one dram
	Alcohol	one ounce
	Oil of clove	ten drops
	Oil of cinnamon	ten drops

Mix and apply as needed.

When ulceration has taken place cleanse the sores with hot water and castile soap, then apply to them the carbolized ointment as above, or dress with powdered aristol or iodoform.

VII.—BOILS AND FURUNCLES.

Boils are troublesome local swellings or inflammations, which originate in the cellular tissue under the skin. The surrounding tissues are hard and form a circular, elevated lump or mass, the center of which becomes the opening point for the discharge of matter or pus when the boil gets ripe. This lump of inflamed tissue presses upon the nerves and other neighboring tissues, causing intense and throbbing pain. The degree of pain depends largely upon the locality and amount of the swelling. Boils upon the neck are especially painful.

The pain increases with the pressure, and is most severe just before the pus is discharged. When left to nature a rupture finally takes place in the center of the swelling, which affords great relief. Through this opening the core is discharged. The center of the swelling is now depressed, but some redness, elevation and hardness, continues for some time about the circumference. This gradually subsides and the process of healing by granulation becomes complete. Boils rarely endanger life, however numerous, but they often occasion great inconvenience and a degree of pain out of proportion to their size and consequence.

CAUSES.

These are not well known. They frequently appear to result in consequence of some debilitated condition of the system, but this cannot be stated as a rule, for they often appear in persons in whom no such condition of debility exists. Sometimes they follow some slight injury, but this is the exception rather than the rule. They are especially common with laborers who work in tanyards and handle the skins of animals; and they are also common with those who breathe the fetid odors of the dissecting room or other fetid animal exhalations. Some have maintained that they result from eating diseased meat, and from various other causes, but in many other instances they appear without any assignable cause. As the skin and cellular tissues hold in their meshes many absorbent vessels and glands, it would seem as though boils are the result of some septic material or poison, introduced into the system from without, by coming into neighboring contact with these sensitive absorbent glands or vessels in the skin, or in some cases by being inhaled and coming into sufficient contact with the absorbent system in the lungs.

TREATMENT.

You can only hope to abort them before the formation of pus, painting the inflamed lump with the tincture of iodine or a strong solution of nitrate of silver checks the process of inflammation, if applied early. The following is the most efficient solution:

℞ Nitrate of silver   twenty grains
    Spts. nitrous ether   one ounce

Mix and apply to the inflamed surface several times.

The external application of camphor or alcohol is also recommended. The best internal remedy is calcium sulphide in pills, each containing one-quarter or one-half of a grain, one pill to be taken three or four times a day.

Persons who suffer from a succession of boils will shortly find relief from the use of this remedy. In debilitated subjects tonic remedies are beneficial, also a change of air, or a residence by the seaside. When pus has formed, abortive treatment is useless. If the tension and pain are severe, hot poultices afford some relief and hasten the process of suppuration. As soon as the boil is soft in the center and shows the pus through the skin on pressure of the finger, it should be opened or lanced. A little strong carbolic acid introduced into the central opening destroys the septic process and hastens the recovery.

VIII.—CARBUNCLES.

A carbuncle, instead of having one central opening like a boil, has several or many, for more tissue is involved and it is in every way a more serious affection.

It always occurs in debilitated persons, in those whose system has been depleted by disease or by chronic alcoholism, or who are otherwise enfeebled. The neck and back are the favorite locations for this tedious and painful affection. It is a hard, angry looking inflammation, sometimes as large as a saucer. It is tedious and painful, and taxes the vitality to a remarkable degree, often endangering life. It is sometimes called by the laity an ant heap, because of its fancied resemblance. It is an elevation containing many little openings through which the pus escapes, the tissue under the skin being honeycombed by the sloughing process. The danger is from exhaustion and blood poisoning or Pyæmia, which see.

TREATMENT.

At an early stage preventive treatment may be of service.
Apply the following externally.

℞	Spirits of camphor	three drams
	Carbolic acid	one dram

Mix and use three or four times a day.

In the meantime take calcium sulphide in pills as recommended in treatment for boils.

When the carbuncle is well advanced, the following method of treatment has proved eminently satisfactory.

Inject carbolic acid into the diseased tissue. If little openings exist, the carbolic acid may be introduced on the point of a silver probe into each opening. The object of this treatment is to convert a septic, ulcerating mass into a healthy, granulating sore.

A more thorough destruction of the diseased tissue may be attempted by making a central opening into the carbuncle scraping out the putrid mass, or by inserting a piece of caustic potash about the size of a pea, or by pushing a small piece into each opening. This caustic treatment should be followed by poultices to hasten the separation of the diseased slough, afterward a dressing of carbolized vaseline; twenty grains of acid to an ounce of vaseline should be used.

Perfect cleanliness must be observed. The patient's strength should be looked after, and the physical vigor maintained.

IX.—MALIGNANT PUSTULE, OR ANTHRAX.

This, fortunately, is a disease we seldom see. It is a very dangerous affection, having its origin in the introduction into the human system of a specific animal poison of bacterial origin.

Any material which has been in contact with the disease is capable of transmitting it as well as the diseased animal, or eating the flesh of an animal diseased with the poison.

The usual site of the disease is some exposed part of the body, as the hands or face. It commences as a small, red, inflamed spot, which itches and contains a black point in the center. In a few hours a vesicle is formed. On the second day other vesicles form about the central vesicle, and the area of inflammation is enlarged and more swollen, with a black or brown spot in the center. The whole lump of diseased tissue forms a dry, gangrenous slough. The whole progress of the disease is rapid, and the mortality is great, varying from fifty to seventy-five per cent. The disease begins with a chill, vomiting, cold sweat, great depression and anxiety, and ends with fever, delirium, muscular spasms and death.

TREATMENT.

The treatment should be prompt and energetic. Local treatment is often successful if it is early enough to prevent the poison from being absorbed into the system. The involved tissue should be destroyed by caustic before absorption and blood poisoning take place. Make an opening into the center of the pustule and insert a piece of caustic potash as large as a pea, or introduce enough strong carbolic acid to penetrate the diseased tissues. Either method is good treatment.

A poultice should then be applied to separate the slough, and the wound heals, as any healthy sore, by granulations. The destruction of the diseased tissue must be thorough.

When the patient's condition becomes desperate before treatment is entered upon, the tendency to death must be counteracted by stimulants and other well-known means. Quinine should be given internally and the sore dressed with carbolized vaseline. A case so desperate should be entrusted to competent medical supervision.

X.—GLANDERS.

Glanders is a disease of the equine or horse family, of bacterial origin, and communicated to man and other animals by inoculation.

When the disease affects the mucous membrane of the horse, it is known as glanders, and when confined to the skin, it is known as farcy.

The disease is characterized by a lump or tubercles the size of a pea or less. These ulcerate and discharge pus or matter streaked with blood. These ulcers may be numerous and show no tendency to heal.

When the mucous membrane is the seat of the disease, pus streaked with blood is discharged from the nostrils. When the skin is the seat of the disease, the lumps known as farcy buds, ulcerate forming abscesses.

CAUSE.

Glanders are due to contagion or poison introduced into the system by inoculation. Man is not very susceptible to the disease, but it may be communicated to him by a horse which is suffering from it.

When the horse snorts, contagious particles of matter are liable to be thrown upon any one who is near by entering the eye, mouth or nose or some abrasion of the skin upon the face or hands. The disease shows first at the point of inoculation. The period of incubation is from one to three days.

SYMPTOMS.

These are chills, followed by fever, pain in the joints and muscles, lameness, profuse perspiration and dark colored urine. The swellings are painful, dark red, and look like the inflammation of erysipelas. The neighboring lymphatic glands are red, large and tender, and show a tendency to inflammation and ulceration.

The constitutional symptoms which intervene are headache, chills, fever, pain in the limbs and joints, nausea, vomiting, diarrhœa, and a discharge from the nose which is first watery, but afterwards it becomes a viscid catarrh, streaked with blood and of a greenish color.

The mouth and throat are involved, the eyes are inflamed, the eruption upon the face becomes a spreading ulcer, and abscesses may form in other parts of the body. The later symptoms are of a typhoid character, as prostration, delirium, stupor and death.

In some cases the lungs are noticeably involved. The breathing is affected, the voice is altered, there is a cough, accompanied by expectoration streaked with blood and the breath is fetid.

TREATMENT.

The diseased tissues must be destroyed as far as possible with carbolic acid, corrosive sublimate, or a hot iron. Nasal ulcers are to be treated with creosote, carbolic acid and iodoform. Nitrate of silver and permanganate of potash are also used.

Tonics and stimulants are also needed. This is a horrible disease in man, and no effort or expense should be spared to prevent it.

XI.—HYDROPHOBIA OR RABIES.

In the human race this is a dreaded disease.

CAUSE.

It is caused by the bite of a rabid or mad animal, usually a dog. The poison is contained in the saliva of the rabid animal, and the person bitten is inoculated with it. Unfortunately the mad dog has a biting propensity. In order to introduce the poison or contagion into the system there must be an abrasion of the skin.

The period between the inoculation and the appearance of the disease is not clearly defined, but from one to two months is given as one extreme, and from six months to one or more years as the other. The great majority of cases develop inside of three months. Moral impressions, as fear, fatigue and excesses, seem to favor the outbreak of this disease. It has been thought by many that those cases occurring after several years are influenced by fear and the imagination.

SYMPTOMS.

The first symptom usually noticed is a sad or melancholy state. The nervous system is disturbed and depressed, and the sleep is broken. The victim is annoyed by sounds or noises, is petulant, fidgety, ill-tempered, unusually irritable, and avoids society. Later all these symptoms are exaggerated. An itching or pain is experienced at the site of the wound, the pulse is rapid, the skin hot and dry, the appetite is lost and the bowels are constipated. Slight convulsions of the muscles take place, the breathing is sighing in character. Pain is experienced in the region of the heart, and delirium may come on.

The neck gets stiff, free movement of the head is checked, there is a peculiar feeling in the throat, swallowing becomes difficult, and at length impossible, the sight of water is distressing and brings on shuddering or spasms. The sufferer experiences an intense thirst, but upon attempting to drink spasms occur. The countenance is anxious and terror stricken, the eyes project and seem to be staring, the limbs tremble, the victim looks fierce and strange, and makes a desperate attempt to swallow but cannot.

As the disease advances all these symptoms are intensified, until the sight of water or a breath of air brings on a renewal of the convulsions. The mouth is so parched and dry that the noise made in attempting to raise and eject the viscid mucous is compared to the barking of a dog. As the thirst becomes more urgent the inability to swallow increases. During the paroxysms, which become more frequent and severe, the patient is violent toward every one about him, acts insanely, and has to be restrained. Finally a fatal paroxysm takes place and the scene of awful suffering and agony is closed. The disease runs its whole course in about three days, usually progressing to a fatal termination.

There are cases where the whole trouble seems to result from an extremely sensitive condition of the nervous system; hence in some cases, fear of hydrophobia seems to be the only assignable cause of the attack. Listening to the details of this disease may have an unhappy effect upon a person whose nervous system is easily excited, and hence such a person should be spared the rehearsal of these frightful details. There is danger of bringing on hysteria, which if not so serious as hydrophobia, is, to say the least, bad enough.

TREATMENT.

Preventive treatment is worthy of consideration. Moral suasion and even firmness must sometimes be used in the management of those who have groundless fears.

The bite of a rabid animal or wound should be cauterized promptly and thoroughly with nitrate of silver stick, or the chloride of zinc, to prevent the absorption of the poison.

When the bite is on the limb, it may be corded above the wound to prevent inoculation, and the poison withdrawn by immediately sucking the wound. The mouth ought to be washed with carbolic acid solution immediately before and after the process, but such deliberate action is hardly to be expected on such an exciting occasion.

Ammonia and alcoholic stimulants may be made to saturate the system so as to retard the absorption of the poison. For a small wound the corrosive sublimate solution is appropriate. Dissolve one tablet, such as is used by surgeons and kept by all druggists, in a pint of warm water, and thoroughly cleanse and saturate the wound with the solution. If this could be done promptly enough, it would avert all danger. The patient needs to have confidence in whatever treatment is adopted for the sake of the moral effect on the nervous system.

For a fully developed case of hydrophobia, place the patient in a dark room and keep him quiet. The spasms may be controlled by the cautious inhalation of choloform. Chloral, morphine and the bromide of soda are valuable antispasmodics, and may be judiciously used. When it is known that a person has been bitten by a rabid animal, the advisability of sending the victim to a Pasteur institute for treatment by inoculations should be entertained and proper medical advice sought in relation to the same.

The superstition that a person, who has been bitten by a dog, which afterwards goes mad, will have hydrophobia is utterly unworthy of confidence.

XII.—TUMORS.

A tumor is a general name applied to a class of enlargements or growths of great variety. They may be composed of various kinds of tissue, as muscle, fat, cartilage, bone or blood. They may invade any portion of the body, and usually manifest a disposition to grow larger, but to this there are exceptions. Tumors seldom, if ever, change from one kind to another, and some may occasion no trouble or inconvenience. They may grow for awhile perhaps slowly, cease to enlarge, and afterwards remain stationary. Such tumors are known as benign, or innocent.

The subject of tumors has been surrounded by considerable obscurity. The microscope has aided much in their diagnosis and classification.

Tumors differ very much in their structure. The benign, or innocent tumors, are composed of muscle, cartilage, bone, fat and sebaceous matter. The sebaceous tumors of the scalp, generally known as wens, are specimens of innocent tumors. They are often called cancers by self-styled doctors and impostors, who add to their reputation by their successful removal.

Of all tumors, cancers are the most important, because of their malignant character. They not only extend, but they destroy the surrounding tissues to such an extent that they eventually destroy life.

When a cancer is removed there is danger of its returning at the same place or in some distant organ. Cancers may occur anywhere and involve any tissue of the human body. The most common site of their activities is the female breast. A cancer is to be contemplated always with dread, for in its worst form the sight is hideous, the smell offensive, and the suffering occasioned intense.

Their cause is unknown. Soft cancers sometimes follow an injury, but a large majority of injuries are unattended by such unfortunate results.

TREATMENT.

There are no internal remedies which can be relied upon to effect a cure. Some tumors can be let alone, others should be removed at an early date. When removal is decided upon, it should be thorough. There are two recognized methods of removal. One is by corrosive applications, and the other is by the surgeon's knife.

Before a malignant tumor can be cured, the entire growth must be destroyed. Unless all the diseased tissue is removed, the disease not only breaks out afresh, but is scattered throughout the system to reappear in other organs.

A cancerous growth, that is superficial, can be effectually cured by means of a caustic paste, but for a deep seated cancer of the breast or other parts, such treatment is unsuitable, because so much destruction of tissue must take place before the diseased growth is reached, that inflammatory processes are awakened and the cancerous growth is inflamed and aggravated. The destruction can neither be rapid nor complete, and causes a great amount of pain. Paste and plasters are suitable only for skin cancers known as epithelial growths.

The method by external application is as follows: First the surface is denuded with caustic potash, combined with other remedies as follows:

R Cocaine thirty grains
  Caustic potash ninety grains
  Vaseline one-fourth of a dram

Mix. Apply to one square inch of surface only at a time. This produces a denuded surface, to which Marsden's paste should be applied.

℞ Arsenious acid   two parts
  Mucilage of acacia   one part

Mix into a paste too thick to run. Spread upon the denuded surface of the cancer and over it put some dry lint.

Dr. Marsden has treated over six thousand cases in the London Cancer Hospital and is considered excellent authority. Numerous pastes are used, containing arsenic or chloride of zinc and pulverized blood-root, but such treatment cannot be advised for household practice.

These pastes contain arsenic. They are to be left on from one to three days, until considerable inflammation is produced. Following the application of the paste, a warm poultice is used, until the slough separates, a process requiring about a week, then apply vaseline ointment, containing a dram of aristol to an ounce of vaseline, for the healing of the wound.

For cancer in the breast the surgeon's knife is the best remedy. It should be applied early, for no treatment will atone for neglect, after the cancer has broken out upon the surface and the surrounding glands are involved. Any treatment will then prove disappointing.

Sebaceous tumors of the scalp should be slit open and the contents removed together with the sack or cyst. The same treatment avails for the little tumors or cysts upon the eyelids. Tumors about the neck and under the ear should be removed with caution, as the large vessels in these regions render surgical operations unusually hazardous.

Soft cancers may develop as the result of some injury. Their growth is usually rapid, and successful treatment is unusually difficult.

Birth marks are vascular tumors, composed of enlarged blood vessels, often situated about the face, and their removal risks a scar or disfigurement as unsightly as the red or purple spot itself. Sometimes they have been treated by the injection of iron or ergot, with the hope of obliterating them. Their removal has also been suggested by making them the site of a vaccination.

CHAPTER XXXII.

MARRIAGE AND MATERNITY.

I.—Marriage. II.—Reproduction. III.—Symptoms of Pregnancy. IV.—Diseases of Pregnancy. V.—Advice to the Pregnant. VI.—Miscarriage. VII.—Labor, Stages and Management. VIII.—Management of Infants. IX.—Care and Education of Children.

I.—MARRIAGE.

THE subject of marriage in its relation to the maintenance and transmission of sound health is of such vital importance as to deserve more than a passing notice.

Many say that poverty burdens life with anxiety, fills it with drudgery, and renders a fruitful marriage, especially oppressive; but the courage, hope and love, of a properly wedded pair can easily outlive and overcome such an objection.

Poverty is to be feared but little in comparison with some of the hereditary and destructive diseases, as syphilis, which continues down through the ages never outlived and never overcome, a perpetual blight and curse, the transmission of which is but the prolongation of the wail of weakness and sorrow. Any one can see, too, that wealth more often fails to produce happiness for the married state than its opposite. Even where there exists the possession of all that money can buy, there must also be the disposition of mutual helpfulness, that delicate sympathy, that indescribable relation or condition, without which there can be no charm, no happiness, and no home. Idle indulgence, rich food, and various luxuries, become tiresome, desire fails, the appetite fails, and life is full of lassitude and complaining.

It is the busy mother, surrounded by her fresh, rosy and interesting group of children, with no time for weariness, no reason for complaint, hands full, heart full, life full, of all that is beautiful, noble and inspiring, who is to be envied rather than the complaining daughter of wealth, who appears to be satisfied with a poodle.

To contemplate marriage simply for support, or to be relieved from labor, without any intention of contributing to the success of the enterprise will prove disappointing.

The young man who casts love aside and contracts an unsuitable commercial marriage, consenting to be a sort of genteel servant in order to be shielded from the struggle of earning a living, deserves little sympathy and usually gets less.

The woman who marries with mercenary or wrong motives is sure to find a place for repentance with many tears. Much depends upon the wife in that subtle process of home making, and however limited the means, she must be able to fill the heart of her husband with satisfaction. If he is allowed to toil without sympathy and his earnings are carelessly squandered, sooner or later he will lose his courage, and for such a wife disaster is in store.

Marriage implies that earnest attention should be given to those matters which have a bearing upon the important subject of reproduction. Those persons ought not to marry who are unwilling to fulfill to a reasonable degree the obligations involved. The legitimate consequences of marriage should be previously understood, and manfully and heroically undertaken. Marriage is justly termed the foundation of society, because it has in view the constant renewal of the race and hence its perpetuity. Human beings ought to live and act wisely both for their own and for posterity's sake. Children are the most precious gifts bestowed upon lawful wedlock. They ought to be strong enough to outlive their parents, and virtuous enough to perpetuate and improve upon their moral qualities.

Fitness for marriage, compatibility with each other and surplus vitality to transmit, are some of the necessary considerations which outweigh in their importance, such other minor considerations as wealth, station or social position.

We are frequently told that the modern requirements of refined society are so exaggerated that it requires a fortune to raise a single child, and a very extensive one to raise a group of children. These exactions are so emphasized, that there appears to be some reason for believing that there is good excuse for thwarting the results of wedlock, on the part of those who say that they cannot afford a family. There is but little ground for such frivolous excuses. It is not necessary to conform to all the whims, fashions and foibles of modern society. The standards which it maintains are often artificial and detrimental, if not suicidal, to the welfare of the race. Many of the most brilliant and talented persons which the world has ever known, have been strangers, at least in early life, to the luxuries now so common and considered so essential. They were not born in houses with a brown stone front nor surfeited with Porter-house steak.

A measure of struggle and hardship is favorable to life and its best development, while idleness and luxury are unfavorable and often destructive. Inertia is death both physical and moral. Activity is the law of life, and when coupled with a vigorous struggle, it develops self-reliance and a strength of character such as was never dandled in the lap of ease.

Much fault is found with our unequal social conditions, and there is much murmuring and complaint. Vast accumulations in the hands of a few, resulting from speculation in food products, questionable shrewdness and combines to squeeze the people, are unfortunate and deplorable. They foster envy and a growing discontent on the part of the masses.

No wonder they think the world is out of joint, when some millionaire in a great city spends a thousand dollars upon a dog house, while the unfortunate child goes barefoot and sleeps in a dry-goods box. But it is to be remembered that fortune is so fickle that the same barefooted boy may become wealthy and the millionaire spendthrift may close his life in an almshouse.

Perhaps these inequalities will be remedied in the future and the excessive accumulations of wealth be prevented by legislation. As specific remedies are found to check the devastation of contagious diseases, so we may hope that the intelligence and enterprise of our young nation will be able to devise just methods to check the growth of all its evils.

At any rate these things do not render it necessary for an industrious man and woman to work so hard for shelter, warmth, food and clothing, that they are obliged to turn their backs frowningly upon the best gift that God ever bestowed upon a married pair. This is a broad and productive land, and there is no such grinding poverty here as in the old world. The vast accumulations, that make people envious, often render the posterity of the rich physically and morally effeminate and tend to the obliteration of their name and place, so that their wealth is again scattered. Admitting the truthfulness of every complaint, our social conditions are not depressing enough to deter young people from marriage who are strong and brave, and with whom the current of love is deep, clear and pure.

The simpler life is made, and the more it is conformed to natural laws the more satisfactory it is in the end.

The modern drift from the country to the city is unfortunate, unnecessary and unwise. Many are allured by the attractions of the city to leave the old homestead and become toilers in the shops and mills. They pay as much for a contracted lot of a few feet front as the farm and its buildings included if sold would bring. A few of the more fortunate perhaps better their condition, but the majority surrender their independence and enter upon a struggle just for their daily bread. The pleasure and independence of country life ought to be emphasized. It is the favored place for making a home. The air and the water are pure and free, restraints are less burdensome and living is more natural and simple. It is the ideal place for children. They thrive better, are more healthy, hardy and moral, and make better men. They cost less to raise, and if less polished they have greater physical endurance, and are not wanting in the necessary refinements of mature years.

Marriage at an age as early as is consistent with the ability to provide a home and the necessities of home comfort should in every way be encouraged. The suitable age for the young man is somewhere in the vicinity of twenty-five years, and for the woman it may be from three to five years younger. At these ages young men and women are sufficiently mature to enter upon the responsibilities of married life, and are much more likely to make it a success than if married earlier or later. Marriage, following long engagements or numerous courtships, does not promise as well for obvious reasons as when entered upon during the freshness and enthusiasm of early life. Hence early marriages should be encouraged in every possible way as the basis of good society. There is no more pleasant or invigorating struggle, than that of battling with the world, for the purpose of getting ahead in it, with necessity impelling you, and hope beckoning you forward. The requirements of life should be so simplified that the young man and woman may have courage to start in that delightful process of home building with every promise of success.

The so-called social evil is a blighting curse, destructive to morals and every virtue. It should obtain no license, and toward it no protecting hand should be extended. It boastfully soils with its touch the innocence and modesty of either sex, never satisfied till it has wrought their degradation and ruin.

Whether single or married self-control and self-mastery should be acquired and practiced in the exercise of the sexual functions. Their only disclosed object, the perpetuity of the race, should be faithfully considered. Apart from this they are scarcely necessary. Their exercise is neither essential to health nor enjoyment. Little if any harm results from holding the sexual activities in abeyance even for a life time, and under the favoring conditions offered by marriage, great moderation is alike conducive to health and happiness.

. The perversion of this instinct is fatal alike to purity and peace, for it disturbs the nervous equilibrium, undermines the health, sours the disposition, fills life with suffering, and digs an early grave. It often leads the unmarried to the gateway of destruction and the married to divorce and degradation.

II.—REPRODUCTION.

The product of conception is carried in the womb for about two hundred and eighty days, during which time it is perfected and developed so as to maintain subsequent to birth an independent existence. This is the period of pregnancy; its commencement is conception, and its termination labor.

This period usually begins with the close of the last menstruation or monthly sickness, and ends in about nine calender months, or to be more precise, in two hundred and eighty days. Living beings thus reproduce themselves, for the perpetuity of the race could not otherwise be maintained.

The process is sexual, and requires the energizing force of both the male and the female. The female has two ovaries, one on each side of the uterus, each about the size and shape of an almond. The ovaries produce at stated intervals of about twenty-eight days a little ovum or egg, so small that two hundred of them would measure but little over an inch in diameter. When the egg is matured it bursts the outer covering of the ovary and is carried along a little tube so small that its central opening will admit only a common bristle. This is known as the Fallopian tube or oviduct, and opens one on each upper side of the womb. The matured egg passes slowly along this tube till it reaches the womb. If conception takes place during its journey it attaches itself to the womb and draws nourishment from it until the development of a human being is accomplished. Otherwise it perishes.

These different stages of development are of great interest to a scientific mind, but must be passed over here for the most part, as the details of reproduction are too extensive and complex except for a technical work. Coincident with the escape of an egg from the ovary, a discharge of blood from the interior of the womb takes place. This occurs once a month in a healthy mature female, and is known as menstruation, or the monthly flow. In order that conception may take place it is necessary that spermatozoa, which are contained in the semen secreted by the male, should come in contact with the egg somewhere on its passage from the ovary to the uterus. Seminal fluid is secreted by the testicle of the male and contains large numbers of micro-organisms called spermatozoa. These little agents are active and capable of rapid movement, and if supplied with warmth and moisture retain their vitality for a number of days. If these little bodies are deposited anywhere within, or near the vagina, they are likely to find their way into the womb and the Fallopian tube in search for the egg.

Having found the little ovum or egg, they penetrate it with great energy. Their mission is then completed, and conception takes place. Conception may take place at any time during the month, but is most likely to occur just before or soon after menstruation. The impregnated ovum goes through a series of rapid changes. First there is division and subdivision of the egg, until it resembles a mulberry, then layers of membrane are formed, some of which begin to organize into a rudimentary being, and others form a sac to surround and protect it. A placenta is formed with its cord, fluid surrounds the perfectly formed embryonic child, and all this mysterious work is accomplished by the end of the third month. From this time onward to delivery, constant growth of the fœtus takes place, and the womb enlarges correspondingly to meet the growing demands of its occupant. The umbilical cord when fully developed is about twenty inches long and about the size of an adult finger in the diameter. It connects the growing fœtus to the placenta and contains a vein and two arteries for transporting blood to and from the fœtus. It is in the placenta that the fœtal blood is oxygenized and rendered fit to be returned to the fœtus for further nourishment. The fœtus and cord are protected from pressure and injury by the amniotic fluid which the membranous sac contains.

When the term of pregnancy is completed, labor takes place, and a new being is born into the world. Labor is accompanied with pains and an uncomfortable bearing down sensation. These pains are not continuous, but come on at intervals. The early pains of labor are due to the dilation of the mouth of the womb. If its muscular tissue is rigid, they may continue for a long time, and may be especially severe and annoying. At birth a well-developed child measures about twenty-two inches in length and weighs from six to seven pounds, although they sometimes weigh much less or considerably more in individual cases.

III.—SYMPTOMS OF PREGNANCY.

The early symptoms of pregnancy are largely probabilities, but when great interests are at stake a skillful practitioner will be able to give even in these cases satisfactory opinions and counsel.

The first and best known symptom of pregnancy is suppression of the monthly sickness. This is the rule, and exceptions are rare. If there is a previous history of good health, and the woman has heretofore been regular, and nothing has occurred of sufficient moment to otherwise account for the cessation, the probability of pregnancy is strong.

Nausea and vomiting are often annoying symptoms during early pregnancy, usually commencing about the fourth week and ending during the second month. This symptom is commonly known among women as morning sickness. Sometimes the patient feels hungry and eats heartily, vomiting immediately after, without discomfort. There are cases where this symptom does not appear at all, and others where it is only slight, and still others where it is very severe and aggravated, continuing on through consecutive weeks, both day and night, until it threatens life.

Ptyalism, or an increased flow of saliva, is sometimes troublesome during pregnancy, the secretion of the salivary glands being very greatly increased above the normal.

Enlargement of the veins of the legs is one of the early symptoms of pregnancy, owing to the increased tension of the blood vessels during this condition.

Changes take place also in the breasts. They become enlarged, tender, and somewhat painful. The circles called the areola, around the breasts, become darker, and when a secretion of milk is discovered there is very strong evidence of the pregnant condition.

The abdomen, after the second month, gradually enlarges, and this symptom is so well understood as to require no explanation.

At the end of about four months the prospective mother begins to feel the movements of the fœtus. These movements, known as quickening, are at first feeble, but constantly become stronger. It is a great error to suppose that life does not exist prior to quickening. This symptom is usually considered a positive sign of the pregnant condition, and unless such movement is imagined or feigned, should be so regarded.

There are some other symptoms, as the sounds of the fœtal heart, ballotement, the uterine souffle, etc., which are of interest only to professional persons, and need not be described at this point. The obscure symptoms require attention from the skillful ear and hand of the physician.

In general, time unveils obscurities and brings to light and explains many mysterious secrets. Unless for some reason it is necessary to at once recognize the fact of pregnancy, a little judicious waiting is recommended.

IV.—DISEASES OF PREGNANCY.

The diseases of pregnancy are in some cases simply an exaggeration of the symptoms already mentioned, as nausea and vomiting, varicose veins, dropsy of the feet and legs, and hemorrhoids or piles.

Nausea and vomiting are among the most common troubles of pregnancy, and they sometimes persist till the vomited matter is streaked with blood, and the stomach manifests symptoms of inflammation. When the nausea is constant, the patient loses flesh, looks haggard, and the mere sight or odor of food is sufficient to provoke renewed attacks.

The mild cases require but little treatment, for the symptoms pass off with the forenoon, and in a few weeks all traces of sickness disappear. A cup of coffee and a slice of toast taken each morning in bed will frequently afford relief. If there is an acid condition of the stomach, a dessert spoonful of the granular citrate of magnesia dissolved in water will be beneficial. A mustard plaster applied over the pit of the stomach will often afford relief in aggravated cases.

When other nourishment cannot be retained, equal parts of lime water and milk may be tried. The following powders are excellent and have usually afforded relief in the author's practice.

℞	Cocaine muriate	two grains
	Bismuth subnitrate	forty grains
	Cerium oxalate	forty grains
	Pepsin pure	forty grains

Mix. Make into twenty powders. Take one powder after each meal or after vomiting.

Sometimes the vomiting is so severe that the hypodermic injection of morphia for a time, in one-eighth grain doses, is essential to produce rest. This treatment, however, should only be attempted by those possessing professional skill.

If constipation is troublesome, and is not relieved by using fruits and vegetables in the diet, the citrate of magnesia or a Seidlitz powder each morning, or a teaspoonful of the compound liquorice powder may be taken each night on going to bed. If the tongue is furred, the breath foul and the skin sallow, some more energetic remedy to act upon the liver may be required, and for this purpose the following is recommended.

℞	Podophyllin	one grain
	Solid ext. nux vomica	four grains
	Ext. taraxacum	twenty grains
	Ext. cascara sagrada	twenty grains
	Pulv. zingiber	ten grains

Mix. Make twenty pills, take one each night, until the bowels act naturally.

Piles or hemorrhoids are sometimes caused by the pressure of the gravid womb upon the veins, and also the increased blood pressure due to this condition. A suppository pushed into the rectum, after the bowels move, or one each night and morning, will afford relief.

The following is recommended:

℞	Cocaine muriate	two grains
	Ext. hyoscyamus	five grains
	Pulv. opii	five grains
	Tannin	ten grains
	Cacao butter q. s. to make	ten suppositories

Use as indicated. An ointment made of galls and opium often affords relief. Sometimes hot fomentations are soothing to piles that are inflamed.

For an excessive flow of saliva use an astringent wash, containing alum and tincture of myrrh as follows:

℞ Alum   twenty grains
    Rose water   two ounces
    Tinct. of myrrh   one dram

Mix. Use to rinse the mouth as needed.

The enlarged veins of the lower extremities may be emptied and relieved by taking the recumbent position frequently and having the limbs raised higher than the head, or placing the feet in a chair when sitting. If the limbs persistently swell, attended with headache, the urine should be examined to see if albumen is present.

When there is a large amount of albumen in the urine of a pregnant woman she needs medical attention, otherwise puerperal convulsions are likely to come on before, during, or after labor.

Neuralgia, due to decayed teeth or from some other obscure cause, is of common occurrence, and is often persistent and troublesome. To extract the painful tooth rarely gives relief, as some other tooth is likely to continue the torment. Hot applications may be applied to the seat of the pain. Menthol liniment may afford relief or chloroform applied locally. If neuralgia is due to anæmia and an impoverished condition of the nerves, tonic treatment internally will yield better results than external applications.

℞ Quinine sulph.   one-half dram
    Ext. nux vomica   four grains
    Dried sulphate of iron ten grains
    Ext. hyoscyamus   ten grains

Mix. Make into twenty pills. Dose one at night and repeat in four or six hours if not relieved, taking three a day until improvement takes place.

Fainting sometimes occurs and is due to emotion, excitement or weakness. The patient should be placed carefully upon a bed or lounge, the clothing loosened and ammonia or spirits of camphor inhaled. A teaspoonful of the aromatic spirits of ammonia, diluted with water, should be given internally, and may be repeated at intervals till the tendency to fainting is relieved.

The pregnant woman often experiences a great variety of distressing nervous symptoms, as insomnia, irritable temper, headache and cough or difficult breathing. Unless these symptoms are aggravated, they pass off in due time and require but little treatment.

Chorea sometimes occurs as a complication of pregnancy, and when it does, requires professional advice, as it is rather an unfavorable accompaniment. It is best treated with the bromide of iron and Fowler's solution.

Where there is irritation of the bladder, or inability to hold the water in the pregnant condition, it is due to the pressure of the womb upon the bladder or upon the urethra, or a too-acid condition of the water. Relief is afforded by the reclining position, and by alkaline drinks, as bicarbonate of soda or the granular citrate of potash.

Other rare derangements may occur in pregnancy, rendering it necessary to seek medical advice.

V.—ADVICE TO THE PREGNANT.

A pregnant woman ought to desire that method of life which will best prepare her for the trials of maternity. She should consult not only her own health and comfort, but also pursue such a course as will be likely to insure the birth of a healthy offspring.

In regard to exercise, only that of a moderate type should be entertained. Physical and mental fatigue should be avoided. Fresh air and sunshine are healthful, and the pregnant woman should be encouraged to go out of doors daily. The occupation of the mind with domestic duties is natural and invigorating. A cheerful and hopeful disposition should be cultivated, and friends should do their part to contribute to this result.

Excitements should be avoided, as well as excessive weariness. Late hours, public entertainments, dancing, horseback riding and fatiguing journeys, involve too much risk and ought to be indulged in, if at all, very cautiously. Any indication of hemorrhage or pain, or premonition of miscarriage, should at once suggest the necessity of absolute rest.

The food should be simple, varied, nutritious, and sufficient in quantity and quality to satisfy the appetite. New demands are made upon the system which must be met by an increased amount of nutrition, otherwise the strength will be impaired. A proper attention to the diet will keep the bowels free and the health up to a vigorous standard.

Fruits are excellent. Nearly all kinds are healthful in their season, and if used freely tend to prevent those unnatural cravings which are sometimes a source of considerable anxiety. Highly seasoned foods and alcoholic stimulants should be rigidly excluded.

Regularity in all the habits of life should be maintained as far as possible, and sufficient sleep secured. Personal cleanliness should be observed, and every tendency to despondency overcome by a cheerful spirit, pleasant and agreeable occupation for the mind, and a life of activity and hope.

To employ the mind frequently in literary pursuits is preferable to giving way to melancholy. In this way the stamp of greater intelligence may be affixed to the offspring and hope kept foremost in the prospective mother's contemplations. Remember that although maternity is often a severe trial, it is the crown and glory of womanhood. Every true gentleman or lady will treat a woman in the pregnant condition with the utmost kindness, courtesy and respect.

During pregnancy loose and comfortable garments should be worn, and in every known way health, cheerfulness and comfort, should be secured. Let reason preside over the passions. It ought not to be necessary to observe that intercourse during pregnancy is unnatural and often productive of much harm. At such a time reason and prudence should prevail, and neither a woman nor her offspring should be imperiled to gratify any instinct which has already received its full accomplishment in the pregnant condition.

VI.—MISCARRIAGE.

For various reasons, miscarriages are liable to occur at any time during pregnancy, anywhere between conception and the seventh month.

Where labor occurs between the seventh and ninth month, it is known as premature labor, but the child, though requiring more care, is mature enough to live and maintain a separate existence. Previous to the seventh month a child is rarely known to live. A woman who is pregnant for the first time is not as likely to miscarry as one who has borne several children. Very fleshy women and those who menstruate profusely are more likely to miscarry than others.

The causes of miscarriage are numerous. Some of the more common are an attack of some acute disease, as measles, scarlet fever, pneumonia, typhoid fever, intermittent fever, dysentery; some excessive emotion or excitement, violent exercise, falls, blows, inflammation of the womb, intercourse, violent purgative medicines; these or similar causes may provoke miscarriage.

Syphilis is a very common cause of miscarriage. Lead poisoning sometimes leads to the same result. The author has found syphilis and fatty placenta most frequently the cause.

The first symptoms of an approaching miscarriage is hemorrhage. This may be slight or profuse. When pain and hemorrhage are both present, a miscarriage is most likely to take place. An attempt should be made to ward off a threatened miscarriage by perfect rest in bed and an unstimulating diet. Cold drinks should be used and a sedative taken as a five-grain Dover's powder. This may be repeated two or three times if needed at intervals of four hours.

After the third month miscarriages often result in an incomplete emptying of the womb. Should any portion of a placenta be retained, it is likely to occasion troublesome hemorrhage and suggests another danger, blood poisoning, from the decomposition of this retained debris. Miscarriages are often attended with a large degree of pain sometimes equal to that of labor at full term.

Miscarriages are common at the close of the first month of pregnancy, and are more frequently overlooked than recognized, as the only symptom is bloodclots and an increased amount of hemorrhage.

Miscarriages criminally procured are to be deprecated, and any man or woman carrying on such unrighteous business, should be dealt with as a base criminal. The principles to be observed in a threatened miscarriage are rest, cold drinks and cold applications to check hemorrhage. If hemorrhage and pain persist, a physician will be needed to manage the case.

After a miscarriage has taken place, rest should still be enjoined as after labor at term, in order to avoid the many risks which follow. Hemorrhage, inflammation, uterine weakness and displacements are some of the consequences which may follow, when rest is not properly enjoined or when the injunction fails to be obeyed.

VII.—LABOR, STAGES AND MANAGEMENT.

Labor is a natural or physiological process. It terminates the period of pregnancy after about two hundred and eighty days.

Sometimes it commences abruptly, but more often there are various premonitions. During the last two weeks of pregnancy the abdomen seems to settle down somewhat, so that there is less interference with the act of breathing, and walking about is performed with less discomfort. Toward the termination of pregnancy uterine contractions take place. At first these are painless and scarcely noticed, but after a time they begin to become painful, and when they take place and continue at regular intervals, labor has commenced. These pains are caused by the muscular contraction of the uterine fibers. Spurious pains may take place, and are often caused by indigestion, constipation, or colic from a collection of gas in the bowels. Spurious pains may be relieved by hot or carminative drinks, a dose of castor oil, or some other mild cathartic.

The beginning of labor is usually distinguished by a discharge of bloody mucous, which results from the expansion or stretching of the mouth of the womb. As labor progresses the pains become harder and more regular. In order to fully understand this important subject, it is customary to describe it under three distinct stages.

The first stage of labor is often quite lengthy and tedious, and lasts till the mouth of the womb is fully extended, so as to permit the expulsion of its contents. This is often the most trying portion of labor, the pains are usually aggravating, the patient is uneasy, fretful and nervous, and forebodes evil. She seeks for rest or comfort in a changed position, but finds it not. If the mouth of the womb is inelastic and reluctant to distend, this stage of labor is correspondingly prolonged. During a pain a portion of the enveloping sac, filled with fluid, is pressed into the mouth of the womb, and seems to assist favorably the dilating process, for it is often noticed that when this sac ruptures and the amniotic fluid escapes early, the progress of labor is retarded, and the first stage is not only longer, but more tedious.

Near the completion of the first stage of labor the bag of waters ruptures and the fluid pours out with a gush. The completion of the first stage is often attended with shivering, slight nervous chills and vomiting. These are of no special consequence and should not be regarded as unfavorable.

The second stage lasts from the complete dilation of the mouth of the womb to the expulsion of the child. The head descends quite rapidly into the pelvic cavity. The bag of waters having ruptured, the womb is able to contract with more energy. The woman now becomes possessed of more courage and is inclined to grasp hold of some object with her hands and pull. Meantime she holds her breath and bears down, thus assisting herself by the voluntary contraction of the abdominal muscles. During this period of labor cramps of the legs sometimes occur, and the back feels as if it would break, but these are relieved, the former by rubbing and the latter by pressing the hand hard over the portion of the back where the pain is experienced.

Powerful uterine contraction takes place, followed by intervals during which a little rest is obtained. Unless there is some impediment or obstruction to labor, the head, which commonly presents, is soon born and the child's body easily follows, completing the second stage of labor.

The third stage consists in the delivery of the placenta or after birth which generally follows labor in fifteen or twenty minutes, and causes but little suffering. The uterus after the birth of the child, contracts upon the placenta and detaches it from its temporary location. Failure of the womb to contract firmly, allows free hemorrhage to take place, and is one of the greatest dangers following child birth, which the experienced physician always guards against. The womb when firmly contracted after delivery can be felt through the abdominal wall, as a hard round ball, about the size of the child's head. The delivery of the after-birth and contraction of the womb, terminates the third stage of labor.

Most cases of labor are easily managed, and when no troublesome emergencies arise, no especial skill is demanded. Labor is a natural process, and the majority of cases could be left to nature without risk. If it was not for exceptional cases, a nurse or midwife could manage a case of labor as well as a physician. Labor is, however, sometimes associated with unexpected accidents and unforeseen emergencies, and if no provision is taken to prepare for any possible difficulty or peril, a valuable life may be sacrificed in consequence.

It is safe and better for all concerned to have a reliable physician engaged, so as to be prepared to meet promptly any unfavorable events. A seasonable engagement enables the physician to ward off any threatening dangers by timely and appropriate attention.

There are no medicines which can be given in advance to ensure an easy and safe delivery, although such specifics are unscrupulously advertised and offered to human credulity.

The room selected by the prospective mother should be quiet, away from confusing noise of the street or household. One of the best qualifications a nurse can possess is good sense, coupled with a quiet and cheerful spirit. The patient should not be kept in bed during the first stage of labor, as sitting up or walking about, favors the descent of the fœtus into the pelvic cavity. The physician can judge quite accurately from the condition of the mouth of the womb, whether or not labor is much advanced, and whether it will be easy or difficult and tedious. Often the greatest hindrance to labor is the rigidity of the mouth of the womb.

Rectal injections of warm water, castile soap and olive oil should be given if the bowels are loaded. Bearing down does no good in the early stage of labor and ought not to be encouraged as it dissipates the strength which will be needed later.

If the bag of waters is not ruptured by the completion of the first stage of labor, the membrane should be broken by the finger nail or in some other appropriate way. When the patient enters upon the second stage of labor it is time for her to take the bed, a mattress is preferable to a feather bed.

The necessary preparations are a rubber cloth under the hips and over this, a folded quilt and sheet, to absorb the discharges. The nightdress and other clothing should be drawn up under the arms. The position most favorable for labor is lying upon the left side or upon the back, as is most comfortable.

Whether it is necessary to use ether or chloroform during the second stage of labor, must be left to the discretion of the attending physician. The judicious use of these agents, in the hands of an experienced practitioner, are never attended by any untoward results. To obtain rest between the pains is of great importance to the patient and should be encouraged.

Drinks to relieve thirst, or for the purpose of nourishment, may be administered as the condition of the patient requires. Everything which will be needed should be in readiness, so that there may be no haste or confusion, as a silk or strong cotton cord, scissors, hot water, and a warm blanket or woolen shawl to wrap about the infant.

The cord is sometimes twisted about the child's neck. It should be drawn down gently and slipped over the head. When the child is born it must be placed in a position favorable for breathing. The cord ought not to be tied, till it has nearly stopped pulsating, and it may be left for some time in perfect safety if the expected physician has not arrived. Firm pressure can be made over the womb by an experienced nurse, which will aid the uterine contractions, prevent hemorrhage and assist in the delivery of the after birth. If the placenta does not follow in a few minutes after the birth of the child, the womb should be grasped in the hand through the abdominal wall, and sufficient pressure made to press out the after birth. Sometimes, though rarely, it is necessary to introduce the hand into the womb in order to separate it. Strong traction upon the cord should not be made, as injury might be done in this way. When all of the above suggestions have been completed, the soiled clothing should be removed, the woman sponged off and dry, warm sheets and napkins should be made use of, to make her comfortable, and additional covering should then be thrown over her, when she should be allowed to rest.

If a bandage is made use of it should extend well down on to the hips and be fastened tightly enough to afford support without being uncomfortable. If there is a tendency to excessive hemorrhage the head of the patient should be lowered, a clean muslin handkerchief, wet in equal parts of vinegar and water, pushed into the vaginal space, and a half teaspoonful of the fluid extract of ergot should be given internally.

A desire for food on the part of the delivered woman should be gratified by some nourishing drink; much depending upon previous habit as to the character of food which may be allowed. She certainly should not be starved, nor on the other hand over fed. She must not be treated as a criminal, with bread and water diet, but must have food sufficiently nutritious to strengthen her exhausted forces.

Attention may be given to the nipples before labor, to harden them and to prevent their cracking or becoming sore, the result of nursing an infant. The glycerite of tannic acid which is simply tannin, dissolved in glycerine by the aid of heat, may be applied daily for three or four weeks before labor which will toughen them. Should they become sore from the lack of such precaution, the same remedy may be applied to heal them. Before the infant nurses, the breasts should be carefully washed, as the remedy is very bitter. After the infant has nursed, the nipples should be washed again and dried before applying the remedy.

When a child is still born, or fails to survive, the secretion of the mother's milk is sometimes excessive and troublesome. In most cases, if the breasts are let alone, nature will absorb it without any harm resulting. It is well to avoid liquids as much as possible, and take a tablet of $\frac{1}{100}$ of a grain of atropia three times a day to check the secretion of milk, and belladonna breast plasters may also be used.

VIII.—MANAGEMENT OF INFANTS.

The infant is the mother's greatest and best gift. It brings a large amount of love along with it, and awakens new thoughts, and broadens the plans and outlook of the parents. A new world of being springs into activity, involving new thoughts, broader action and sweeter and purer life. The happy pair have now a human being, a part of themselves to live for and to love in common. This gives to life a new zest and a wider outlook. Mother love is strong and pure; it is the safeguard of the little stranger. Mother instinct has anticipated the arrival, and prepared for its advent warm flannels, blankets, slips, napkins, and whatever else she has learned will be needed in order that the welcome of the newcomer may be hearty and fitting.

Sometimes it happens that the baby enters the world before the arrival of the expected doctor; when this occurs, it need cause no excitement. It must be remembered that a new-born child must be able to breathe. It must have air, and hence must be lifted up into a position favorable for respiration. The cord ought not to be tied for two or three minutes, and need not be for some time, not until the infant has breatned, has cried lustily, and the pulsation of the cord has nearly ceased. Take a strong string and tie the cord tightly about two inches from the body of the child, at about three inches place another tie, and sever the cord between the two knots with a pair of scissors. The cord should be wrapped in a piece of absorbent cotton and laid over the left side of the child and held in place by a band. Before this is done it should be washed in the following manner: Rub it over quickly and thoroughly with warm sweet oil or vaseline which has been poured upon the palm of the hand, then rub it quickly again with a piece of soft muslin, and arrange and put on the clothes. The oil renders the skin soft and natural. The head, face and eyes, should be washed clean with a sponge or soft cloth and warm water, after the baby has been dressed. This method in winter prevents taking cold, from too great reduction of the temperature.

When the body of the child is washed in water, which may be done in summer if preferred, it should be done by immersing the infant in a warm bath, keeping only the head out of the water, scrubbing it briskly meantime with the hand. After the bath it should be rolled up in a woolen shawl or blanket. Care must be exercised to ascertain if the circulation of the newly-born child has been properly established, and to see that its temperature is high enough. Infants need to be kept warm, and only the face should be exposed, as is needful for the purpose of respiration.

Should it appear to be feeble from any cause, and not seem warm to the hand, a bottle of hot water should be placed near it in bed. Warmth is essential to its life, and should it fail to generate sufficient animal heat the deficiency must be made up artificially. This is of especial importance in children born prematurely.

It may be necessary to moisten the cotton enclosing the decaying cord with mild carbolic acid solution to prevent odor before the separation occurs. The cord separates in from five to seven days, leaving a partially healed stump, which may be dressed with carbolized vaseline or a powder of boric acid or aristol.

The band should not be pinned too tightly about the child's body just snug enough to be comfortable, and in dressing an infant safety pins should always be used.

All things considered, the best nourishment for a baby is that secreted by the mother's breasts. After labor and the mother and child have rested a few hours, it should be allowed the breast, which contains a secretion intended to act as a mild cathartic, and cleanses the child internally. Feeding a new-born child is generally needless and harmful. Perhaps a little pure water should be allowed to rinse out the mouth, but beyond this the supply provided by nature is sufficient. The infant should be allowed to nurse occasionally to encourage it, and to stimulate the milk glands of the mother, so that there may be a sufficient secretion. In from about forty to fifty hours, the full flow of milk is usually established, and by this time the infant gets thoroughly hungry and enjoys nursing. A newly born infant needs to nurse about every two hours throughout the daytime. It does not need to nurse so often during the night, two or three times being sufficient.

It is much better for a child to lie down than to be rocked, and carrying it about the house is a bad and needless habit, which soon spoils the best baby.

When, for any reason, the mother cannot nurse her child the subject of artificial feeding must be considered. As the death rate among infants artificially fed is much greater than among those nursed by the mother, it should be regarded as a misfortune to be obliged to raise it upon a bottle. Artificial feeding, to be successful, requires a large amount of care. It is not by any means an impossibility to raise a healthy child without the breast. A very young infant should have rich, pure milk, one part; mixed with pure water, three parts. A small amount of salt should be added and the whole sweetened with milk sugar and given warm. The addition of a little cream makes the resemblance to human milk closer. The added water, if not absolutely pure, should have been boiled and cooled before using.

Great care must be taken with the nursing bottle to have it scrupulously clean. When not in use it may stand filled with water, to which some baking soda has been added. When the mother nurses her infant she needs to be careful of her own diet, lest by carelessness the little one's stomach and bowels are disordered.

Babies ought not to be dosed with paregoric, soothing syrups, or patent medicines, to produce sleep. A healthy child does not need to be lulled to sleep by narcotic drugs. Mothers are little aware of the harm they do when they drug their children to sleep, and of the liability of producing life-long injuries. Sleep ought to be natural, and the baby can do no more natural thing than to sleep. While soothing syrups produce sleep, it is not natural sleep. The nervous system is powerfully impressed, and the child jumps and starts while sleeping, or awakens startled and frightened. Never, as you value the life of your infant, should you unnecessarily give it carminatives, soothing syrups, cordials or sleeping drops. When, it frets and does not sleep see that tight bandages are loosened. A child ought to be put to bed regularly and taught to go to sleep without even being held or rocked. The clothing, especially at night, should be light and loose, and afford free play for the limbs. A young child should be first undressed and sponged over with warm water, then put on a loose slip and see that the diapers are dry, soft and clean. It should sleep in a crib or cradle by itself, and if properly prepared for sleep, and it still frets, it is probably hungry. After a baby is three or four months old, barley gruel, made by boiling barley for a long time in water, is good to add to the milk if the bowels incline to be loose. When constipation is troublesome thin oatmeal gruel added to the milk will be admirable to correct such a tendency.

Do not give a small child cake or candy to quiet it. Such things produce disordered stomach, loose bowels and other troubles. Tea and coffee are too stimulating, and hence unsuitable to be given to an infant. When it nurses from the breast it should be removed to its own place after it falls asleep. It is not considered a good plan for a mother to nurse a child when she is overheated or when greatly fatigued. As the salivary glands are inactive in young infants, a little pure water should be regularly given to allay thirst.

When a baby is so constipated that oatmeal gruel does not relieve such a condition, a few drops of castor oil may be administered, or frequently an injection containing glycerine, or a glycerine suppository may be used occasionally as needed. Castor oil is a valuable and safe physic. It should be given in small doses and repeated till action ensues. But when the diet of a baby is properly regulated physic will be needed very rarely, if at all. When vomiting occurs, unless from overfeeding, add a tablespoonful of lime water to each nurse till the stomach is again regulated.

It should be remembered that hot weather diminishes the digestive ability of the stomach, when the food should receive increased attention. In very hot weather diminish the amount of food, and avoid its being too hearty. When a child approaches teething, which begins about the seventh, eighth or ninth month, or sometimes sooner, a severe ordeal is often encountered, especially if the weather is hot and the stomach is weak and disordered. This is frequently a trying time for the baby, and results in disturbing either the nervous system, and the child worries, frets, is irritable, and in some cases there may be convulsions, or the stomach is upset and the bowels are loose. A baby that nurses ought not to be weaned just before or during hot weather. When it drools, protect the chest by bibs, and if a tendency to bite is manifested, provide a rubber ring. The gums may be rubbed with the finger, and in some cases they may be bathed with a soothing lotion containing a small amount of cocaine. When they are very sensitive and appear to be painful, the following will afford relief:

℞	Cocaine muriate	two grains
	Tinct. crocus	fifteen drops
	Syr. tolu	three drams

Mix and apply a little to the gums several times a day with the fingers.

When the gums are red, inflamed and painful, the physician may decide to lance them, to relieve the nervous system and prevent convulsions. Should convulsions occur, place the child in a warm bath, apply cold to the head and give a mild laxative if necessary.

The following prescription has relieved many cases of convulsions:

℞ Bromide of soda   one dram
   Chloral hydrate   one-fourth of a dram
   Syrup of tolu   one ounce
   Anise water   one ounce

Mix and give one teaspoonful every hour till relief and rest are produced. This dose is suitable for a child from six to nine months old. For older children a larger dose can be used. In all these cases the benefits of pure air, especially the pure air of the country, should not be forgotten. A change of air has sometimes seemed to be the main factor in saving the life, where teething, debility, hot and impure air all combined to thwart the remedies employed.

A little account of the process of teething will doubtless prove interesting. The teeth come in pairs. The two lower front teeth usually appear first, but sometimes the two upper ones precede them. These are the four incisors or cutting teeth, and in a majority of cases they appear between the seventh and ninth month. The next teeth to appear are called the lateral incisors, one on each side of the pairs already mentioned, so that by the time the child is one year old, there are eight front teeth, four upper and four under. Between the twelfth and sixteenth month four molars appear, two upper and two under. Between the fourteenth and twentieth month the four canines are cut through. These are also known as the eye or stomach teeth. Between the ages of one and a half and three years the second set of molars appear and this completes the set of milk or shedding teeth. The foregoing order is the usual one, but variations frequently occur. The roots of the temporary teeth are absorbed by the approach of the permanent set underneath. The temporary teeth appear designed to last only until the permanent set is ready to appear.

The permanent teeth are thirty-two in number, sixteen upper and sixteen under. They begin to appear usually between the sixth and seventh year, and the set is completed by the appearance of the wisdom teeth, which are tardy in arrival being delayed until somewhere about twenty years of age. At the time of the coming of the permanent teeth the mouth and gums have enlarged, and the temporary teeth loosen or fall out or should be extracted so that the permanent teeth may appear in their proper places. The temporary teeth ought not to be extracted too early, as their loss may cause contraction of the jaw so that the permanent teeth will be irregular or crowded. The coming of the wisdom teeth often causes considerable inconvenience and in some cases suffering enabling one to sympathize with the tedious ordeal through which an infant passes in teething. The wisdom teeth, though last to appear, are often the first to decay and require removal.

The care of the teeth is always important, and in their care cleanliness is the word to be emphasized, and even children should be taught the daily and proper use of a suitable toothbrush. The decay of the teeth is caused by particles of food between them which decompose and which ought to be removed after each meal. Even when the temporary teeth decay early, they should be preserved by temporary filling.

It is apparent to the medical man that a close relation exists between sound health and sound teeth, for the latter are essential to the proper mastication and preparation of the food for digestion, a work which must be done in the mouth, and which will be poorly done if the teeth are decayed and sensitive. The permanent teeth are frequently attacked by tartar which is deposited around the gum. It sometimes extends below the gums, destroying the sockets of the teeth and causing them to loosen. This accumulation of tartar causes the teeth to be sensitive, affects the breath unfavorably and frequently the general health, as when it causes neuralgia and similar troubles. It is a fact that a great many young persons neglect their teeth. There is nothing which causes them to appear more unfavorably. A foul mouth is often the only acquaintance and introduction with the neglectful that a neat person would desire. The teeth should be brushed up and down twice a day, after breakfast and before retiring; remaining particles of food should be removed by a toothpick or soft silk thread passed between them. The following is an excellent tooth powder, and may be used once a day in the interests of a clean mouth.

   ℞ Precipitated chalk   one ounce
    Pulv. castile soap   one ounce
    Pulv. orris root   one ounce

The above may be mixed and flavored with wintergreen, sassafras or rose to suit the taste of the person for whom it is prepared.

The following antiseptic wash is harmless and can be used as required to cleanse the mouth, and it will also keep the gums in a healthy condition:

℞ Carbolic acid — one dram
Antisepsine — one ounce
Alcohol — one ounce
Glycerine — half an ounce
Oil of Wintergreen — two drops

Mix. Add a teaspoonful of this mixture to a wine glass full of water and use to rinse the mouth as needed.

When the gums bleed easily, it indicates that the teeth need attention and the tartar around them should be removed, after which the foregoing wash is appropriate.

The teeth of some are much softer than those of others, and decay earlier, there being a deficiency in the organic matter which they contain. The teeth are unfavorably affected by sickness, by pregnancy and by the taking of unsuitable medicines. Medicines which affect the teeth should either be administered in pill form or else taken through a glass tube, and afterward the mouth should be rinsed with a solution of bicarbonate of soda, (common cooking soda.)

Caries or decay of the teeth is a common affection, and causes severe pain after the cavity has extended so as to expose the sensitive nerve to the air. A little oil of clove placed in the cavity usually gives temporary relief from toothache. Other substances used for this purpose are laudanum, chloroform, ether and creosote. The last should be used with great caution as it may corrode the surrounding tissues and produce a sore mouth.

IX.—CARE AND EDUCATION OF CHILDREN.

In the care of children of all ages the regulation of their diet is a matter worthy of special attention. A liberal supply of well cooked food has much to do with the promotion of their well being, the bulk of which should consist of such simple articles as milk with the cereals, together with fruits. When meat is allowed, the quantity must not be too abundant, and the avoidance of too hearty suppers will prevent many attacks of sudden sickness and disturbance at night coupled with anxious solicitude.

Those children who are physically frail, need to have still more attention paid to the important subject of their diet, so as to have in view an improvement of their bodily health and physical development. Not only must their food be nutritious and wholesome, but it must contain sufficient variety to satisfy the demands of nature and tempt a sluggish appetite.

Life in the city is not so favorable for the growth and moral development of young children as the country, but what is lacking may be supplied if appropriate attention is given to their welfare. Exercise and recreation need to be provided at all seasons of the year. This fact is receiving more adequate recognition than formerly, and is deserving of still more even than it is now receiving.

Young children who are especially bright, smart and wise for their years need to be restrained or held back. Such children ought not to be sent to school before they are six or seven years old. The brain of the young child is often inclined to excessive activity, and fond mothers and other members of the family sometimes take delight in teaching a bright infant to say and do many things which tend to over-tax the mental capacity and over-stimulate the brain. Caution in this respect ought not to go unheeded. Small children ought to be kept free from excitement, especially of an emotional nature. Birthday parties, late hours or aping the ways of older people are all objectionable.

Simple methods of instruction for young children are especially appropriate, such as used in the kindergarten schools, where attention is given to learning language, form, color, etc., in natural and attractive ways, and even this kind of training ought not to be too forcing in its character.

The moral education of children should not be overlooked. The mother will be repaid for giving proper attention to this side of the child's nature. She must learn to interpret the wants, anticipate the fears and discover the defects of the children, so as to direct them aright. She must restrain and encourage, as the nature of each requires, and she will experience great pleasure and satisfaction in so doing. She must especially teach them truth, gentleness and affection, by precept and by example, at an early age. A mother possessing patience, gentleness and affection can assist in the development of these desirable qualities to a surprising degree. The restraints interposed by the mother should be firm but kind and calculated to improve the physical and moral well being of her children. Members of the same family vary in disposition and the training must vary so as to adapt itself to the requirements of each child. The best system of education at home or at school is that which draws out and develops the strength and vigor of each individual mind. Dull scholars should not be despised and held up to ridicule before their schoolmates. Such scholars, in the long run, often outdistance those of greater promise, as they mature slowly.

There is no good reason why boys and girls should not be educated together. Brothers and sisters are brought up together in the same homes, and there is no valid reason why they should not be educated together in the same schools or colleges. Where coeducation has been tried it has proved eminently satisfactory. The idea that the education of a girl or young woman can be more superficial or less thorough and extensive than that of her brother is not a good one, and ought not to prevail in the future. Prominent educators are recognizing these facts, and colleges are opening their doors with a more friendly welcome to the female student than formerly.

Prizes for the brightest scholars are unjust. It is not the bright scholar, who can commit to memory easily, who needs encouragement, but the dull one. All who do well should share in whatever honors and prizes may be offered.

The brain of the student cannot do good work without sufficient rest and nourishment. Over-feeding, lack of sleep, want of exercise, and too much or the wrong emotional excitement, are some of the things which interfere with the progress of education. No system of education should be allowed to seriously interfere with the health. All students need compulsory and systematic exercise.

Instruction upon those delicate matters which may excite the curiosity of the young, ought not to be omitted or left to chance. Too much reserve and secrecy is possible, for this will increase rather than diminish the desire of the young for knowledge. Hence this should be imparted, carefully and truthfully. The teaching of elementary anatomy and physiology in the schools is important; the functions of the heart and stomach are explained, and in a suitable time and way, the other functions of the organs may be so explained as to satisfy the youthful mind without arousing its passions. It is easy and natural to pass from the study of plants to animal, and from the functions of one organ to that of another, and such information, wisely imparted, is far better than that learned from suspicious books or persons of doubtful morals. The mother should keep the confidence of her boys and girls so that she may impart to them such instruction with respect to themselves as will satisfy their desire for increasing knowledge, and be productive of sound health and good morals.

CHAPTER XXXIII.

NURSING. DIET FOR THE SICK AND HOW TO PREPARE IT.

I.—Nursing. II.—Diet for the Sick and its Preparation.

I.—NURSING.

THE success of medical treatment depends more upon proper nursing than is generally supposed. In the great majority of functional diseases nature would be able to perform the miracle of healing without medicine if only suitable attention were given to the diet. Many of the functional, and some of the organic diseases, result from faulty nutrition. The diet may be too scanty, too abundant, or inappropriate. In either case nature is misused and the process of recovery may be impeded.

Much has already been said in the body of this work about diet and nutrition in connection with the treatment of various diseases and does not need to be repeated. A few practical matters, referring more directly to the nurse, male or female, remain for our consideration.

Good nurses of either sex are often in demand for the care of the sick. They are more easy to find, and as a class, better qualified, than formerly. So much attention has been devoted to the important subject of training nurses, by physicians and hospitals, that many have been induced and have found it profitable to fully equip themselves for professional nursing. A good nurse possesses such requisites as a cheerful disposition, good health, quiet manners and sound judgment. The need of a cheerful disposition in the sick room is obvious. Good nature is communicated from one to another. Like some diseases it is always contagious, but unlike them, its effects upon the patient are always favorable.

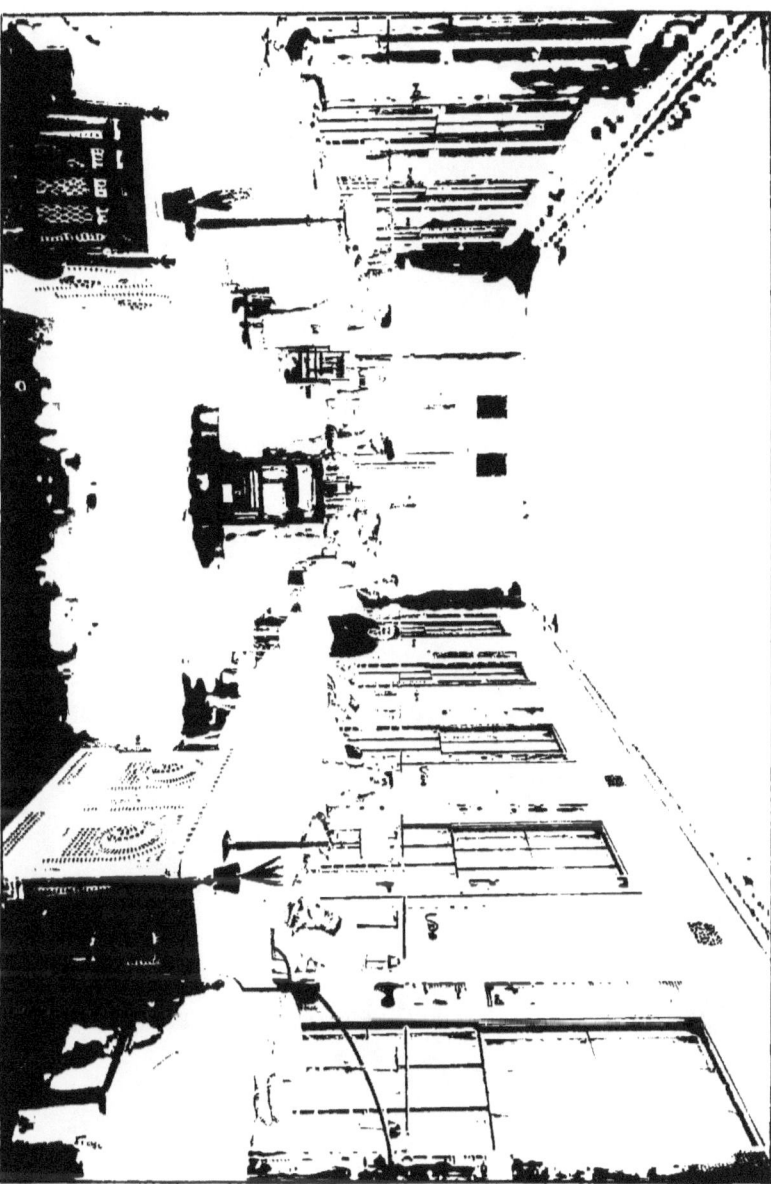

WARD B.—BOSTON CITY HOSPITAL.

It is no easy task to do faithful nursing, for the customary rest is more or less disturbed. To satisfy the exacting demands of the sick, who are frequently difficult to manage and unwilling to be pleased, is often a heavy tax upon the vitality of the nurse. A frail person, or one with impaired health, will not be able to endure such a trying ordeal. The people who employ a nurse are often unsympathetic and do not care to listen to complaints, for their minds being occupied with one invalid, they have no place for another, and hence a person in poor health should not attempt nursing.

A quiet manner is especially a desirable quality in a nurse. It is difficult to think of a requisite which is so constant and important. Sick people ought not to be disturbed too frequently. Noise, talking and commotion, are often very wearying to them. Fussiness, meddling with the pillows, and raising the patient's head, may be carried to such an extent as to be a constant torment. The noise of a rocking chair is often sufficient to distract a patient beyond telling. If the pillow needs fixing or the head of the patient needs raising, the nurse should do it quietly, at a proper time and in a gentle manner. Some nurses indulge in talk about other patients in whom they have been interested, how they looked, what they said, and how they died. A nurse must not mention any such experiences, and if cases are mentioned by another should answer civilly any question asked without volunteering to give any details.

A competent nurse does not need to attempt in any way to impress the fact of her qualifications upon a physician or others. Deeds, not words, form the standard by which one is correctly estimated. There is no one thing which more fully recommends a nurse for her difficult work than a refined and quiet manner.

A nurse requires good judgment because so many important matters demand attention. The sick room must be ventilated without endangering the patient. A nurse who "must have air" even though the patient catches a death cold from the direct draught of an open window is too inconsiderate or too obstinate to be desirable. A nurse should know how to regulate the temperature of a sick room and should be provided with a thermometer, an inexpensive article which will relieve of all anxiety in this respect. A nurse ought to be able to keep an accurate account of the patient's temperature, and hence it is necessary to be familiar with the use of a fever thermometer. A nurse ought to know how to give an enema properly, either rectal or vaginal, how to pass a catheter, how to introduce a suppository, how to make a mustard or flaxseed poultice, flaxseed tea or cream of tartar lemonade, as well as the various methods of preparing suitable and palatable dishes for the sick.

A good nurse will dress tidily, paying suitable attention to herself as well as the patient. The bedding needs to be frequently changed and in some diseases daily and to this she must give appropriate attention. Sick people are fastidious, hence fragments of food should not be left around in sight of the patient, but are to be carried away as soon as possible. When food is brought, it should look inviting. No old messes, unattractive, dirty, or rumpled napkin should be used. A nurse ought to know thoroughly the following facts. In sickness food has to be adapted to the altered condition of the system. The careless administration of food may do much harm, especially in recovery from fevers. Loss of appetite and inability to digest food are symptoms in many acute diseases, but in recovery from fevers the appetite is usually strong, sometimes ravenous, and such conditions require the exercise of much good judgment.

It was customary in fevers formerly to allow only a small amount of food or drink but the present method, in which a free use of water, milk, malt and the various preparations of beef are allowed, yields better results. In fevers there is great waste of the bodily tissues and a generous supply of liquid food is indicated. In some cases small quantities of liquid food should be given like medicine hourly. Milk is the best food in fevers. It is a complete food in itself, containing all the nutritious principles, is cheap, easy to obtain and generally relished by the great majority of cases. When it disagrees or fails to be digested properly, it may be mixed with toast water, lime water or seltzer water occasionally where an aperient effect is desired or the alkaline mineral waters as Vichy. The use of the two latter waters with milk may be alternated with pleasant results. Whey, though not very nutritious, is pleasant and often useful, and when milk disagrees, it may be made for a time to take its place. Ordinarily food should not be forced upon the sick, and only as much should be allowed as can be utilized without causing distress or doing harm. In the use of food as with medicines it is not a large amount which is needed but the right kinds.

During recovery from typhoid fever the diet needs to be still more generous, but it should consist of such simple articles as milk, rice well cooked, tapioca, custard, baked apples, fruit jellies, and some have advised raw meat chopped or pounded fine, or eggs added to soup and in this way they are easily digested and nutritious.

A few fresh flowers may be allowed in the room, for they often brighten and cheer the patient. They can do no harm unless their odor is offensive and they otherwise annoy the patient which is unusual.

II.—DIET FOR THE SICK AND ITS PREPARATION.

Toast Water.—Toast a slice of stale bread till it is nicely browned, without burning it. Pour over it in a dish one pint of boiling water. It may be flavored with grated nutmeg. Let it cool, and strain. This makes a simple and pleasant drink.

Rice Water.—Wash half a cupful of rice, put it on, in three pints of water, and boil for two hours. A little nutmeg, stick of cinnamon, or a shred of orange or lemon peel, may be boiled with it to flavor. Strain, season, and use in diarrhœal diseases.

Barley Water.—Wash half a cup of pearl barley, put it on in three pints of cold water to boil for two or three hours. Then strain, season, and flavor with extract of lemon.

Oatmeal Water.—Put a tablespoonful of coarse oatmeal in a pitcher containing a pint of water. Stir, and after a while strain and use to make lemonade or for a nourishing drink.

Jelly Water.—Stir a teaspoonful of any acid jelly into a goblet of water and sweeten to taste. Currant, cranberry, plum, barberry, quince, strawberry, raspberry or blackberry jelly may be used in this way, all of which make pleasant drinks.

Tamarind Water.—Into a glass of water stir a tablespoonful of preserved tamarinds.

Lime Water.—Over a piece of unslacked lime, the size of a cubic inch, pour a pint of boiling water. Let it stand and settle, turn off this first water and add a quart of pure cold water. Stir together and let it settle again. Then pour this off and bottle for use as an antacid. Use a tablespoonful of lime water to half a pint of milk.

Herb Drinks.—These are made by pouring boiling water over a small handful of the herb, as catnip, pennyroyal, camomile, etc. Strain after standing a few minutes, and sweeten to taste.

Apple Water.—Boil a large juicy apple, which has been pared and cored, in a pint of water until the apple is cooked very soft. Strain and press out all the juice from the pulp. Sweeten and drink after it is cold.

Gum Arabic Water.—Dissolve one ounce of gum and one tablespoonful of sugar in one quart of cold water. Flavor with lemon. This makes a pleasant demulcent drink good for irritation in the throat, or to allay a cough.

Flaxseed Tea.—Take one ounce of flaxseed, one tablespoonful of white sugar, half an ounce of liquorice root and the juice of one lemon. Add one quart of boiling water, and after standing four or five hours strain.

Flaxseed Lemonade.—Cover two ounces of flaxseed with a pint of hot water and let it stand for two hours. Strain, add lemon juice and sweeten to taste. This is a good drink in fevers.

Cream of Tartar Lemonade.—Put one teaspoonful of cream of tartar into a bowl and add one pint boiling water. Squeeze in the juice of a lemon and sweeten to taste. This is an excellent drink in all febrile conditions.

Slippery Elm Tea.—Take one ounce of slippery elm bark and break into small pieces. Pour over it a pint of water and let it stand for several hours. This makes a useful demulcent drink.

Sage Tea.—Take half an ounce of sage leaves, a tablespoonful of sugar and the peel of half a lemon cut up fine. Cover with a pint or more of boiling water. After standing half an hour strain. This may be used hot or cold.

Arrow Root.—Mix a tablespoonful of arrow root with sufficient water to make a paste. Stir this into a pint of boiling water or milk. Orange peel may be used to flavor. It may be sweetened or seasoned to a taste.

Slippery Elm Jelly—Take four ounces of slippery elm bark, pour over it a quart of cold water and let it stand over night. Add the juice and peel of one lemon, and let it simmer on the stove for fifteen minutes. Strain into a mould.

Orange Jelly.—Take one ounce of gelatin, one pint of orange juice, and let them soak together half an hour. Add half a cup of sugar, one pint of boiling water, and stir until all are dissolved, then strain into a mould.

Tapioca Jelly.—Soak two tablespoonfuls of tapioca in a teacupful of cold water for two or three hours. Then stir in a pint of boiling water. Keep it stirring and boil gently. Sweeten and pour into a mould. A little wine may be added if needed.

Lemon Sauce.—Boil half a cup of sugar in two cups of water. Make a paste of a tablespoonful of cornstarch and cold water. Stir together and boil ten minutes. Add the juice of one lemon.

Boiled Custard.—To one quart of boiling milk add two tablespoonfuls of cornstarch made into a paste with milk. Add three eggs well beaten, stir continually. Sweeten and flavor to taste and add a pinch of salt. The whites of the eggs may be beaten to a froth separately and put on the top of the custard.

Tapioca Cream.—Soak three tablespoonfuls of tapioca in water over night. Pour off the water and add one quart of milk. Bring it to a boil and stir in the yolks of three eggs, one tablespoonful of sugar and a little salt. Flavor with lemon or vanilla. Frost with the whites of the eggs, beaten to a froth, and brown in the oven.

Lemon Jelly.—Soak half a package of gelatin in half a pint of cold water for an hour, add a pint of boiling water, the juice of a lemon and two tablespoonfuls of sugar. Stir until the gelatin is dissolved and strain into a mould.

Apple Souffle.—Bake half a dozen sour apples, scrape out the pulp, sweeten, add the whites of two eggs beaten to a froth, flavor to taste and bake a few minutes in an oven.

Blanc Mange.—Take two tablespoonfuls of cornstarch and make a paste of it by adding a little cold milk. Stir this paste into a pint of milk, boiling it for three or four minutes. Pour into moulds or cups to cool.

Iceland Moss Blanc Mange.—Wash an ounce of moss in cold water, then put it into a lace bag and put it on to boil in half a pint of water and the same amount of milk. Sweeten, flavor with vanilla and pour into moulds when it begins to thicken.

Koumiss.—Take one quart of warm, fresh milk, add a tablespoonful of sugar and one-half of a compressed yeast cake dissolved in warm water or a tablespoonful of brewer's yeast. Let it stand till foamy. Put into stout bottles, use corks that have been soaked soft in boiling water, and tie them down with a stout string and put in a cool place or ice chest. Open the bottle by means of a champagne tap.

Peptonized Milk.—See page 446.

Thickened Milk.—Take one pint of hot milk, stir into it a paste made of one tablespoonful of flour, cornstarch or arrow root and a little cold water. Add a little salt, boil three or four minutes, stirring constantly. Flavor with extract of lemon, cinnamon or grated nutmeg.

Whey.—Put a teaspoonful of liquid rennet or a teaspoonful of dry pepsin powder into a pint of warm milk. Let it stand till the curd evaporates and then strain.

Wine Whey.—Take a wineglassful of sherry and add it to half a pint of boiling milk. After standing a while strain it to separate the whey. It may be flavored with grated nutmeg.

Egg Nog, No. 1.—Beat up thoroughly a fresh egg, add sugar, then add a cup of milk, a tablespoonful of brandy and grated nutmeg. Whip well.

Egg Nog, No. 2.—Brandy two ounces, cinnamon water two ounces. Rub up the yolks of two eggs with a tablespoonful of sugar, then add the brandy and cinnamon water. Stir in the whites of the eggs whipped to a froth.

Egg Cordial.—Whip the white of an egg to a froth, add a teaspoonful of sugar, one tablespoonful of cream and whip together, then add by degrees one tablespoonful of brandy and mix all thoroughly.

Milk and Egg.—Beat up a fresh egg and stir it into a half-pint of boiling milk, stir constantly and drink while hot.

Milk Punch.—Mix a tumbler of milk and two tablespoonfuls of brandy, sweeten and flavor with grated nutmeg.

Vegetable Soup.—Take two potatoes, one tomato and a slice of stale bread. Turn over them a quart of water and boil it down to a pint. Season with salt and flavor with celery. Strain it for use.

Egg Broth.—Soak two ounces of pearl sago for half an hour in half a pint of water. Beat the yolks of four eggs in one-half cup of cream or milk, add one quart of beef tea and stir the whole together. A little wine may be added if required.

Chicken Broth.—Clean a chicken, remove the skin, put into a quart or more of water, depending upon the size of the chicken. Add a tablespoonful of washed rice, a little salt and a sprig of parsley. Boil three hours. Skim off particles of fat.

Beef Tea.—Cut up one pound of lean beef, put into a preserve jar with half a pint of cold water. After it has stood awhile put it into a kettle of hot water and simmer for three hours. Season the broth in the jar to taste. Strain through a coarse cloth.

Beef Tea.—Cut up a pound of lean beef, add a pint of cold water, set it on the back part of the stove and let it stand for an hour, then bring it forward and to a boil. Remove any fat from the top, season to taste and pour off.

Beef Essence.—Place one pound of lean steak in a hot frying pan and turn after a minute. Let it simply heat through, then press the juice out of it with a lemon squeezer.

Meat Juice. Concentrated.—Put one pound of lean beef cut up into pieces into a preserve jar, add a little salt, two tablespoonfuls of water and screw on the cover. Place the jar in a kettle of water, bring to a boil and boil for two hours. Press the juice out of the beef after it gets cold and skim off all particles of fat. This makes a concentrated food which may be used in small quantities.

Meat Juice, Raw.—Cut up a pound of lean beef and add half a pint of cold water. Soak it all day occasionally shaking it. Press out the juice with a lemon squeezer and season.

Mutton Broth—One pound of loin of mutton, water three pints. Boil till tender, add salt and a little pepper, and when cold skim off the fat.

Beef Broth and Oatmeal Gruel.—Mix half a cup of oatmeal gruel and a pint of beef tea, heat to the boiling point and stir meantime. Skim off any particles of fat.

Oysters, Roasted.—Place one dozen fresh oysters in the shell in an oven till they open slightly. Remove the oysters and serve with pepper and salt. Oysters thus cooked are very digestible.

Clam Broth.—Wash and boil a dozen clams, strain the broth over some crackers.

Ice for the Sick Room.—Bind with a tape a piece of flannel to the top of a tumbler so that it will form a bag extending half way to the bottom, fill with pieces of ice, cover the top with a second piece of flannel. The ice will keep for a long time, because the melted water passes away from the ice to the bottom of the tumbler.

AUTHOR.—SEE FRONTISPIECE.

MANY readers of THE NEW MEDICAL WORLD will doubtless like to know something about the author and his qualifications for the preparation of such a work and so the publishers have compiled this brief sketch from "Stone's Biography of Eminent Physicians and Surgeons" and "The Biographical Review of Hampden County."—born North Stonington, Ct., Sept. 29th, 1845,—father, a clergyman of strong character, possessing varied gifts,—mother, Almira Miner of Stonington, Ct., descended from old Colonial ancestry, —educated in the public schools of his native town,—prepared for college at Suffield, Ct.,—graduated from Brown University 1870,— belongs to the famous class of which President Andrews is a member, —received the degree of A. M. from Brown in 1873,—studied medicine with Prof. Albert VanderVeer,—received the degree of M. D. at the completion of a course in the Albany Medical College,—one of the prominent physicians and surgeons of Springfield, Mass,—is a man of literary tastes,—qualified both by education and experience for the preparation of such a work,—the commendations received already from eminent sources confirm our views. The Dr. belongs to various medical and other societies,—ex-President of Hampden District Medical Soc.,—fellow of American Academy of Political and Social Science, etc.

THE PUBLISHERS.

A FEW REPRESENTATIVE MEDICAL CELEBRITIES.

THE pictures of a few representative medical celebrities, American and foreign, are included in this work. No effort has been made to include more than a few of the many eminent men of the profession who are already recorded upon the roll of honor. It was intended to make the selection chiefly on the ground of original work in some particular line of medicine or surgery, but owing to popular interest in certain well-known men a few exceptions to the original plan have been made. It will be noticed that the outline given of the life work of each is much condensed and briefly recalls only a few biographical facts.

WILLIAM HARVEY, M. D.,—born in England in 1578,—died in 1657,—everywhere honored as the discoverer of the circulation of the blood,—after receiving his medical degrees, he settled in London,—appointed lecturer at the College of Physicians, and in 1628 gave his views upon the circulation of the blood to the world after having taught them for nine years,—was physician to James I and also Charles I,—was the most eminent medical man of his age.

EDWARD JENNER, M. D.,—born in England in 1749,—died in 1823,—celebrated for the discovery of vaccination,—many honors were conferred upon him by foreign courts and the learned societies of Europe. Parliament in two grants voted him a total of 30,000 pounds. His discovery has been of great service and is practiced successfully throughout the civilized world rendering his name immortal.

SIR ASTLEY COOPER, BART.—born in England in 1768,—died in 1841,—widely celebrated as a surgeon and occupied chairs as a lecturer upon both anatomy and surgery,—an enthusiast in his profession,—author of the first great work upon Hernia, also a celebrated work upon Fractures and Dislocations,—removed a tumor from the head of Geo. IV and received from him in return a baronetcy. His practice is said to have reached the enormous sum of 21,000 pounds annually.

EPHRAIM McDOWELL, M. D.,—born in Virginia in 1771,—died in 1830,—studied medicine at Edinburgh,—settled at Danville, Ky, where in 1809 he performed the first ovariotomy, without anæsthetics, with a mob about his office threatening to lynch him if his patient, (a Mrs. Crawford,) did not survive the operation,—also a celebrated lithotomist,—operated successfully upon James K. Polk, who afterward became President of the U. S.,—a pioneer in abdominal surgery who earned the distinguished title, "FATHER OF OVARIOTOMY."

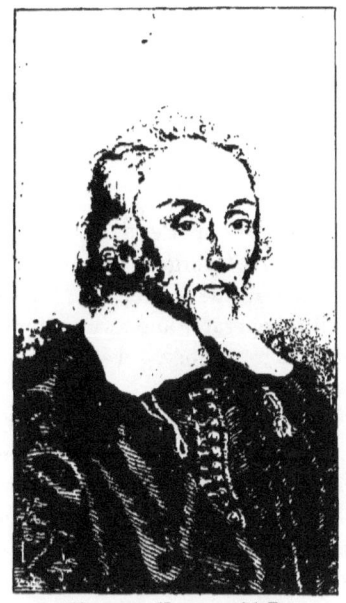

WILLIAM HARVEY, M.D.

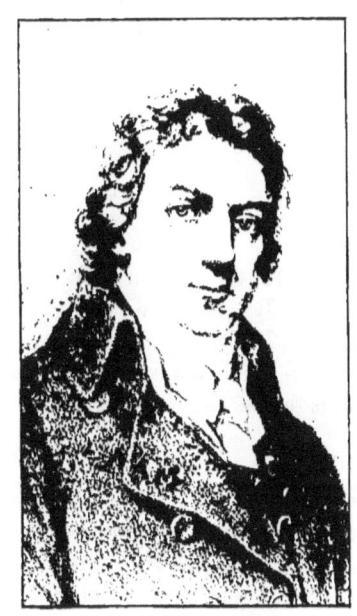

EDWARD JENNER, M.D.

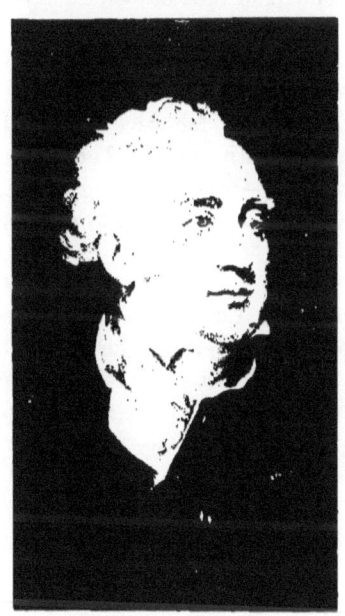

SIR ASTLEY COOPER, BART.

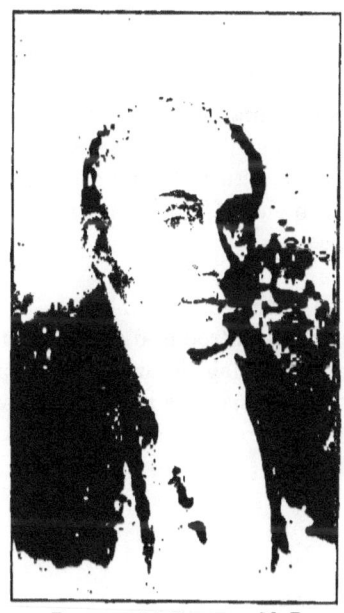

EPHRAIM McDOWELL, M.D.

SAMUEL D. GROSS, M. D., LL.D.,—born in Penn. in 1805,—died in 1884,—occupied chairs as professor of surgery in Louisville College, Ky., the University of New York, the Jefferson Medical College, Phila,—a noted surgeon, a skillful operator and a voluminous author,—made many original contributions to surgery,—was regarded in his day as the greatest living surgeon.

OLIVER WENDELL HOLMES, M. D., LL.D.,—born in Mass. in 1809,—died in 1894,—a skilled physician, celebrated anatomist, popular lecturer, voluminous author,—occupied chairs as professor in Dartmouth and Harvard Colleges, filling the latter for 39 years,—great fame due to a peculiar genius as a writer of both prose and poetry,—possessed a great diversity of talent,—works exhibit a wide range of thought,—was one of the founders of the *Atlantic Monthly*.

PHILIP RICORD, M. D.,—born in 1810 at Baltimore, Md,—died in 1891,—a French physician and surgeon who won in Paris a worldwide reputation and had a very extensive and lucrative practice,—reputation due to his resources, his inventiveness and dexterity coupled with wide and accurate knowledge,—was consulting surgeon to Napoleon III,—wrote numerous medical works,—specialty venereal diseases.

J. MARION SIMS, M. D.,—born in South Carolina in 1813,—died in 1883,—introduced the use of the silver-wire suture,—instrumental in establishing the women's hospital in N. Y. city,—received many honors abroad,—a member of learned societies in Europe and America,—author of a standard work on female surgery,—a monument has been erected to his memory by physicians.

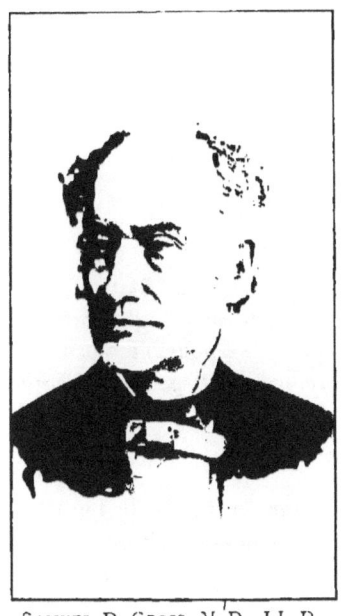
Samuel D. Gross, M. D., LL. D.

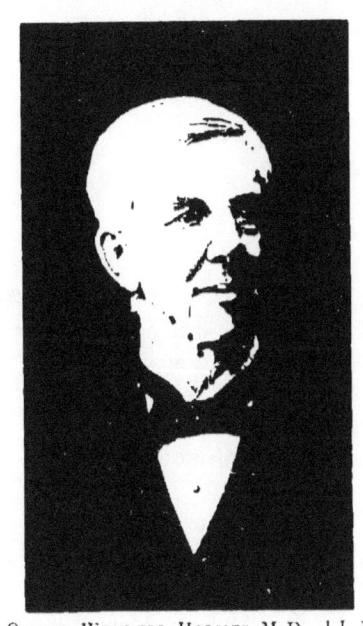
Oliver Wendell Holmes, M. D., LL. D.

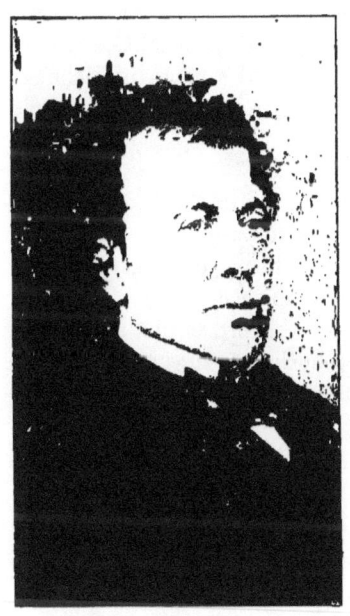
Philip Ricord, M. D.

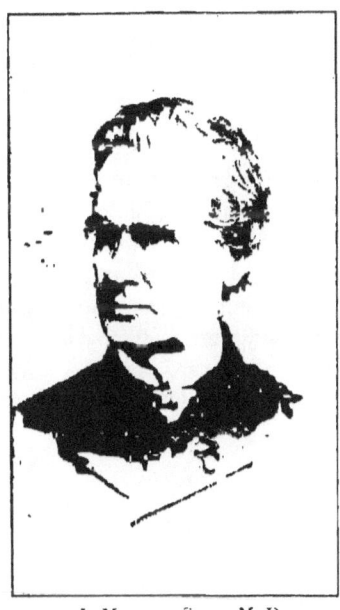
J. Marion Sims, M. D.

N. S. DAVIS, M. D., LL. D., Chicago, Ill.,—born in State of New York in 1817,—has done pioneer work in the cause of higher medical education,—written much,—has filled many responsible positions,—has occupied chairs in the Rush Medical College and Northwestern University, the latter of which he was instrumental in organizing,—also dean of latter.

D. HAYES AGNEW, M. D.,—born in Penn. in 1818,—died in 1892,—prof. of surgery in the University of Penn.—widely known for surgical inventions and work upon surgery,—called to Washington, D. C., to attend Pres. Garfield after he was shot.

FORDYCE BARKER, M. D.,—born in Maine in 1819,—died in 1891, occupied chairs as professor in Bowdoin, N. Y. Medical College and professor of clinical midwifery and diseases of women in Bellevue,—had extensive private practice,—wrote a treatise on puerperal diseases.

PROF. LOUIS PASTEUR,—born in France in 1822,—died in 1895,—celebrated chemist, biologist, scientific investigator, etc.,—regarded as the foremost representative of the germ theory of disease,—paved the way for the antiseptic methods now so successfully used in surgery,—invented successful treatment for the prevention and cure of hydrophobia, etc.,—turned his attention untiringly to searching out the causes of disease,—in 1874 was granted a pension by the French government of 20,000 francs.

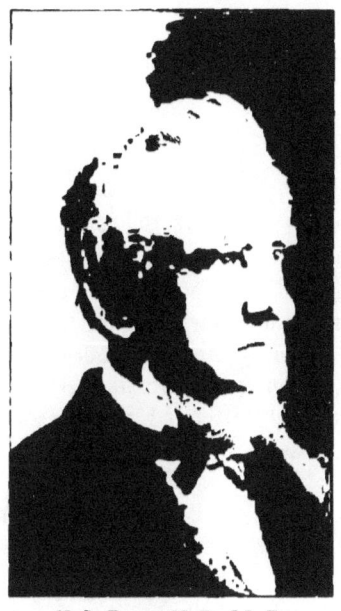

N. S. DAVIS, M. D., LL. D.

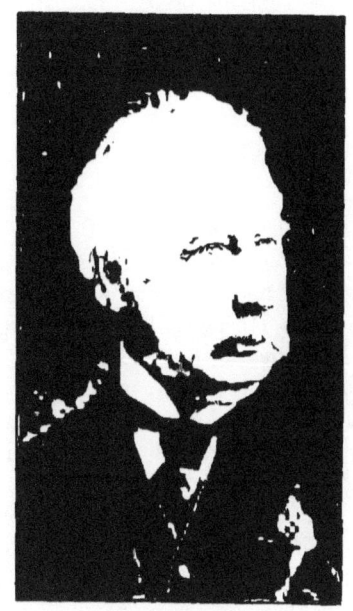

D. HAYES AGNEW, M. D.

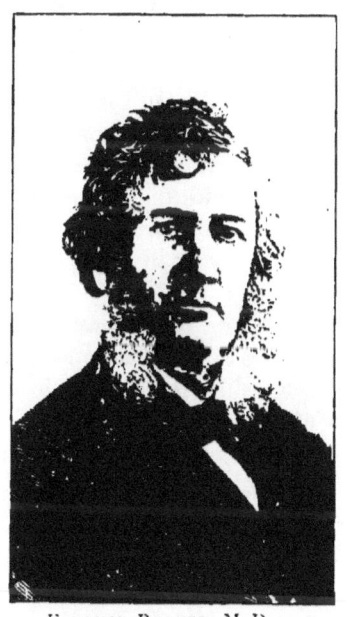

FORDYCE BARKER, M. D.

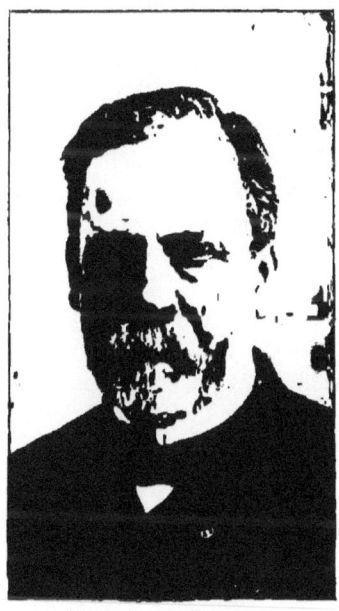

PROF. LOUIS PASTEUR.

SIR JOSEPH LISTER, BART.—born in England in 1827,—has been connected with several universities at Edinburgh, Glasgow, etc.,—as lecturer and professor upon surgery,—professor of surgery at Kings College Hospital, London,—surgeon-extraordinary to the Queen,—established antiseptic surgery or Listerism by the use of germicides, thus reducing the mortality in hospitals in a wonderful degree and annihilating the danger which had formerly attended operative surgery. He is the pioneer of applied antiseptics.

PROF. THEODOR BILLROTH,—born in 1829 on the Island of Rugen,—professor of surgery at Vienna,—a master of surgical technique,—has given special attention to the healing of wounds,—has had remarkable success in plastic operations,—is much admired for his courage,—has made himself famous by the performance of difficult and dangerous operations,—one of the most celebrated surgeons in the world.

SIR MORRELL MACKENZIE, BART.—born in England in 1837 and died in 1892,—in 1863, founded a hospital for the treatment of diseases of the throat,—summoned to attend the Crown Prince of Germany and obtained great notoriety for his disagreement with the German physicians,—possessed of skill and great fertility of resources,—operated with dexterity and acquired distinguished success in his specialty.

ROBERT KOCH, M. D.,—born in Germany in 1847,—professor of hygiene at the University of Berlin,—famous for studies concerning the contagia of consumption and cholera,—discovered the tubercle bacillus, the germ which causes consumption,—has been awarded 100,000 marks by the German government for this service.

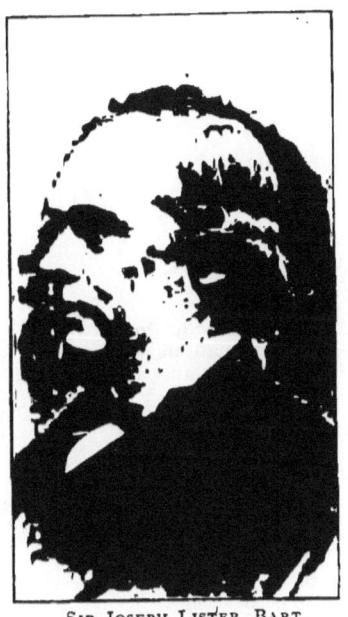
Sir Joseph Lister, Bart.

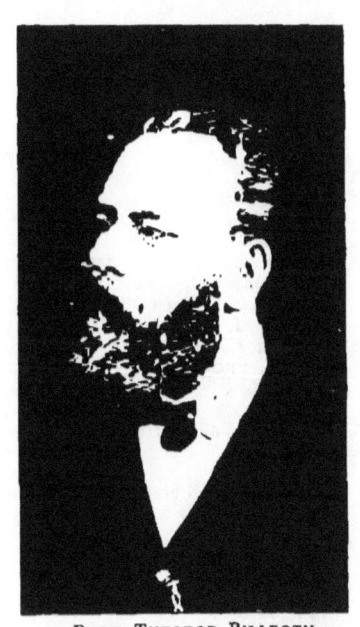
Prof. Theodor Billroth.

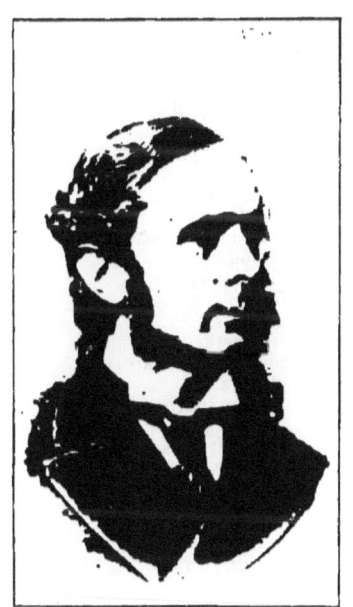
Sir Morrell Mackenzie, Bart.

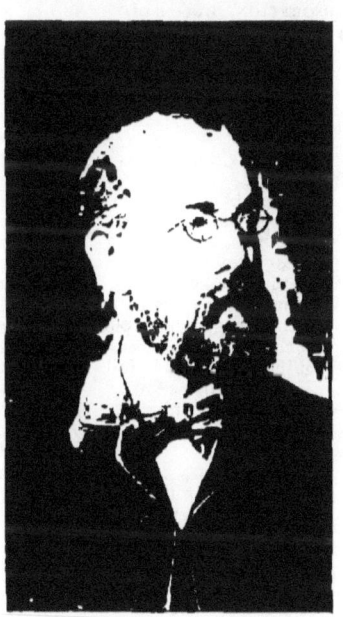
Robert Koch, M.D.

INDEX.

	PAGE.
ABDOMEN,	161
bandage of,	535
contents of,	161
distention of,	387
dropsy of,	349, 363, 401
enlargement of,	526
in disease of spleen,	352
tapping of,	349
ABDOMINAL CAVITY,	368
ABNORMAL PRODUCTS,	398
in blood,	179, 180, 183, 184
in urine,	399
ABORTION (see miscarriage),	530
ABSCESSES,	504
of antrum,	300
of alveola (gum boil),	301
of brain,	253
of kidney,	400
of lachrymal sac,	280
of liver,	350
of lungs,	322
of rectum,	372
in septicæmia,	184
ABSORBENT VESSELS,	369
ABSORPTION, process of,	369
ACCIDENTS (see Chap. VI.),	111
bite of mad dog,	91, 515
bite of serpents,	120
burns and scalds,	85, 113
dislocations,	176
dog bite,	122, 123
drowning,	111
fainting,	112
foreign bodies in ear,	284
foreign bodies in eye,	92, 273
fractures,	171
frost bite,	119
getting choked,	85, 306, 312, 328
hemorrhage from ear,	145
hemorrhage from wounds,	124
incised wounds,	126
injuries of spine in falls,	159
lightning stroke,	116
poison gases, inhaled,	100
poisoned wounds,	122
poisons,	88
scalp wounds,	127
sprains and bruises,	116
stings of insects,	121

	PAGE.
ACETANILIDE,	71
dose,	77
in high temperature,	478
in la grippe,	469, 470
in rheumatism,	77
ACETABULUM, THE,	163
ACIDS (poisons),	88
ACID, ACETIC,	93
ACID, CARBOLIC (poison),	92
ACID, CARBOLIC (antidote),	92
ACID, CARBOLIC (dose),	77
in abscess,	505
in burns and scalds,	115
in carbuncles,	511
in chilblains,	508
in eczema,	219
in hay fever,	297
in itching,	216
for lice,	224
for leucorrhœa,	438
in mouth wash,	542
in nettle rash,	221
in scarlet fever,	458
in shingles,	217
in small pox,	499
in vaginal wash,	478
in vomiting,	77, 337, 447
ACID, CARBOLIC OINTMENT,	85
for burns, chapped hands, cracked lips, cold sores, itching of skin, etc.,	85
ACID, HYDRIODIC SYRUP,	77
in asthma,	77
in enlarged spleen,	353
in hay fever,	296
ACIDS, MINERAL (poison),	91
antidotes,	91
aid digestion,	330, 335
in fevers,	465
in gastritis,	335
injure teeth,	491
ACID, SULPHURIC, AROMATIC,	382
in cholera,	382
in cholera morbus,	381
ACID, OXALIC (poison),	92
ACID, PRUSSIC (poison),	93
ACID, SALICYLIC (dose),	77
in corns,	230
in rheumatism,	493

INDEX.

	PAGE.
ACIDITY of gastric juice,	330
of stomach remedy for.	448
of stomach in pregnancy,	526
of urine,	398, 412
of urine in pregnancy.	529
ACNE,	212
ACONITE, as poison,	98
dose of	77
as household remedy,	81
how to give,	70
in pleurisy,	322
in acute diseases (early stages of),	65
ACUTE YELLOW ATROPHY,	
of liver,	352
ADAM'S APPLE (see larynx),	306
ADDISON'S DISEASE,	405
AGE, affects pulse,	141
affects respiration,	142
affects action of medicine,	60, 76
AGES, doses for different,	76
best for marriage,	522
of first menstruation,	433
of teething,	540
of turn of life,	434
best for weaning the baby,	446
AGNEW D. HAYES, M. D.,	560
ALBUMEN,	398, 399
in Bright's disease,	401
in scarlet fever,	458
ALCOHOL, its use and abuse,	102
antiseptic mouth wash,	542
externally in baldness,	212
externally in scarlet fever,	458
as stimulant,	69
ALCOHOLISM, CHRONIC,	104
ALIMENTARY CANAL,	299
ALIMENTATION (see food),	31
children, diet of,	542
rectal,	336, 376
sick, diet for,	549
ALKALIES (see antacids),	57, 91
in rheumatism,	493
ALKALINITY, of blood,	179
of urine,	398
of pancreatic secretions,	191
ALOPECIA (see baldness),	209
ALTERATIVES,	71
ALUM, dose of,	77
emetic in croup,	61, 82, 442
in filtering water,	30
in glossitis,	305
mouth wash,	528
for excessive perspiration,	206
ALVEOLAR ABSCESS	301
AMENORRHŒA,	
see menstruation, cessation of,	434
symptom of pregnancy,	525
AMMONIA, as poison,	93
dose of,	77
in bronchitis,	317, 318

	PAGE.
AMMONIA, in fainting,	112
in headache,	247
in hydrophobia,	516
in hysteria.	482
in pneumonia,	322
as stimulant,	82
AMNESIA,	253
AMYLOID LIVER,	351
ANAEMIA,	171
cause of headache,	246
cause of heart murmur,	361
tongue in,	139
ANÆSTHETICS	72
discoverer of use,	2
in labor,	534
ANATOMY,	149
of bones,	153
of brain,	233
of bladder,	407
of blood vessels,	366
of cranial nerves,	235
of ear,	281
of eye,	257
of face,	155
of female organs,	430
of gall bladder,	344
of heart,	354
of intestine, large,	370
of intestine, small,	368
of joints,	166
of kidneys,	396
of liver,	341
of lower extremities,	163
of lungs,	313
of male organs,	417
of mouth,	298
of muscles.	166
of rectum,	371
of skull,	153
of spinal column,	157
of spleen,	352
of stomach,	328
of throat,	306
of trachea,	312
of upper extremities,	160
ANATOMY, relation of to physiology,	151
to be taught to young how,	544
ANEURISM,	396
ANGINA PECTORIS,	363
ANIMAL FOOD,	33
ANISE, dose and use of,	77, 78
in colic of infants,	389
ANODYNES,	72
ANTACIDS (see alkalies),	57, 59
bicarbonate of soda,	80
bicarbonate of potash,	415
chalk mixture,	78
lime water,	79
ANTHELMINTICS,	72
ANTHRAX.	512

INDEX.

	PAGE.
ANTIDOTES, to poisons,	90
ANTIFERMENT (see pepsin),	330
ANTIPERIODICS (see quinine),	84
ANTIPYRETICS,	71
ANTISEPSINE,	542
ANTISEPTICS,	16, 71
solutions of,	185, 125
ANTISPASMODICS,	68, 483
ANTITOXINE (serum),	450
how prepared, foot note,	450
ANTRUM, THE,	300
ANUS (see rectum),	370, 371
cancer of,	376
deformity of,	371
fissure and ulcer of,	372
fistula and abscess of,	372
injuries of,	371
itching of,	373
piles of,	374
stricture of,	375
AORTA, THE,	355, 356, 357
APERIENTS (see cathartics),	61
APHASIA,	253
APHONIA,	309
APHRODISIACS,	73
APHTHOUS, sore mouth (see canker),	302
APOPLEXY,	251
APPENDICITIS,	384, 385
APPENDIX VERMIFORM,	370
APPETITE,	140
loss of,	338
prescription for,	339
unnatural,	339
worms, cause,	339
APPLE SOUFFLE,	551
APPLE WATER,	550
AQUEOUS HUMOR,	259
ARACHNOID, THE,	234
AREOLA, THE,	525
ARISTOL, surgical powder,	123, 126, 127, 537
in catarrh,	295
ARM, THE,	160
bones of	162
joints of,	160, 161, 166
muscles of,	168, 169
ARNICA, dose and use of,	78, 82
in bruises,	119
ARROW ROOT, in diet for sick,	550
ARSENIC, as poison,	94
antidote,	94
pigments of,	25
as medicine,	74
in acne,	213
in cancer,	518
in consumption,	324
for corns,	231
for headache,	247
for psoriasis,	222
(see Fowler's solution,)	

	PAGE.
ARTERIES,	366
aneurism of,	366
degeneration of,	367
ARTICULATIONS, (see joints,)	166
ASCENDING COLON,	370
ASCITES, (see dropsy,)	349, 363
ASPHYXIA, see drowning,)	111
(see inhalation of gases,)	100
ASSAFŒTIDA, in hysteria,	482
ASTHENIA, (see weakness,)	181
(see emaciation,)	445
ASTHMA,	142, 314
prescriptions for,	315
remedies and doses for,	77, 79
ASTIGMATISM,	263, 264
ASTRINGENTS,	58, 66
ATLAS, THE,	158
ATMOSPHERE,	24, 29
(see air and ventilation,)	24, 26
polluted,	28, 29
change of, in disease,	446
ATOMIZER, spray,	296
in catarrh,	294
in hay fever,	297
in whooping cough,	461
ATROPHY, acute yellow of liver,	352
of muscles, (see wasting,)	323
of consumption,	323
from loss of appetite,	339
ATROPIA, (see belladonna,)	81
doses of,	78
with aconite and morphia,	82
in aphonia,	309
in cholera,	382
in cholera morbus,	381
in corneal ulcer,	274
in hay fever,	296
in night sweats,	325
in peritonitis,	388
in wetting bed,	412
in whooping cough,	461
to check secretion of milk,	82, 536
ATTACHMENTS, muscular,	159, 167
AUDITORY CANAL,	281, 282, 283
AURICLE, (see external ear,)	281
of heart,	356, 357
AUSCULTATION,	
(see ear over chest,	319, 321
AUTHOR, (see frontispiece,)	555
(see preface,)	iii-iv
AXIS, THE,	158
BABY, (see infants,)	536
anodynes, bad for,	72, 538
born before doctor arrives,	536
tying cord,	536
band for,	537
barley gruel for,	446
bath for,	201, 537
circulation of,	537

INDEX.

	PAGE.
BABY, clothing for,	538
cow's milk for,	538
excitement bad for,	543
impure air, bad for,	29
mortality of,	29, 133
need water,	539
nurse how often,	537
nurse how old,	446
peptonized milk for,	446
soothing lotion for gums,	539
teething of,	540
warmth for,	537
weight and size of,	525
BACK, pain in, (lumbago,)	243
in pyelitis,	400
in Bright's disease,	401
BACTERIA, in air,	21, 131
in blood,	448
in milk,	465
in water,	24, 32, 382, 474
in disease,	321, 448
cause all contagious diseases,	11, 13
BALDNESS,	209
prevention of,	211
BANDAGE, after labor,	535
BARBER'S ITCH,	226
BARKER, FORDYCE, M. D.,	560
BARLEY GRUEL,	446, 538
BARLEY WATER,	549
BATH for infants,	201, 537
BATHING,	136, 201
BED for labor,	534
BED SORES, (see ulcers,)	205
treatment of same as burns and ulcers,	115
BEEF ESSENCE,	553
BEEF TEA,	553
BEE STINGS, (see stings of insects,)	121
BELLADONNA, tincture of,	81
causes redness of face,	204
externally for itching,	218
leaves in asthma,	315
BELLY ACHE, (see stomach ache,)	337
BELLY BAND,	537
BETHESDA WATER,	64
BEVERAGE, Water as,	29, 50
BICEPS MUSCLE,	168
BICYCLE RIDING,	46
BIFURCATION OF TRACHEA,	312, 313
BILE,	343
in blood,	346
in bowels,	346
in urine,	148, 398
BILIOUS COLIC,	349
BILIOUS FEVER,	464
BILIOUSNESS,	344
remedies for,	345, 346
BILLROTH, THEODOR, PROF.,	562
BIOLOGIST,	560
BISMUTH, dose and uses,	78

	PAGE.
BISMUTH, in cholera infantum,	447
in gastric ulcer,	336
in intestinal catarrh,	334
in pregnancy,	527
BITES OF ANIMALS,	122
rabid animals,	514
dogs,	123
insects,	121
scorpions,	122
serpents,	120
spiders,	122
BLACKBERRY ROOT,	66
BLACK EYE, (ecchymosis),	271
remedy for,	271
BLACK VOMIT,	476
BLADDER, GALL,	344
calculi in,	344, 350
urinary,	407
obscure affections of	416
stone in,	413, 414
BLANC MANGE,	551
BLEEDING, (see hemorrhage),	145, 253
from bowels,	145, 473
from brain,	251
from ear,	145
from lungs,	323, 325
from nose,	292, 293
from stomach,	335, 338
from uterus,	146, 531, 535
from wounds,	124, 126, 127
BLEPHARITIS,	270
BLINDNESS,	277
from cataract,	278
from corneal ulcers,	274
from glaucoma,	276
purulent ophthalmia,	272
BLISTERS,	3, 60
in jaundice,	347
BLOOD, circulation of,	357
diseases of,	179
in urine,	146, 148, 400
poisoning,	186
vomit of,	145, 335
BLOODY FLUX, (in dysentery),	378
BLOOD TONICS,	79
BLOOD VESSELS,	366
diseases of,	366, 367
intemperance affects,	106
of skin,	198
BLUSHING,	204
BOILED custard,	551
milk in dysentery,	379
water in disease,	30, 31
BOILS,	509
remedy for	510
BONE, composition of,	149
crepitus in fracture of,	117
syphilis causes ulceration of,	424
pain in,	423
BONES, their number,	153

	PAGE
BONES, their form,	151
of face,	155
of skull,	153
of spinal column,	158
of pelvis,	163
of lower extremities,	165
of upper extremities,	162
of skeleton,	150
BOTTLE FEEDING,	538
BOWELS, obstruction of,	383
BRAIN, THE,	233
abscess of,	253
deformity of,	255
tobacco affects,	109
tumors of,	253
BRANDY, in cholera infantum,	446
iced, in gastritis,	335
BREAKBONE FEVER, (see neuralgic fever),	470
BREASTS,	525, 535
care of,	535
milk of,	526, 537
BREATH, bad,	28, 305
BREECH, (see hernia),	385
BRIGHT, DR. RICHARD,	400
BRIGHT'S DISEASE,	400
BROMIDE, of arsenic,	222
of potash,	248, 461
of soda,	482, 485, 487, 540
BRONCHITIS,	315
BRONCHITIS, CAPILLARY,	317
BROTH, beef and oatmeal,	554
chicken,	553
egg,	553
mutton,	553
BRUISES,	116, 118
may cause abscess,	119
BUBO,	427
BUCHU,	64
BUNIONS,	231
BURNS AND SCALDS,	12, 113
CÆCUM, THE,	370, 384
CACHEXIA, in cancer,	138
CAFFEINE, dose of,	78
in dropsy,	64, 366
in heart disease,	363
in Bright's disease,	402
CALCULI of gall bladder,	344
CALCULUS, salivary,	303
vesical,	413
CALOMEL, in vomiting,	337
in worms,	395
CAMPHOR,	78
in chordee,	428
in fainting,	528
in gastritis,	335
CAMPHOR LINIMENT,	83
CAMPHOR LINIMENT COMPOUND,	83
in neuralgia,	244

	PAGE
CAMPHOR, SPIRITS OF,	82
CANAL, alimentary,	299
auditory,	282
CANCER,	138
of breasts,	434, 518
of kidneys,	400
of liver,	351
of pancreas,	193
of penis,	419
of rectum,	376
of stomach,	338
of testicle,	421
of womb,	434, 438
CANCRUM ORIS,	302
CANKER,	302
CAPILLARIES,	366
CAPILLARY BRONCHITIS.	317
CAPSULES	73
CARBOLIC ACID, poison. (See acid carbolic),	92
strength of solution,	217
CARBOLIZED OINTMENT,	85
CARBUNCLES,	511
CARLSBAD MINERAL WATER,	404
CARMINATIVES,	72
CARE of breasts,	535
of eyes,	268
during menstruation,	435
of skin,	200
CARPUS, (see wrist),	161, 162
CASTOR OIL,	62, 78, 83
in cholera infantum,	447
CATALEPSY,	482
CATARACT,	277
CATARRH of ear, chronic,	285
nasal, chronic,	293
Southern California in,	41
summer,	295
CATARRHAL STOMATITIS,	301
CATHARTICS,	61, 63
CATHETER,	409, 410, 415
CAUSES OF DISEASE, general,	9
special,	11
CELEBRITIES, MEDICAL,	555
CELLARS, ventilation of,	22
CELLS, epithelial,	401
CEREBELLUM, THE,	235
CEREBO SPINAL MENINGITIS,	241
CERUMEN, (see wax in ear),	283
CEREBRUM, THE,	234
CHANCRE,	421
CHANCROID,	421
CHANGE OF LIFE,	434
CHEEKS, THE,	299
CHEERFULNESS,	49, 546
CHICKEN BROTH,	553
CHICKEN POX,	440
CHILBLAINS,	508
CHILDREN, care and education of,	542
easily affected by medicine,	60

INDEX.

	Page
CHILDREN not to sleep with old people,	190
CHILLS AND FEVER,	401, 464, 466
CHLORAL HYDRATE, (poison),	97
in asthma,	315
in bronchitis,	317
in convulsions,	487
in corea,	485
in croup,	444
habit,	107
in diphtheria,	449
in teething,	540
in whooping cough,	461
CHLORINE MIXTURE,	310, 449
CHLOROFORM, dose,	78
in cholera,	383
in convulsions,	487
in cough mixture,	86
in earache,	286
in hernia,	386
in labor,	534
in neuralgia,	244
in tapeworm,	393
CHLOROFORM LINIMENT,	83, 118
CHLOROSIS,	182
CHOICE OF A HOME,	17
CHOKING, (see accidents),	85
CHOLERA, ASIATIC,	381
CHOLERA INFANTUM,	133, 444
CHOLERA MORBUS,	379
CHORDEE,	428
CHOREA,	484
CHOROID, THE,	258
inflammation of,	276
CHRONIC ALCOHOLISM,	104
CHRONIC SORE THROAT,	308
CHYLE,	187, 192
CILIARY MUSCLE,	259
CILIARY PROCESS,	259
CIRCULATION, THE,	357
CIRRHOSIS OF LIVER,	348
CITRATE OF POTASH,	415
CLAM BROTH,	554
CLAP, (see gonorrhœa),	425
CLARK, DR. ALONZO	388
CLAVICLE, THE,	150, 160
fracture of,	175
CLAVUS, (see corns)	229
CLEANLINESS,	422
in gonorrhœa,	439
CLEFT PALATE, (see hare lip),	304
CLERGYMAN'S SORE THROAT,	308
(see chronic sore throat).	
CLIMACTERIC,	434
CLIMATE,	40, 42
CLOTHING,	36, 39
of infants,	536
COCAINE AND CHLORAL HABIT,	107
COCAINE in burns,	115
in cancer,	517

	Page
COCAINE in dysentery,	379
in itching,	216
in nausea and vomiting of pregnancy,	527
in teething,	539
COD LIVER OIL EMULSION,	68
in scrofula,	191
COFFEE, bad for children,	36
COLD, taking,	307
in the head,	290
COLD SORES, (see herpes),	85, 217, 465
COLD WATER, dressings,	293, 242
in fainting,	113
COLIC,	388
bilious,	349
renal,	399
COLLAR BONE, (see clavicle),	150, 160
fracture of,	175
COLLES FRACTURE,	161
COLON, THE,	371
COMA,	146
COMEDO, (see acne),	212
COMMON ABBREVIATIONS,	73
COMMON SENSE, MEDICAL,	8
COMPOSITION TEA,	65
CONCEPTION,	523, 524
CONFINEMENT, (see labor),	531
CONGENITAL DEFECTS,	255
of brain,	240, 255
of ear,	287
of genital organs,	418
of mouth and hard palate,	304
of rectum,	371
CONGESTION, (of brain),	245, 251
treatment of,	86
of liver,	345
of lungs,	321
CONJUNCTIVITIS,	271
CONSTIPATION,	147, 389
CONSUMPTION,	322, 325
cessation of monthly flow in,	323
CONSUMPTIVES climate for,	42
CONTAGION,	27
CONTAGIOUS DISEASES,	11
CONVULSIONS,	486
in Bright's disease,	402
in hydrophobia,	515, 516
in scarlet fever,	458
in teething,	540
in worms,	391, 393
COOKING, (see diet for sick),	549
COOPER, SIR ASTLEY,	556
COPPER, salts of poison,	95
CORD, umbilical,	524, 534, 536
spinal,	238
CORNEA,	258
inflammation of	273
ulcers of	274
CORNEAL OPACITIES,	274
CORNS,	229

INDEX.

	PAGE
CORONARY ARTERIES,	356
CORPUSCLES OF BLOOD,	179
CORROSIVE SUBLIMATE,	71
poison,	95
antiseptic tablets of,	125
in diphtheria,	450
in blood poisoning,	185
in freckles,	228
in lice,	224
lotion of,	208
CORYZA, ACUTE,	290
COSMETICS,	202
COUGH,	143, 325
COUGH MIXTURE,	86, 453
COUNTENANCE, THE,	137
COVERINGS OF BRAIN,	233
COWPER'S GLANDS,	408
COW POX,	500
CRAMPS,	380
CRANIAL NERVES,	235
CRAZY BONE,	160
CREAM OF TARTAR,	221
CREAM OF TARTAR LEMONADE,	550
CREOSOTE, poison,	92
in consumption,	324
CROOKES TUBE,	5
CROSS EYE,	279
CROUP,	441, 443
CRUSTS,	205
CYANOSIS,	138
CYSTITIS, acute and chronic,	408
DAMP LOCATIONS, unhealthy,	19, 28
DANDRUFF,	207
DAVIS, DR. N. S.,	560
DEAD ANIMALS AND BODIES, danger from,	122
DEAD, KISSING THE, danger from,	136
DEAFNESS,	282
congenital,	287
DEATH, causes of,	11, 23, 132, 133
from consumption,	325
signs of,	135, 146, 148
DECAYING VEGETABLES, unhealthy,	27
DELIRIUM,	135, 146
DELIRIUM TREMENS, (see chronic alcoholism),	104
DELTOID muscle, the,	168, 169
DELUSION of insanity,	250
DELUSIONS, strange,	53
DEMENTIA of insanity,	251
DENGUE, (see neuralgic fever),	470
DENTITION, (see teething),	540
DIABETES,	403
DIAPHRAGM,	328, 340, 341
DIARRHŒA,	66, 444
in cholera,	380, 382
mixture,	86
in typhoid fever,	472

	PAGE
DIASTOLE	355
DIET, (see food),	32
in Bright's disease,	462
in constipation,	390
in diabetes,	404
regulation of,	62
when nursing infant,	538
for the sick,	549
(see typhoid fever),	473, 548
DIGESTION,	329, 369
alcohol deranges,	105
emotions disturb,	49
heat impairs,	444
tonics aid,	67
DIGITALIS,	69, 64, 363, 366, 402
DIPHTHERIA,	348, 461
DIRECTIONS for testing the eyes,	264
DISEASE, functional and organic,	131
DISEASE, GENERAL CAUSES OF,	9
bathing in relation to,	136
germs of,	11, 12
kissing in relation to,	135
mastoid,	287
special causes of,	7, 11
symptoms of,	137
temperature in relation to,	133
the skin in relation to,	146
DISEASES of the bladder,	408
of the blood,	180
of the blood vessels,	366
of the brain,	240
of female genital organs,	436
of the ear,	282
of the eye,	270
of the glands,	189
of the heart,	359
of the kidneys,	398
of the liver,	344
of the lungs and trachea,	314
of the male genital organs,	418
of the mouth and tongue,	301
of the nose,	289
of the pancreas,	192
of the rectum,	371
of the skin,	202
of the stomach,	331
of the spleen,	352
of the throat and larynx,	306
venereal,	421
DISINFECTION,	461, 463
of typhoid stools,	474
DISLOCATIONS,	176, 177
DISORDERS, of menstruation,	433
DIURETICS,	63
DIZZINESS,	247
DOG BITES,	122, 123
DOSES, always adult,	76
rules for,	75
DOSE TABLE,	77
DOVER'S POWDER,	72, 78, 320, 531

	PAGE.
DRAINAGE,	21
DRESS, (see clothing),	36
DRINK, most healthful,	30
DROPSY. of brain,	240
in Bright's disease,	401
in heart disease,	363
DROWNING,	111
DRUGGISTS. danger from prescribing,	429
DRUM OF EAR,	282
DUODENUM,	368, 370, 192
DURA MATER,	233
DUST, in the house,	20, 27
DUSTING POWDER,	207
DYSENTERY,	378
DYSMENORRHŒA, (see menstruation),	433
DYSPEPSIA.	331
DYSPHAGIA,	140
EAR ACHE,	285
EAR ANATOMY OF,	281
defects of,	287
diseases of,	282, 285, 287
foreign bodies in,	284
inflation of,	287
EAR SYMPTOMS.	147
EAR WAX,	283
EATING, (see food),	33
time for,	49
ECCHYMOSIS,	271
ECSTACY,	483
ECZEMA,	218
EDUCATION, of children,	542
EFFECTS of tobacco, the,	109
EGG BROTH,	553
EGG NOG,	552
ELBOW, THE,	166
ELECTRICITY,	3, 253
ELIMINATIVES,	58
EMACIATION,	445
EMBOLISM,	254
EMBOLUS,	362
EMETICS,	61
EMMENAGOGUES,	72
EMPYEMA. (see pus in plural cavity),	320, 505
ENDOCARDITIS,	361
ENLARGED. blood vessels,	348
heart,	365
liver,	348, 351
prostate,	414
spleen,	353
veins in pregnancy,	525
ENTERALGIA. (see colic),	388
ENTERIC FEVER, (see typhoid).	471
ENURESIS, (see wetting the bed).	412
EPIDEMIC.	468
EPIDEMICS, destruction of.	23, 381, 474, 477

	PAGE.
EPIDERMIS,	194, 196
EPIGLOTTIS,	307, 443
EPILEPSY,	479
EPISTAXIS,(see nasal hemorrhage),	292, 293
ERGOT,	66
fluid extract, dose,	79
in hemorrhage of lungs.	325
in hemorrhage of womb,	535
ERRORS OF REFRACTION,	262
ERYSIPELAS,	490
ERYTHEMA,	204
ESCHAROTICS,	71
ETHER,	2, 487, 534
ETHMOID BONE, THE,	154
EUSTACHIAN TUBE,	282
EXANTHEM, (see eruption)	457, 498
EXCESSES, hurtful,	50
EXCORIATIONS,	205
EXERCISE,	43, 141, 406, 543
EXERTION. immoderate hurtful,	46
EXHAUSTION,	46, 49
EXPECTORANTS,	70
EXTENSION IN FRACTURES,	174
EXTRACTS. FLUID,	
EXTREMITIES, bones of lower.	150, 153, 155
bones of upper.	153, 162
EYEBALL.	257, 260
EYEBROW,	260
EYE, care of,	268
diseases of,	270
examination of,	262
inner canthus of,	261
interior of,	259
normal,	268, 256
in old age.	261
squint or cross eye,	279
symptoms,	147
EYELASH.	261
EYELIDS.	260
EYESIGHT, directions for testing,	264
FACE, bones of,	155
expressions of,	157
muscles of,	157
pimples of,	212
FACIAL PARALYSIS,	254
FAINTING,	112
in pregnancy,	528
FALLING OF THE BOWEL,	375
(see prolapse of rectum).	
FALLING SICKNESS, (see epilepsy),	479
FALLOPIAN TUBES,	431, 523
FARCY, (see glanders),	513
FAR SIGHT. (see hypermetropia).	262
FATS. (see carbo-hydrates),	34, 36
FATTY DEGENERATION of heart.	365
of liver,	351
FAVUS,	227

INDEX.

	Page
FEEBLE CHILDREN,	537
FEET, suffer from neglect,	230
FELON,	505
FEMALE, genital organs,	430
pelvis,	430
FEMUR, THE,	163, 165
fractures of,	175
FETID BREATH,	305
FEVERS,	464
temperature in,	134
FEVER, SCARLET,	456
FEVER SORES,	217
FIBRIN,	179, 180
FIBULA, THE,	165
FINGER, dislocation of,	177
FISSURE, of rectum,	372
FISSURES, in the skin,	205
FISTULA, rectal,	372
salivary,	303
FITS,	486
FLATULENCE,	333
FLAXSEED, tea,	409, 550
lemonade,	550
FLESH,	34
FLEXORS,	168
FLOODING, (see uterine hemorrhage)	434
FLORIDA, climate of,	42
FLOWERS, in sick room,	549
FŒTUS,	524
movement of,	526
FOLLICLES, (see villi).	369
of stomach (see glands),	330
FONTANELLE	154, 489
FOOD,	32
animal,	33
in Bright's disease,	462
for children,	542
in constipation,	390
in cholera infantum,	446
in diabetes,	404
for infants,	537, 538, 539
after labor,	535
in pregnancy,	529
in rickets,	488
for the sick,	549
FOOT, THE,	165
FOREARM,	160, 161, 162
fracture of,	175
FOREIGN BODIES, in ear,	284
in eye,	733
in nose,	291
FORESKIN, (see phimosis),	418
FOUL, breath,	28, 140
mouth,	541
odors,	28, 29, 291
odors, signals of danger,	24
FOWLER'S SOLUTION, dose,	219
in chorea,	485
in chronic diarrhœa,	377
in eczema,	219

	Page
FOWLER'S SOLUTION, in nervous disorders,	374
in psoriasis,	222
FRACTURES,	171
symptoms of,	172
treatment of,	173
FRANCE, for invalids,	42
FRECKLES,	227
FRENCH HEEL, an abomination,	230
FRIGHT, bad for children,	484, 486
FROSTBITE,	119
FRUIT, valuable in diet,	530
FURUNCLES, (see boils),	509
GALL, (see bile),	343, 346
bladder,	342, 344
stones,	349
GALVANISM, (see electricity),	277
GANGLIA, (see brain substance), 234, 238
GANGLIONIC MASSES,	239
GANGRENE, of lungs,	140
of mouth,	302
GARFIELD, death of,	184
GARGLES,	308, 310, 311, 449, 456
GASES, poison,	100
sewer,	22, 100
GASTRALGIA,	337
GASTRIC FEVER,	334
ulcer,	335
GASTRIC JUICE,	330
GELSEMIUM,	70
GENITAL ORGANS, female,	430
male,	417
GERMAN MEASLES,	453
soap,	214, 222
GIN DRINKERS' LIVER,	348
GLANDERS,	513
(see poisoned wounds,)	122
GLANDS, THE, (see liver, pancreas and spleen,	191, 352
of groin	423, 427
of intestines	368
of lips	304
lymphatic,	187, 188
Meibomian of eyelids,	261
parotid,	299, 454
of skin,	195, 196, 205, 207
sub-maxillary and sub-lingual,	299
supra-renal,	397, 405
GLANDS, THE, tonsilar,	310
in diphtheria,	448
in scrofula,	189
sebaceous disorders of,	207, 208
sudorific disorders of,	209
GLASSES, use of,	264, 265
GLAUCOMA,	276
GLEET,	428
GLOSSITIS,	304
GYMNASTICS, (see exercise).	45

	PAGE.
GLUTEN FLOUR,	169
GLYCOGEN,	342
GLYCOGENIC, function of liver,	342
GONORRHŒA,	425
GONORRHŒAL, rheumatism,	428
GOUT,	494
GRAHAM BREAD,	390
GRANULAR LIDS,	272
GRAVEL,	399
GREEN SICKNESS, (see chlorosis),	182
GROSS, SAMUEL D., M. D.,	558
GROWTHS,	279, 303
GUM ARABIC, (see acacia),	447
water,	550
GUMBOIL,	301
GUMS,	300
lancing or cutting,	540
lotion for,	539
unhealthy,	541
HAIR,	155
cleansing, directions for,	210
dandruff,	207, 210
lice in,	223
loss of,	209
restoratives containing lead poison,	210
remedies to prevent loss of hair,	211
HAIR DYES,	99
HALLUCINATION,	250
HAND, bones of,	150, 151, 161
muscles of,	168
training of,	43
HARE LIP,	304
HARVEY, WILLIAM, M.D.,	556
HAVERSIAN CANALS,	151
HAY FEVER,	295
HEAD, (see brain),	233
(see cranial nerves),	235
bones of,	153, 155
cleanliness of,	201
HEADACHE,	241, 245
HEARING, acuteness of,	283
HEART, action of,	141, 357, 358
degeneration of,	365
clot of blood in,	362
description of,	354
dilitation of,	361
enlargement of,	365
inflammation of sac,	360
murmur of,	361
neuralgia of,	363
nourishment of,	356
overwork of,	359
palpitation of,	365
sac of,	359
valves of,	356
valvular disease of,	361
work of,	354
HEARTBURN,	333

	PAGE.
HEAT,	12
debilitates stomach,	444
destroys disease germs,	16, 30
not favorable to development of race,	41
sweating relieves heat,	196
HEBRIDES ISLANDS,	29
HEEL, bone of,	164
HEMIPLEGIA,	254
HEMISPHERES, of brain,	233
HEMORRHAGE,	145
of bowels,	115
of brain,	251
of ear,	145
in eye,	277
after labor,	533, 535
of lungs,	145, 323
in miscarriage,	531
of nose,	292
of stomach,	335
in typhoid fever,	473
uterine,	434
from wounds,	124
HEMORRHOIDS, (see piles),	374
HENBANE, doses and use,	79
in pregnancy,	527
HERB DRINKS,	549, 65
HERNIA,	385
HERPES, of lips,	217
of genitals,	217
zoster,	216
HICCOUGH,	340
in peritonitis,	387
HIP, dislocation of,	177
fracture of,	175
HIVES, (see nettle rash),	220
HOBNAIL, liver,	348
HOLMES, DR. OLIVER WENDELL,	558
HOMEOPATHIC, treatment,	9
HORSEBACK RIDING,	46
HOT WATER, general uses of,	86
for eyes,	269
HOUSE, choice of location,	17, 19
furnishings of,	20
drainage and sewerage of,	21, 22
ventilation of,	24 to 29
water supply of,	29 to 32
HUMERUS, THE,	160, 162
fracture of,	172
HYDATID DISEASE,	352
of kidneys,	400
of liver,	352
HYDROCELE,	420
HYDROCEPHALUS,	240
HYDROPHOBIA,	15, 514
HYGIENE, (see sanitary subjects),	17, 26, 29
HYOID BONE,	157
HYOSCYAMUS, (see henbane),	79
HYPODERMIC USE OF MEDICINE,	59

INDEX.

	PAGE
HYPODERMIC USE OF MEDICINE,	
in asthma,	314
in peritonitis,	388
HYPERMETROPIA, far sight,	262, 264
HYPERTROPHY, (see enlargement)	
of heart,	365
of liver,	348
HYSTERIA,	480
ICE, in fever,	499
in gastritis,	335
polluted by sewerage,	30
in sick room,	554
ICELAND, infant mortality of,	29
moss, blanc mange,	551
ICTERUS, (see jaundice),	346
ILEO-CÆCAL VALVE,	384
ILEUM, THE,	368
ILIUM, THE,	163
ILLUSIONS of insanity,	250
IMPACTED WAX, in ear,	283
INCISED WOUNDS,	126
INCUBATION STAGE OF DISEASES	15
of measles,	451
of mumps,	454
of scarlet fever,	457
of small pox,	497
of whooping cough,	460
INDIAN MEAL, healthy, (see corn bread),	390
INDIGESTION,	49, 331
food in chronic,	333
of infants,	444
peptonized milk in,	446
INFANT FEEDING, 446, 537, 538,	539
INFANTS, management of,	536
INFLAMMATION,	502
of bowels,	383
of brain,	241
of choroid,	276
of cornea,	273
of ear,	284
of eyelids,	270
of iris,	275
of lungs,	320
of optic nerve,	277
of retina,	277
sympathetic,	276
of tear duct,	279
of tongue,	304
INFLATION, of ear,	287
INFLUENZA, (see la grippe),	468
INFUSIONS,	73
INGROWING NAIL,	507
INNOMINATA, THE,	163
INSANITY,	249
INSECT BITES,	121
INSOMNIA,	248
INSTRUMENTS,	1, 2
INTEMPERANCE,	102, 104

	PAGE
INTERIOR, of eye,	259
INTERMITTENT FEVER,	465
INTERNAL CANTHUS,	261
INTERNAL EAR,	282
INTESTINAL CATARRH,	376
INTESTINES, the large,	370
the small,	368
the coats of,	371
IODINE,	7, 9, 84
in boils,	510
for bunions,	231
for corns,	230
for enlarged glands,	456
for felon,	506
in hay fever,	296
in sore throat,	309
in sprains,	118
IPECAC. dose and uses,	79, 84
emetic,	61
in bronchitis,	318
in croup,	442
in fits,	487
in whooping cough,	460
IRIDECTOMY,	276
IRIS,	258
IRITIS,	275
IRON, dose and use,	79
in acne,	213
in erysipelas,	490
in rickets,	489
in scrofula,	191
tonic,	68
ISCHIUM, THE,	163
ITCH,	224
ITCHING,	215
of anus,	373
in ivy poisoning,	99
troublesome,	436
IVY POISONING,	98
JABORANDI,	65
JAEGER'S TEST TYPE,	265, 268
JAUNDICE,	346
JAWBONE, THE,	156
JEJUNUM, THE,	368
JELLY, lemon, orange, tapioca,	551
slippery elm,	550
water to prepare,	549
JENNER, EDWARD, M. D.,	497, 500, 556
JENNER, SIR WILLIAM,	474
JOINTS, THE,	166
KIDNEYS, THE,	130, 148
description of,	396
diseases of,	399
to preserve the health of,	405
secretions of,	398
section of,	397
situation of, (see plates).	

	PAGE.
KIDNEYS. THE.	. 396
stone in pelvis of.	. 400
KISSING. danger of in disease.	. 135
in syphilis.	423
KNEE CAP. (see patella).	. 164
dislocation of.	. 178
KNEE JOINT.	. 164, 166
KOCH. ROBERT ,M. D..	. 324, 562
KOUMISS.	. 552
in consumption,	. 224
in dyspepsia,	. 333
LABOR.	. 523, 525, 531
management of,	. 533
premature,	. 530
stages of. .	. 532
LABYRINTH. of ear,	. 282
LACHRYMAL SAC,	. 280
LACTEALS.	. 369
LARYNGISMUS.	. 443
LARYNGITIS, .	. 307
LARYNX.	. 306
spasm of, .	. 443
LAUDANUM, dose and use,	. 79
LAXATIVES, (see cathartics),	. 61
LEAD, poison and antidote, .	. 96
in water, .	. 30
in hair dyes.	. 99
LEG. THE, .	. 163, 165, 169
fracture of.	. 173
paralysis of.	. 159
(see paraplegia),	. 254
(see hemiplegia),	. 254
(see locomotor ataxia),	. 254
LEMONADE, flaxseed, cream of tartar. .	. 550
LEMON SAUCE.	. 551
LENTIGO, (see freckles),	. 227
LEPROSY,	. 222
LEUCORRHŒA.	. 437
LEUKÆMIA, .	. 183
LICE,	. 223
LIGHT, for reading,	. 268, 269
LIGHTNING STROKE, .	. 116
LIME WATER AND SWEET OIL,	85, 115
LIME WATER,	. 79, 549
LINES FOR ASTIGMATISM, .	. 263
LINIMENTS, .	. 80, 84
camphor, .	. 83
camphor and chloroform,	. 83
menthol. .	. 84
LISTER, SIR JOSEPH, .	. 16, 562
LITMUS PAPER, .	. 179, 398
LIVER, THE, .	. 341
diseases of,	. 344
lobules of,	. 342
LOBELIA, dose.	. 79
antispasmodic.	. 69
in asthma.	. 313

	PAGE.
LOCOMOTOR ATAXIA.	. 254
LOSS OF APPETITE.	. 338
LOWER EXTREMITIES. .	. 163, 165
LUMBAGO.	. 243
LUNGS. THE. .	. 313
diseases of,	. 314, 325
LYMPH, .	187
LYMPHATIC SYSTEM. THE.	. 187
vessels and glands. .	. 188
MACKENZIE SIR. MORRELL.	. 562
MALAR BONES. THE. .	. 156
MALARIA.	. 321, 403
MALARIAL FEVER.	. 463
regions,	. 464
sores.	. 217
typhoid fever. .	. 464
MALE GENITAL ORGANS. THE.	417
affections of	. 418
description of, .	. 417
MALIGNANT PUSTULE.	. 512
diseases, .	. 449 451, 457
ulcers.	. 205
MALLEOLUS. THE. (see ankle).	. 164
MAMMARY GLANDS. (see breasts)	525
cancer of,	. 518
care of,	. 533
MANAGEMENT, of infants, .	. 536
of labor, .	. 531
of skin. .	. 200
MANDRAKE. (see podophyllin),	. 63
MANGE, THE,	. 227
MANIA, (see insanity), .	. 251
MARRIAGE.	. 519
proper age for,	. 522
after syphilis,	. 425
MASSAGE.	. 253, 482
MASSETER MUSCLE.	. 167
MASTOID, disease,	. 287
MASTURBATION. (see evil habits).	418
(see phymosis),	. 418
MATCHES. care of,	. 97
MATERIA MEDICA,(see medicines)	57
MATERNITY.	519, 530
MATRIX. suppuration of. .	. 506
MCDOWELL, EPHRAIM, M. D , .	. 556
MEASLES.	. 431
German. .	. 433
MEASLY. pork, (see larvæ),	. 392
MEASURES, FLUID.	. 75
MEAT,	. 34, 35, 332
causes gout, .	. 34
raw, chopped or pounded,	. 549
to abstain from, when, .	. 426
infected,	. 326
MEAT, juice,	. 553
MEDICAL. Abbreviations,	73, 74, 75
celebrities.	. 555
common sense.	8
progress. .	1

INDEX.

	PAGE
MEDICAL, signs,	75
study fascinating,	6
MEDICINE, doses of,	75, 76, 77
household,	80
methods of giving,	58, 59
size of dose,	9, 57
a popular science,	7
MEDICINES.	57, 87
classes of,	61, 73
how introduced,	359, 60
affect teeth, how given,	191, 542
patent,	55
sometimes work mischief,	8, 470
sore mouth from,	542
MEDULLA OBLONGATA,	235
MEIBOMIAN, glands,	261
MELANCHOLIA,	251
MELANCHOLY,	530
MEMBRANE. mucous,	299, 329
(see mucous coat).	
MEMBRANOUS, croup,	441
MENINGITIS,	241
MENSTRUATION,	433
care during,	435
cessation of,	434
delayed,	433
profuse,	434
MERCURY, in syphilis,	424
METATARSUS,	165
MICRO-ORGANISMS,	13, 524
MICROSCOPE,	1, 13, 401
MILIUM,	215
MILK, (see diet in treatment of),	
Bright's disease,	402
consumption,	324
crust,	218
diabetes,	404
fevers,	473, 475, 548
measles, mumps, etc.,	452, 455
cows for infants,	538
for food,	34
for koumiss,	552
and egg,	552
peptonized,	446
punch,	553
thickened,	552
infected in consumption,	326
medicated by giving to mother,	425
secretion of in pregnancy,	526
secretion excessive,	535
MINERAL ACIDS, (see acids),	91
MINERAL WATERS,	404, 411, 414
MINNESOTA, for consumptives,	42
MISCARRIAGE,	530
MITRAL VALVE,	356
MOIST FEET AND HANDS,	206
MOLES,	228
MORAL, education of children,	543
MORNING SICKNESS,	525
MOSQUITO BITES,	122

	PAGE
MOTHER, to instruct children,	545
MOTHERS' MARKS, (see birth marks),	518
MOUTH, the description of,	298, 306
cleansing of,	28
diseases of,	301
foul,	541
glands of,	299
(see red gum),	207
washes for,	302, 545
MUCOUS COAT, action of alcohol on,	105
of alimentary canal,	299
catarrh of,	376
of eye,	261
of intestines,	368, 371
medicines in inflammation of	66
œsophagus,	328
of mouth and nose,	289, 299
rectum,	371
stomach,	299, 329, 332
throat,	306, 307
urethra and vagina,	425, 437
MUMPS,	454
orchitis from,	420
(see secondary inflammation),	455
MUSCLES,	149, 166, 169
of eyeball,	168
of face,	157
MUSCULAR, action in fractures,	172, 175
in respiration,	39
fiber,	152, 167
MUSTARD, plaster,	470
liniment,	244, 447, 493
poultice,	59
MUTTON,	34, 333
broth,	553
MYOPIA.	262, 264, 268
NÆVUS, (see birth marks),	518
NAIL. ingrowing,	507
NASAL BONES, (see bones of face)	155
catarrh acute, (see cold in head)	290
catarrh chronic,	293
cavities description of,	289
cavities lining of,	289
cavities ulcers in,	291
NAUSEA,	143, 336
in appendicitis,	385
in cholera infantum,	445
in gastritis,	334
in hernia,	366
in peritonitis,	387
in pregnancy,	525, 526
NAVEL STRING, (see cord)	534, 536
dressing for,	537
stump of,	527
NEAR SIGHT, (see myopia)	262, 264, 268
NERVES, THE,	238, 239

INDEX. 577

	PAGE.		PAGE.
NERVES, cerebro spinal,	238	OPIUM, as poison,	97
cranial,	235, 237	as sudorific,	65
of motion and sensation,	240	OPTIC NERVE, THE,	236, 258, 226
sympathetic,	238	commissure,	360
of skin,	198	division of,	258
of touch,	198, 238	foramen,	257
NARCOTICS,	58	inflammation of,	277
NERVOUS DISEASES,	479	ORANGE JELLY,	551
NETTLE RASH, (see urticaria),	220	ORBITS, THE,	257
NEURALGIA,	144, 242, 217	ORCHITIS,	420, 427
NEURALGIC FEVER,	470	OS CALCIS,	164
NIPPLES, (see breasts),	525, 535	OSSICLES, THE,	282
NITRATE OF SILVER,	96, 506	OSSIFICATION, centers of,	149
NITROGEN, in the air,	24	OTITIS MEDIA,	285
NOG, EGG,	552	OVARIAN, neuralgia,	242
NOSE, THE,	289	OVARIES, THE,	430, 432
catarrh of,	295	situation and size of,	523
growths in,	292	OVULATION,	431
hemorrhage from,	145, 293	OVUM, THE,	431
NOSTRILS, (see nasal cavities),	289	OXALIC ACID, poison,	92
NUMBNESS,	254	OXYGEN,	88, 130
NURSES, qualifications of,	546	OYSTERS, in diabetes,	404
NURSING,	546	roasted,	554
(see cholera infantum),	444		
rules for baby,	537	PAIN, (see neuralgia),	143, 72
		agonizing, how relieved,	3
OATMEAL, in constipation,	390	in stomach and bowels, 337, 380, 388	
gruel in constipation of infants,	539	in eyeball,	275, 276
gruel with beef broth,	554	in colic,	388, 399, 349
OBESITY, (see food),	32, 496	in other diseases, 445, 400, 420, 433	
OBSTRUCTION, of bowels,	383	471, 387, 409, 413, 493, 469, 495, etc.	
OCCIPITAL BONE, THE,	154	PALATE, bones,	155, 156
ŒSOPHAGUS, THE,	328, 329	cleft (see hare lip)	304
OIL, almonds, sweet,	208	hard and soft,	300
bergamot,	208	PALPITATION,	360
cajuput,	337	PANCREAS, THE,	191
castor,	78, 83	diseases of,	192
clove,	85	PANCREATIN,	191
mustard,	244, 447, 493	PAPILLÆ, of skin,	199
sweet or olive,	85, 92, 350	of tongue,	300
OINTMENTS,		PARALYSIS,	146
85, 115, 211, 214, 216, 219, 223, 227, etc.		of eyelids,	270
OLD SIGHT,	264	facial,	254
OLECRANON, THE,	160	following apoplexy,	252
OLFACTORY, nerves and bulbs,		following diphtheria,	450
	235, 236	of one side of body,	251
ONYCHIA,	506	spinal,	159
ONYXIS, (see ingrowing nail),	507	PARA PHIMOSIS,	418
OPACITIES, corneal,	274	PARAPLEGIA,	254
of lens,	278	PARASITES,	391, 393, 394
OPHTHALMIA, (see conjunctivitis),	271	of beard,	226
granular,	272	in scalp,	227
purulent,	429, 272	of skin,	229
OPIATES, care in use,	66	PAREGORIC,	79, 87, 381
caution in use,	72	caution about,	538
OPIUM, dose and use, (see morphia)	79	PARIETAL BONES,	153, 156
anodyne,	72	PAROTID GLANDS, THE,	299
in bilious colic,	350	PAROTIDITIS, (see mumps),	454
in cough and diarrhœa mixture,	86	PASTEUR, PROF. LOUIS,	16, 560
in other affections,	410, 388, 415	PATELLA, THE,	164

INDEX.

	Page
Pectoris, Angina,	363
Pediculosis, (see lice),	223
Pelvis, The,	161, 163
Penis, The,	417
Pepsin,	330
Peptonized Milk,	446
Pericarditis,	360
Pericardium, The,	359
Periosteum, The,	153
Peritoneum, The,	387
Peritonitis,	387
Permanganate of Potash,	30
(use in water).	
Perspiration, (see sweating),	197
absence of,	205
excessive,	206
Pertussis, (see whooping cough),	459
Phalanges, The,	150, 161
Pharyngitis, (see acute sore throat),	307
Pharynx, The,	306
Phenacetine,	71, 79, 185, 469, 470, 474
Phimosis,	418
Phosphorus, poison,	96
Phthisis, (see consumption),	322
Physiology,	151, 152
Pia Mater, The,	234
Pigment, of skin,	195
of eye,	258
Piles,	374
Pills, for bad tasting medicine,	73
cathartic,	63
for constipation,	391
Pimples, face,	212
Pink Root, for worms,	395
Placenta, The,	524, 533
retained,	531
Plague, desolations of,	23
Plaster, mustard,	470
of Paris splints,	174
Pleura, The,	313, 318
Pleurisy,	318
Pneumonia,	52, 320
Podophyllin,	63
Poison, gases,	100
ivy,	98
Poisoned, wounds,	122
(see hydrophobia),	514
(see anthrax),	512
Poisoning, how to treat,	90
chronic,	99
Poisons,	88
vegetable,	98
Pokeroot, for obesity,	497
Polypi, of ear,	285
of nose,	292
of rectum,	375
Pons Varolii, The,	235
Pork, cause of tape worm,	392

	Page
Potatoes, in scurvy,	232
Poultice,	59, 185, 320
flaxseed and mustard,	322, 478
sweet oil in,	86
warm with laudanum,	493
Powders,	73
Pregnancy, caution in medicine, during,	60
clothing during,	530
diseases of,	526
symptoms of,	525
termination of,	531
termination of, (criminal),	531
Pregnant, advice for,	529
first time,	530
Presbyopia, (see old sight),	264
Prescribing, home,	52
Prevention, of disease,	12, 130
of cholera infantum,	445
of consumption,	325
of small pox,	500
Privies, (see water-closets),	19, 24
Prolapse of Rectum,	375
(see displacement),	39, 431
Prostate Gland, The,	408
enlarged,	414
Pruritus, (see prurigo),	215
of genital organs,	436
of anus or rectum,	373
Psoriasis,	221
Ptyalism,	525
Puerperal Fever,	477
Pulmonary Artery,	358
Pulsatilla, in orchitis,	427
Pulse, what can be learned from,	140
quick in acute diseases and fevers,	322, 323, 472
slow in apoplexy and diseases of brain,	141, 242
Pupil, The, (see iris),	258
in brain disease, contracted,	241, 97
in acute diseases, enlarged,	457
Purgatives, (see cathartics),	61
Pustule, malignant,	512
Pustules,	204, 498
Pyæmia,	183
Pyloric End, of stomach,	329
Quickening,	525
Quick Lime,	93
Quinine, dose and uses,	79, 84
in acute disease,	65
in pleurisy,	320
in malaria,	68, 467
in quinsy,	310
in remittent fever,	465
Quinsy, (see tonsilitis),	309
Rabies, (see hydrophobia),	514
Rachitis, (see rickets),	488

	PAGE.
RADIAL ARTERY,	140
RADIUS, THE,	160, 161, 162
RECTAL, alimentation,	336, 376
injections,	534
medication,	60
RECTUM, THE,	370
diseases of,	371
REDUCED IRON,	213, 309
REFLEX ACTION,	239
REFRACTION, errors of,	262
REMEDIES, household,	264
RENAL COLIC,	399
REPRODUCTION,	523
RESPIRATION,	97, 142, 313, 358
artificial,	111
failure of,	97
ribs rise and fall in,	161
RESPIRATORY ORGANS,	313
muscle of, (see diaphragm),	39
REST, after labor,	537, 531
after miscarriage,	531
during menstruation,	435
RETENTION OF URINE,	411
RETINA,	259
rods and cones of,	277
RE-VACCINATION,	499, 500
RHEUMATISM,	491
allied to gout,	494
gonorrhœal,	428
RIBS,	161
RICE, as food,	34
water,	549
water stools,	445
RICKETS,	488
RICORD, PHILIP, M. D.,	558
RIDING, (see exercise),	43
bicycle and horseback,	46
RIGIDITY, of womb in labor,	534
RINGWORM,	226
ROOM, suitable for confinement,	533
ROSE COLD, (see hay fever),	295
ROSEOLA, (see German measles),	453
ROUND WORMS,	394
ROWING, (see exercise),	46
RUBEOLA, (see measles),	451
RUPTURE, (see hernia),	385
SACRUM, THE,	163
SAGE TEA,	65, 550
SALINE, mineral waters,	345
SALINES, (see Epsom salts),	62, 78
SALIVA, action on food,	36, 330
excessive flow of,	528, 139
from mercurials,	139
in mumps,	455
in pregnancy,	525
SALIVARY, fistula, glands,	299
SALOL, use,	410, 379, 465, 474
SALT, (see chloride of sodium),	34
antidote to nitrate of silver,	96

	PAGE.
SALT, for eyes, inflammation of,	269
emetic, use of,	61
good in bath,	50, 136
in gastric juice,	330
for hemorrhage,	325
in nasal catarrh,	291, 294
is poison,	88
in vomiting,	337
SALTISH TASTE, of blood,	179
SALT RHEUM, (see eczema,)	218
Fowler's solution in,	219
SALTS, EPSOM, (sulphate of magnesia),	62, 78, 93
antidote in lead poison,	96
use in appendicitis,	385
in peritonitis,	388
SALT WATER, bathing in,	50, 136
SANTONINE, for worms,	394, 395
SAUCE, lemon,	551
SCAB, (see crusts),	205, 498
SCABIES, (see itch),	224
SCALES,	204, 208, 210
SCALP, to clean,	201, 210
dandruff in,	210, 211
eczema of,	218
in favus,	227
lice in,	223
ringworm of,	226
tumors of,	208
wounds of,	127
SCAPULA, THE,	160, 162
SCAR,	125, 205, 498, 500
SCARFSKIN,	194, 195, 196, 199
injury of, (see burns and scalds)	113
SCARLATINA, (see scarlet fever),	456
convulsions in,	486
otitis media from,	286
pulse rapid in,	141
skin paralyzed in,	204
strawberry tongue in,	138
temperature high in,	135
vomiting symptom of,	137
SCHOOL, children, food of,	326
co-education in,	544
age to begin to go to,	543
football too vigorous for,	46
kindergarten methods in,	543
physical culture in,	45
SCHOOLROOMS, ventilation of,	26, 27
to be looked after,	190
SCIATICA, (see neuralgia),	243
SCLEROTIC, THE,	258
SCROFULA,	189
SCROTUM, THE,	419, 420
SCURVY,	231
SEA AIR, beneficial,	50
SEA SICKNESS, (see nausea and vomiting),	143
remedies for,	336
SEA VOYAGES, in consumption,	324, 326

INDEX.

	PAGE
SEA VOYAGES, for hay fever,	296
in overwork,	248
SEBACEOUS, glands,	195, 196
(see seborrhea),	207
tumors or wens,	208, 518
SEDATIVES,	69, 70
SELF REGULATION,	48
SEMINAL FLUID,	524
SENILE BALDNESS,	209
SEPTICÆMIA,	183
SERPENTS, bites of,	120
SERUM,	113, 180, 510
SEWERAGE,	21
SEWER GAS,	16, 30, 100
SHINGLES, (see herpes zoster),	216
SHOCK,	114, 137
SHOES, bad fitting cause corns,	230
cause bunions,	231
SHORT BREATH, (see respiration),	142
SHORT SIGHT, (see myopia),	262
SHOULDER,	160, 166
dislocation of,	177
in fracture of clavicle,	175
SIGHT, loss of, (see blindness),	277
dim in old age,	262
far, (see hypermetropia),	262
loss of from cataract,	278
loss from corneal ulcer,	274
loss from glaucoma,	276
loss from purulent ophthalmia,	272
loss from sympathetic disease,	276
near, (see myopia),	262
old (see presbyopia),	264
SIGMOID FLEXURE OF COLON,	371
SIMS, J MARION, M. D.,	558
SIZE, of infant at birth,	525
of tumors vary,	204
SKELETON, THE HUMAN,	49, 150
SKIAGRAPH, (see X-Rays),	5
SKIN, THE,	146
bathing of,	137
burns of,	114
care of,	6, 201
cosmetics for,	202
description of,	194
diseases of,	199, 212
diseases to be cured,	201
friction of,	50
general observation about,	202
management of,	200
in scarlet fever,	457, 458
sebaceous glands of,	207
sweat glands of,	205
in syphilis,	423, 425
SKULL, bones of,	153, 156
SLEEP,	49
cure for fatigue,	50
from anodynes bad,	538
in chloral and opium poison,	97
rocking infants to, bad,	538

	PAGE
SLEEP, want of, causes exhaustion,	248
want of, (see insomnia),	248
SLEEPLESSNESS, in insanity,	251
remedies for,	249
(see insomnia),	248
SLIPPERY ELM, tea and jelly,	550
SMALL DOSES,	77
SMALL POX,	497
prevention of,	500
SMELL, sense of,	235, 290
in dog,	197
SNELLEN'S TEST TYPE,	268
SOAP, in cleansing the skin,	201
German in skin diseases	214, 222
SOCIAL EVIL, THE,	522
SODA, bicarb. antacid,	80, 91, 93
bromide of, 80, 246, 480, 482, 485,	487
SOIL, for house,	19
pure,	22
polluted,	23
SORE EYES (see care of eyes),	268
(see diseases of eyes),	270
throat, acute,	307
throat, chronic,	308
throat, quinsy,	309
SOUP, vegetable,	555
SPASMS, (see convulsions),	486
from epilepsy,	480
from strychnia,	98
from teething,	540
SPECIAL SENSE, nerves of,	236
SPECIFIC, (see antitoxine),	451
quinine,	68
SPECTACLES, (see glasses), 264, 265,	268
SPEECH, absence of,	282
(see deafness).	
SPERMATOZOA, (see testicles), 419,	524
SPHENOID BONE,	154
SPHINCTER MUSCLES,	371
SPIDER BITES,	122
SPINA BIFIDA,	255
SPINAL CORD,	238, 239
hardening of	254
injury of,	159
paralysis from,	159, 254, 411
SPINAL COLUMN,	157, 158
SPINE, bones of the,	158
dislocation of,	159
injuries of,	159
SPIRITS, of camphor,	82
SPLEEN, THE,	192, 352
diseases of,	353
SPLINTS,	173, 174
SPORES,	14
SPOTTED FEVER, (see meningitis),	241
SPRAINS,	116
SQUINT, (see cross eye),	279
STARCH, (see food),	34
bad in obesity,	496

INDEX.   581

	PAGE.		PAGE.
STAPHYLOMA,	274	SWEATING, excessive,	206
STARCH, saliva changes,	36, 330	favorable,	147
STERILITY, leucorrhœa may cause,	438	SWEEPING, how to get rid of dust,	27
(see gonorrhœa),	439	SWEET OIL,	83, 350, 536
STERNUM, THE,	161, 162	SYCOSIS, (see barber's itch),	226
STETHOSCOPE,	2	SYMPATHETIC NERVES,	238, 239
STILLBORN,	535	SYMPTOMS, how to interpret,	137
frequent cause of,	425	of dislocations,	176
STIMULANTS,	69	of fracture,	172
(see alcohol),	102, 104	SYPHILIS, acquired,	422
STINGS OF INSECTS,	121	cause of iritis,	275
STOMACH, THE, interior of,	329	cause of miscarriage,	531
cancer of,	338	cause of skin disease,	205
functional disturbance of,	331	hereditary,	424
(see dyspepsia).		causes infant mortality,	425
inflammation of,	334	marriage after,	425
neuralgia of,	337	pollutes all life,	12
ulcer of,	335	tertiary can be prevented,	423
STONE, in bladder,	413	(see venereal affections),	421
in gall bladder,	344	SYRUP, hive,	61, 84
in pelvis of kidney (see pyelitis),	400	ipecac,	84
STRABISMUS, (see cross eye),	279	SYRUPS, defined, use of,	73
STRAMONIUM, in asthma,	315	SYSTOLE, of heart,	355
in shingles,	218		
STRANGE delusions,	53	TAKING COLD,	307
STRANGURY,	148	TAMARIND and toast water,	549
STRICTURE, of urethra,	410, 428	TAPE WORM,	392
of œsophagus,	328	sure cure for,	393
of rectum,	375	TAPIOCA CREAM AND JELLY,	551
STRYCHNIA, dose and use,	80	TARSUS, THE,	150, 164, 165
alkaloid of nux vomica,	98	TARTAR EMETIC,	95
antidote to chloral poison,	98	antidote,	95
antidote to snake poison,	121	TARTAR, to be removed from	
in paralysis of bladder,	411	teeth,	542
nerve stimulant,	255, 277	TASTE, as symptom of disease,	140
in paralysis of diphtheria,	450	TEA, use of,	36
STUPES, turpentine,	478	not good for children,	36
ST. VITUS DANCE, (see chorea,)	484	not good for complexion,	200
STYE,	270	TEA BEEF,	553
STYPTIC,	66	sage and flaxseed,	550
SUBLINGUAL, and submaxillary		slippery elm,	550
glands,	299	TEAR DUCT,	279
SULPHONAL, in sleeplessness,	80	TEETH, decay of,	542
SUNLIGHT, best disinfectant,	29	in digestion,	330
SUNSTROKE, cause of,	12	action of medicine on,	139, 542
SUPPRESSION, of urine dangerous,	148	decayed unhealthy,	139
SUPPURATION of appendix,	384	filthy, pollute atmosphere,	28
of felon,	506	in typhoid fever,	139
of matrix,	506	TEETHING,	540
SUPPOSITORIES,	60	TEMPERANCE, favors longevity,	50
for dysentery,	379	TEMPERATURE, in disease.	133
for enlarged prostate,	415	in pleurisy	319
for inflammation of bladder.	410	in pneumonia,	321
for piles,	371, 527	in quinsy,	310
SUPRA-RENAL CAPSULES,	397, 405	in typhoid fever, etc.,	473
SUTURE, sagittal, the,	153	in health,	34
SUTURES of skull bones,	154	of atmosphere, (see climate).	40
SWEAT GLANDS, sudoriferous		TENESMUS, straining,	413
glands,	196	TESTICLES, THE,	419
SWEATING to break up cold,	65	diseases of,	420, 421

	PAGE
TESTICLES, (see orchitis),	427
TESTING EYESIGHT,	264
TEST LETTERS,	266, 267
TEST TYPE,	265, 268
TESTS, for albumen and sugar in urine,	399
THERMOMETER, fever,	547
THICKENED MILK,	552
THORAX,	161
THREAD WORMS,	393
THROAT, boundaries of,	306
affections of,	306, 307, 308, 309
THROMBOSIS,	362
THYMOL, in acne,	214
TIGHT LACING, effects of	39
TINCTURES,	73
of aconite root,	81
of arnica,	82
of belladonna,	81
of cantharides,	211
of capsicum,	212
of digitalis,	248
of iodine,	84
of Jamaica ginger,	83
TINEA, (see ringworm),	226
how contracted,	227
TOAST WATER,	549
TOBACCO,	12
effects of using,	109, 110
TOE NAILS, ingrowing,	507
TONGUE,	138, 299
beefsteak,	139
diseases of,	301
enlargement of,	304
inflammation of,	304
tongue tie,	304
wounds of,	304
TONICS,	67
TONSILITIS, (see quinsy),	309
to prevent,	311
TONSILS,	306
TOOTHACHE,	85, 542
TOUCH, sense of,	198, 199
TOXIC STOMATITIS,	303
TRACHEA,	312
TRACHEOTOMY,	312
TRAVEL, beneficial,	51, 87
TREATMENT, (see any disease),	
of fractures,	173
TROUBLESOME ITCHING,	436
TRUE CROUP,	441
TRUSS, for congenital hernia,	386
TUBERCLE BACILLUS,	325, 562
TUBERCULIN,	324
TUBERCULOSIS,	322
TULLY'S POWDER,	80
TUMORS,	516
of brain,	253
of breasts,	517, 518
of scalp,	208

	PAGE
TUMORS, of scrotum,	204, 420
TURBINATED BONES,	156
TURKISH BATH,	497
TWINS,	431
TWITCHING OF THE LIDS,	270
TYMPANUM, THE,	282
TYPHOID FEVER,	471
boiling water destroys germs of	16, 30
germs of from drinking water,	32
germs from sewers,	23
where prevalent,	24
to prevent spread of,	474
TYPHUS FEVER,	474
ULCERS, ULCERATION,	205, 302
of bowels from burns,	114
from dysentery,	379
of cornea,	274
of eyelids,	270
malignant,	205
of nasal cavities,	291
of rectum,	372
of stomach,	335
of uterus,	437, 438
(see suppuration of vermiform appendix),	384
varicose,	367
ULNA, THE,	160
UMBILICAL CORD, size of,	524
UNNATURAL APPETITE,	339
UPPER EXTREMITIES,	160, 162
and lower jaw,	155, 156
URÆMIC SYMPTOMS,	401, 402
URATES AND UREA,	148, 358, 398
URETERS, THE,	407
URETHRA,	408
URETHRITIS, (see gonorrhœa),	425
URIC ACID,	148, 495
URINARY ORGANS,	407
diseases of,	408
URINE,	147, 147
abnormal products of,	398
analysis of, important,	398
blood in,	146, 148, 399, 400
highly colored, in sickness,	148, 346, 398
incontinence of,	412
retention of,	410
secreted from blood,	397
suppression of,	397, 148, 411
symptom of disease,	147, 148
tests for albumen and sugar in	399
URINIFEROUS TUBULES,	401
URTICARIA, (see nettle rash),	220
USE OF GLASSES,	261, 264
UTERUS, THE, (see womb),	431, 432
cancer of,	434, 437
contractions of,	533
displacements of,	435, 438

INDEX.

	PAGE
UTERUS, during and after labor,	532, 533
hemorrhage of,	434, 437
labor pains due to,	525
ligaments of,	431, 432
pus from,	437
in reproduction,	523, 524
weakness of from miscarriage,	531
UVULA, (see soft palate),	300

VACCINATION, (see prevention of small pox),	500
how and when to do it,	501
VALERIAN, (in headache),	246
VALVES, of heart,	356, 357, 358
of veins,	366
of lymphatic vessels,	188
VALVULAR DISEASE,	361
rheumatism as cause of,	493
VARICELLA, (see chicken pox),	419
VARICOCELE,	419
VARICOSE, ulcer,	367
veins,	367
VARIOLA, (see small pox),	497
VARIOLOID,	499
VEGETABLE FOODS,	33
prevent scurvy,	232
poisons,	89, 98
soup,	553
VEIN, portal,	369
VEINS, THE,	366, 367
varicose,	367
VENA CAVA, inferior, superior,	356
(see plate),	70
VENTILATION,	26
of schoolrooms,	190
of shops, mills, mines,	326
VENTRICLES, of heart,	356, 357
VERATRUM,	70
VERMICULAR MOTION,	369
VERMIFORM APPENDIX,	370
(see appendicitis),	384
VERTEBRA,	157, 158
VERTIGO,	247
VESICAL CALCULUS,	413
(see stone in bladder),	
VESICLES,	217, 204, 448, 498
VESICULÆ SEMINALES,	408
VESSELS, BLOOD, THE,	366
VICHY WATER, (see Carlsbad),	404
VILLI INTESTINAL,	369
VINEGAR, antidote to ammonia,	93
VIRUS,	501
VISION, description of,	257
indistinct,	262, 264
loss of,	264
VITREOUS HUMOR,	259
VOCAL CORDS, THE,	306, 309

	PAGE
VOICE, THE, loss of,	306, 309
VOMER, THE,	156
VOMITING,	170, 336, 337
in acute diseases,	350, 380, 382, 445
medicines to cause,	61, 84, 85
in obstruction of bowels,	383
in peritonitis,	478
in pregnancy,	525, 526
in poisoning,	90
in rupture,	386
in scarlet fever,	457
as symptom,	143

WALKING, (see exercise),	46
WALKING TYPHOID,	473
WALL PAPER, danger of,	25
WARM BATH, of sweet oil,	536
refreshing,	50
WARMTH, necessary for baby,	537
WARTS,	229, 292
WASTE AND REPAIR, (see food),	32
WATER SUPPLY, THE,	29
WAXY LIVER, (see amyloid),	351
WEAKNESS, (see anæmia),	180
from heat,	445
uterine,	531
WEAK SIGHT, or eyes,	264, 269
WEANING,	446, 539
WEEPING EYE,	279
WEIGHT, of infant,	525
WELLS, in cities danger of,	29, 30
WENS,	208
WHEY,	552
WHITES, THE, (see leucorrhœa),	437
WHITLOW, (see felon),	505
WHOOPING COUGH, (see pertussis)	459
WINE WHEY,	552
WOMB, (see uterus),	431, 432
WORMS,	391
WORRY, MENTAL, danger of,	10, 48
WOUNDS, treatment of,	124
of eyelids,	271
incised,	126
poisoned,	122
of scalp,	127
of tongue,	304
WRIST, bones of,	161
dislocation and fracture of,	161

X-RAYS,	4, 5, 6

YEAST, illustrates septic germs,	15
germs,	14
YELLOW FEVER,	11, 15, 476
germs of,	477
hemorrhage in,	476

ZINC COMPOUNDS, poison,	95

www.ingramcontent.com/pod-product-compliance
Lightning Source LLC
Chambersburg PA
CBHW021228300426
44111CB00007B/458